SOCIOLOGY IN NURSING AND HEALTHCARE

Edited by

Hannah Cooke
BSc MSc(Econ) MSc(Nurs) PhD RN DN RNT
Lecturer, School of Nursing, Midwifery and Social Work
The University of Manchester, Manchester, UK

Susan Philpin
BSc(Econ) MPhil PhD RGN
Senior Lecturer, Head of Centre for Primary Care, Public Health and Older People
School of Health Science, Swansea University, Swansea, UK

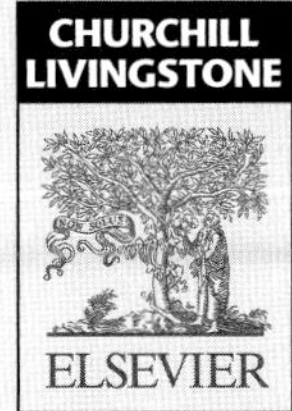

Edinburgh London New York Oxford Philadelphia St Louis Sydney Toronto 2008

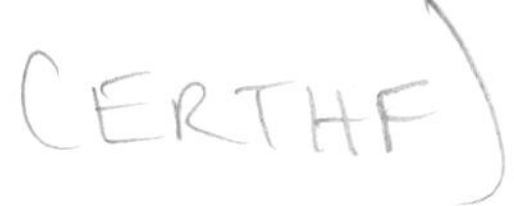

CHURCHILL
LIVINGSTONE
ELSEVIER

An imprint of Elsevier Limited

ISBN 978-0-443-10155-7

British Library Cataloguing in Publication Data
A catalogue record for this book is available from the British Library

Library of Congress Cataloging in Publication Data
A catalog record for this book is available from the Library of Congress

Note
Neither the Publisher nor the Editors assume any responsibility for any loss or injury and/or damage to persons or property arising out of or related to any use of the material contained in this book. It is the responsibility of the treating practitioner, relying on independent expertise and knowledge of the patient, to determine the best treatment and method of application for the patient.

The Publisher

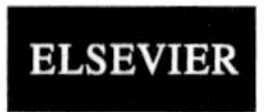

The publisher's policy is to use **paper manufactured from sustainable forests**

Printed in China

SOCIOLOGY IN NURSING AND HEALTHCARE

For Elsevier:

Commissioning Editor: Ninette Premdas
Development Editor: Sheila Black
Project Manager: Anne Dickie
Senior Designer: Sarah Russell

Contents

List of contributors

Lyn Gardner BSc MSc RMN PGCEA
Lecturer, School of Health Science, Swansea University, Swansea, UK

Martin Johnson MSc PhD RN
Professor in Nursing, University of Salford, Salford, UK

Susan Lambert BSc(Econ) PhD
Head of Centre for Health Economics and Policy Studies, School of Health Science, Swansea University, Swansea, UK

Ronnie Moore BSc(Soc Anth, Soc Joint Hons) DPhil PGCE
Schools of Public Health and Population Science & Sociology, University College, Dublin, Ireland

Gillian Olumide BSc(Econ) MA PhD
Lecturer, Centre for Health Economics and Policy Studies, School of Health Science, Swansea University, Swansea, UK

Lindsay Prior BSc(Soc) BSc(Maths) MA PhD
Professor of Sociology, School of Sociology, Social Policy and Social Work, Queen's University, Belfast, UK

Foreword

It is now 30 years since the teaching of sociology was formally identified as part of the nursing and midwifery pre-registration curriculum. Those curricula also introduced the nursing (or midwifery) process as the means of assessing, planning, implementing and regularly reviewing our patients' nursing care. We were required to consider physiological, psychological and sociological needs in formulating our care plans and the teaching of these subjects, 'applied' to nursing, became the norm in schools throughout the UK. Not that they hadn't been taught before, but now we had to demonstrate to General Nursing Council (GNC) Inspectors and students that we were meeting the requirements.

The issues around relating theory to practice are well known, but the application of sociological theory to day-to-day nursing care has never been easy without the use of real examples from practice. Those studying nursing, whether as undergraduates or at a more advanced level, see the value of theory best when they can use that knowledge to empower them to improve patient care. This book does exactly that, using reflection to ensure nurses can incorporate sociological concepts into practice.

I first met sociology as a subject as a Masters student, some 10 years after I had finished pre-registration training. But, although our Sister tutors taught neither sociology nor reflection, they took every opportunity to enhance our understanding of the social construct of the society in which we lived and from where our patients came. We were introduced to the world of anomie by a visit to a local mill. Poverty and the effect it had on the old and young were the lived experience of the back-to-back houses visited with the District Nurse. Assisted by experienced ward sisters, we daily saw the way it aged especially the women who were the mothers and daughters in those communities. Those women also had role conflict, often working, running a home on a low income and caring for grandchildren and an elderly parent. They were experts in addressing the challenges of 'women's work' and were beginning to appreciate the conflicts which would arise as first husbands and then sons joined the long-term unemployed. Sometimes, then as now, the family would become reliant on their wages. As the local authority re-housed Manchester slum dwellers into newly built suburbs, we students realized what social isolation was, although we didn't know its name. All we knew was how little family help was available to support rehabilitation, as elderly parents ended up in tower blocks (with a broken lift) and their children in terraced houses 20 miles away. Social engineering destroyed everything that they had, and the excuse was that they would have better housing and indoor sanitation.

I would have valued more insight. I would have then been able to consider how best to address these issues, minimize them and perhaps avoid them becoming real problems. Students today face similar challenges as they strive to support their patients and clients. Unemployment is now a way of life for our least skilled and poorest educated. Generations of families, especially the men, are unable to find regular work and often the work that is available is soul destroying. Try telling a redundant steel worker that a job making computer parts is 'real work'. Generations of miners' families are trapped within the former pit villages of South Yorkshire and the Welsh valleys, socially isolated (ghettoized?) by a redundancy settlement that reduced their mortgage but gave them un-sellable houses. The role conflict that arises in these communities where two generations of men are in forced dependency on their womenfolk certainly affects their mental and physical health.

The challenges of maintaining and improving health for the poor in society remain a reality. We know the gap between the 'haves' and the 'have-nots' continues to widen and most nursing students of today are living that experience as participant observers. Many are in debt, the bursary has failed to keep pace with the cost of living and much of the original bursary support offered in the 1990s to those who had extra responsibilities, has gone. Access to the social security system is limited and many of them live with debt. Does an understanding of sociology enable them to understand this society better? I believe it does, but I also believe that it gives them the will to do something about it. Certainly they are better fitted to understand the hopelessness our poorer patients have when faced with yet another means test for their income support. Imagine too the role confusion experienced when a nursing student works part-time as a healthcare assistant, especially if on the same unit. Or the role conflict if your part-time job is behind a bar with those very different behaviours and cultural norms.

With the separation of families which started after the Second World War, the elderly and infirm have become much more socially isolated than even the re-housing of the 1960s made them. Then, children were only a bus ride away; now they can be re-located across continents. This change in the social structure of society has a real effect on the rehabilitation and integration in the community of our older people, 'incomers' and those with disabilities. Stigmatization of those who are different is not new, but when an individual is isolated from both family and fellow countrymen, it can become a serious threat to mind and body. As a young, white, well-educated, resident nursing student, I was unaware of how society functioned to support, or indeed discriminated against, the individual or even a group of people. Such ignorance limited the scope of care that I could give.

New challenges face the students of today. While 'the Poor are always with us', this generation has to ensure that poverty as a social construct becomes unacceptable if they are to improve the Health of the Nation. This means understanding society in its widest context, rising to the challenges it throws at us daily as we live a lifestyle that we know damages us. Some people face the old challenges of alcohol and smoking. Young people and the not so young have issues, such as drug addiction to contend with. Women continue to age in relation to their income and obesity continues to be primarily a disease of the poor. Stress comes in all shapes and sizes, but poverty, chronic disease and social isolation make it worse. Our mental health remains fragile and the social stressors that affect it impinge on us all.

We need to understand ourselves and our society better if we are to improve health. Hopefully, the students of today will benefit from the insights this book offers as they strive to address the complexities of care giving in the twenty-first century.

Professor Betty Kershaw DBE FRCN RNT
Emeritus Dean, School of Nursing and Midwifery, University of Sheffield
Past President of the Royal College of Nursing, UK
2008

Acknowledgements

This book has brought together authors from two books previously published by Elsevier, together with four new authors, in order to produce a new work, introducing nurses and other health professionals to sociology.

In Chapters 5 and 6, Ronnie Moore revisits and extends work previously published in Birchenall M and Birchenall P 1998 *'Sociology as applied to nursing and healthcare'* (Chapter 5).

In Chapter 8, Martin Johnson revisits work previously published in Birchenall and Birchenall (Chapter 8).

In Chapters 3, 4 and 15, Hannah Cooke revisits and extends work previously published in Williams A. Cooke H and May C 1998 *'Sociology, nursing and health'* (Chapters 4, 5 and 9).

In chapter 12, Lindsay Prior draws on his own previously published work: 'Repositioning the patient: the implications of being "at risk"' (*Social Science and Medicine* Vol 60 Issue 8, April 2005, Elsevier Ltd) and 'Belief, knowledge and expertise: the emergence of the lay expert in medical sociology' (*Sociology of Health and Illness*. Vol 25 Silver Anniversary Issue 2003). Material from *Sociology of Health and Illness* is reproduced with kind permission of Blackwell Publishing Ltd.

We would like to thank Dame Betty Kershaw for supplying the Foreword and all our contributors for their support and patience.

Hannah Cooke and Susan Philpin
Manchester and Swansea 2008

Dedication

This book is dedicated to the memory of Dr Dorothy Baker (1930–2007).

PART

1

Sociology, nursing and everyday life

CHAPTER

1

Introduction

Hannah Cooke and Susan Philpin

KEY CONCEPTS

- Why do nurses study sociology?
- The idea of the 'sociological imagination'
- How do sociologists work?
- Society and culture
- The structure and content of this book

Why do nurses study sociology?

Nurses in the UK have experienced a period of unprecedented change over recent years. The health service in which they work has been reorganized so often that the process has been described by some analysts as 'continuous revolution'; a term normally associated with Maoist China (Webster 2002). At the same time, nurses have been under intense pressure to take on new roles and responsibilities in a government-inspired programme of workforce reform aimed at breaking down traditional occupational boundaries and creating a flexible labour force (Department of Health 2006). The same is true for many allied professions and for nurses in many other parts of the world. For many individuals caught up in it, this process has been bewildering and many have feared that nursing will lose its professional identity (Shields & Watson 2007). Policy and commentary on nursing range from the government's optimistic promises to 'liberate' nurses (Department of Health 2002) to the deeply pessimistic forecast by some nurses of the 'demise' of nursing (Shields & Watson 2007). What are ordinary nurses to make of all this?

At the same time, it has been suggested that the needs of patients are changing. The government has a very clear narrative about what patients want in a twenty-first century, consumerist society. This narrative supports their political project and includes concepts such as choice and flexibility. However, political rhetoric is constantly changing and does not always reflect reality (see Chapter 7). We also live in a society marked by an ageing population as well as deepening inequality, where considerations of equity may arguably be as important. How are nurses to know whether the decisions being made about the care that they offer are based on evidence? How are they to evaluate the evidence offered to support a particular set of policy choices?

Nursing is a profession that has too often been shaped by other people. Political decisions about healthcare are often made without very much thought being given to the impact on nursing. Traditionally, nurses have just been expected to 'cope' and to get on with the job. Nurses have been educated to apply their knowledge and skills to the care of individual patients and sometimes, this has obscured their vision of the wider context of their work. Big decisions which have affected nursing have thus sometimes been made behind nurses' backs (Hart 2004).

Nursing draws on knowledge from a variety of subjects, such as the biological sciences, sociology, psychology, politics and ethics. In a crowded curriculum, nurses sometimes wonder why they study sociology and the Making a Difference reforms (Department of Health 1999) have threatened its future in some institutions. Our ideas about nursing are situated in a particular social and historical context and we need to understand the way in which that changing context influences current conceptions of our occupation. The authors of this book believe that nurses need to understand the context in which they work in order to practise effectively and in order to have a voice in the future of nursing. Sociology offers an important means to understand this context.

Since the 1990s, there has been lively debate in the nursing press about the role of sociology in the nursing curriculum. This was, in part, instigated by one of the authors who suggested that sociology offered nurses a means to look critically at their own occupation (Cooke 1993). In response, Keith Sharp (1995) suggested that sociology was an unsuitable subject for nurses to study and that while sociologists should study nurses, nurses should not study sociology.

According to Sharp, sociology is *multi-paradigmatic;* by which Sharp meant that sociology is characterized by a variety of different theoretical standpoints and ways of seeing reality. As a result he said, sociology is a *reflexive* discipline; by which he meant that sociologists continually question the grounds upon which sociological knowledge is based. This according to Sharp meant that sociology was an unsuitable subject of study for nurses, since nursing was a practical activity and what nurses needed were 'recipes for action' not questions for debate.

Sharp's papers offended a good many nurses.To paraphrase his arguments, he seemed to imply that sociology was just much too complicated and difficult for nurses who needed to be told what to do and how to do it. Porter (1995) in particular took Sharp to task for his 'old fashioned' and patronising conception of nursing. Porter suggested that Sharp saw nursing as 'women's work' requiring 'little thought or skill'. According to Porter, reflective practice was essential to good nursing and required a knowledge of sociology (1997).

> *'The activity of nursing inevitably involves the social interaction of human individuals. As a consequence, if nurses are to do their job properly, they require an understanding of the nature of those interactions, and of the context in which they take place. In other words, they require a knowledge of sociology'. (Porter 1997: 217)*

Porter (1995, 1997) offered three criteria which nurses could use to evaluate the usefulness of sociological knowledge to nurses:

1. *Pragmatic utility* – the usefulness of sociological ideas to the prosecution of nursing
2. *Philosophical compatibility* – the compatibility of sociological ideas to nursing's internally generated philosophy
3. *Ideological sympathy* – the compatibility of sociological ideas with the values of nursing.

In the following sections, we consider what might distinguish a sociological viewpoint from other ways of looking at the world.

Sociological imagination

Some years ago, a colleague of one of the authors said that she hoped that teaching sociology offered student nurses 'built in crap detectors'. Good sociology should equip students with the intellectual tools to critically question 'official' versions of reality. Too often official versions of reality are presented as natural, inevitable and unquestionable. Official discourse frequently appeals to conceptions of 'human nature' or the 'real world' in order to justify the actions and choices of powerful people. For example, in a recent study, a manager told one of the authors, 'in the real world nurses cannot expect lunch breaks', while another said that it was 'just human nature' for some managers to bully nurses (Cooke 2006). Cowen (1994) suggests that the assertion that something is 'just human nature' is frequently summoned in order to have the last word on the subject. Just like the invocation of the 'real world', it justifies the inevitability of the status quo and fends off demands for change.

According to the sociologist Erving Goffman (1964, cited in 1983), sociology has an important role to play in questioning 'official' versions of reality. This is what he calls the sociologist's 'warrant'.

> *'If one must have warrant addressed to social needs, let it be for unsponsored analyses of the social arrangements enjoyed by those with institutional authority – priests, psychiatrists, school teachers, police, generals, government leaders, parents, males, whites, nationals, media operators, and all the other well-placed persons who are in a position to give official imprint to versions of reality'. (Goffman 1983: 17)*

C. Wright Mills (1959) used the term the 'sociological imagination' to describe the 'promise' of sociology. For Mills 'the sociological imagination enables us to grasp history and biography and the relations between the two in society. That is its task and its promise' (p. 12). Mills explains this in terms of the relationship between private 'troubles' and public 'issues'. 'Troubles' occur within the lives of individuals and their immediate social world. 'Issues' transcend the individual and have to do with public institutions and the larger structures of social and historical life. Too often, people blame themselves for their troubles and fail to see the wider issues involved. This makes people feel powerless. For example illness is a very personal trouble but studies of the social determinants of health have demonstrated that our chances of getting ill are often determined by social circumstances which can be changed (see Chapter 6).

Giddens (1986) says that the sociological imagination should involve an historical, an anthropological and a critical sensitivity. The sociological imagination is historical in that it allows us to understand the distinctive nature of our present society by comparing it with the past. It is anthropological in that it allows us to see the 'kaleidoscope' of different forms of social life that exist in the world. These two dimensions lead us to the third dimension of 'critical sensitivity'. The sociological imagination shows us that existing social relations are not fixed and unquestionable. According to Bauman (1990), sociology has an 'anti-fixating' power.

> *'It renders flexible again the world hitherto oppressive in its apparent fixity; it shows it as a world which could be different from what it is now'. (Bauman 1990: 16)*

and thus it expands our consciousness of the different possibilities for the future.

How do sociologists work?

By its very nature, sociology deals with issues that are very pressing to us all and about which many people (not least journalists and politicians) have vociferous opinions. It confronts problems which are often subjects of major controversy in society such as the relationship between social class and illness, the changing role of religion, the rising divorce rate and the changing nature of work. Perhaps because of its subject matter sociology 'raises hackles that other academic subjects fail to reach' (Giddens 1995: 18). Maybe because we all have our own cherished views on such controversial topics, sociology is often derided as jargon ridden. If commentators agree with it however, it is 'just common sense'.

However sociologists are concerned with understanding society in a 'disciplined' way (Berger 1966), involving both a theoretical understanding of social issues and empirical investigation bound by explicit rules of evidence.

According to Bauman (1990: 12):

> *'sociology (unlike common sense) makes an effort to subordinate itself to the rigorous rules of* ***responsible speech*** *which is assumed to be an attribute of science ... This means that sociologists are expected to take great care to distinguish ... between the statements corroborated by available evidence and such statements as can only claim the status of provisional, untested guess'.*

Bauman also says that sociology also differs from common sense by the **'size of the field'** from which the material for judgement is drawn. Most of us make judgements based on our own life experiences. Sociologists test their theories about the world by collecting empirical data using both qualitative and quantitative research methods. Qualitative methods involve a variety of methods of data collection, such as observations and in depth interviews which allow the researcher to describe the world from the point of view of social actors. Quantitative research is concerned with measurement and with analysing numerical data from sources such as surveys and official statistics which can tell us about wider patterns in society.

Bauman also says that sociology makes us question the world (as we saw earlier) by 'defamiliarizing' the familiar. Sociology invites us to stand back from familiar situations and look at them with fresh eyes (see Chapter 2). This offers the benefits of self awareness:

> *'It may open up new and previously unsuspected possibilities of living one's life with more self awareness, more comprehension-perhaps also with more freedom and control'. (Bauman 1990: 15)*

Society and culture

Sociology, to state the obvious, is engaged in the study of human society – but what do we *mean* by society? Margaret Thatcher (1987) has been famously quoted (or misquoted) as declaring in an interview that '... there is no such thing as society. There are individuals, men and women, and there are families'. A society is generally regarded as a collection of these individuals, but, as Giddens (2001: 22) explains, it is also a 'system of interrelationships which connects individuals together'. It is these interrelationships with which sociology seeks to engage.

It is also in relation to understanding these interrelationships connecting individuals that a core debate in sociology occurs, which will recur throughout the text – that of the primacy of **structure** or **agency.** Here 'structure' refers to social relations in society such as social class, ethnicity and gender which constrain individuals' actions and opportunities. 'Agency' refers to individuals' capacity to act of their own volition, making their own choices and creating the relationships which make up society. The key question is:

> *'Is the community which is society a collection of individuals who, as individuals, actively forge their relationships with one another and create society in the process of doing so? Or do the social relationships which make up society achieve an autonomous identity that establishes them as external conditions which determines the activities of the members of society ...?' (Walsh 1998: 8)*

This debate is at the heart of the 'pluralism' in sociology to which Giddens refers. When the work of key theorists is drawn upon throughout the text, it will be seen that some, such as Durkheim and Marx, take a 'structural' approach whereas others, such as Weber, take an agency or 'action' approach. Many contemporary theorists, such as Giddens (1976) argue that structure and agency are two sides of the same coin in that structures are constituted through action and action is constituted structurally.

Closely connected to society, is the concept of *culture*, which refers to 'the ways of life of the members of a society, or of groups within a society. It includes how they dress, their marriage customs and family life, their patterns of work, religious ceremonies and leisure pursuits' (Giddens 2001: 22). The culture of a social group is comprised of the group's shared *norms* and *values*. Norms refer to expected and accepted ways of behaving within a particular social group; they are specific guidelines as to what is deemed acceptable behaviour in particular social situations and will vary between different cultures. Compliance with social norms is ensured through varying degrees of positive or negative *sanctions*, where adherence to norms is rewarded and deviation is punished. Values could also be viewed as guidelines to behaviour but are more abstract and general than norms, defining what people in particular social groups believe to be worthwhile and as with norms, values are also culturally variable. However, it is important to note that cultural groups are not homogeneous; their members may hold and be influenced by a complex range of different norms and values. In addition, cultural groups are not static; they change and evolve in response to various influences.

The structure and content of this book

The book is presented in three parts. Part 1: *Sociology, nursing and everyday life* introduces the key areas which form the context to everyday life for both nurses and patients, exploring families, work and organizations, religion and belief systems, social class and disadvantaged groups. Part 2: *Healthcare systems and nursing* explores various aspects of healthcare provision, including healthcare policy and organizational change, issues of power and communication, nursing work and partnerships in providing care in the community. Part 3: *The experience of illness* explores patients' perspectives, understandings and experiences of the nature of health and illness.

The three parts are linked by the central purpose of this text, which is to encourage readers to develop their 'sociological imagination' in relation to nursing practice and education, developing sensitivity to the relationship between 'private troubles' and 'public issues' (Mills 1959). A key theme throughout the text concerns the ways in which ideas *change* over time in response to different social contexts, with many chapters taking an historical perspective. The influence of inequalities on health and illness experiences, including the experience of death and dying, is another important recurring theme. In addition, the concept of 'boundaries' in health work, health, illness and dying is considered in a number of chapters. Key theoretical perspectives/major thinkers are introduced (painlessly, we hope) through the substantive topics in appropriate chapters, rather than having a separate chapter on 'sociological perspectives'. The chapters provide references and some have further reading suggestions. Important terms are highlighted in bold or italic.

PART 1 – SOCIOLOGY, NURSING AND EVERYDAY LIFE

In **Chapter 2**, Lyn Gardner continues with the theme of 'thinking sociologically', this time drawing on Bauman's (1990) work and applying it to families. Gardner looks at the various ways of defining families and also the *diversity* of families and family forms. In an attempt to throw some further light onto this diverse picture of family forms, she offers a brief review of the historical development of the family, which reveals additional evidence to challenge the notion of the ubiquity of the nuclear family. She also explores feminist literature which has emerged to challenge the unequal power relationships within families. This chapter also looks at what goes on *inside* families, including the role of families as care providers, and children's perspectives on family life. Key theorists introduced in this chapter include Bauman in relation to thinking sociologically and Parsons in relation to the Functionalist approach to families.

In **Chapter 3**, Hannah Cooke looks at classical and contemporary sociological studies of religion and their application to healthcare and considers how these can help us to understand the complex relationships between religion, society, illness and healthcare in the contemporary world. This chapter introduces relevant (to our understanding of religion) aspects of the work of three of the 'founders' of sociology: Marx, Weber and Durkheim. The chapter looks at the impact of secularization and recent developments in religion, such as fundamentalism and 'new age' religions. It also explores the influence of religion on health and healthcare and nurses' recent interest in spiritual care.

In **Chapter 4**, Hannah Cooke explores the changes in work and organizations from the industrial to the 'post-industrial' age. In doing so, she highlights debates which are underpinned by different values and beliefs which recur throughout our discussion of healthcare and nursing in this book. This chapter introduces and explores many concepts – such as the 'market', bureaucracies, professions, managerialism – which underpin contemporary ideas in health and welfare provision. Key theorists introduced in this chapter include Weber in relation to bureaucracies and Goffman in relation to total institutions.

Chapters 5 and 6 by Ronnie Moore consider the nature of social inequalities and their influence on health. **Chapter 5** sets the scene by exploring the concepts of social class and poverty, drawing on the work of the key theorists in this area. Moore starts with an historical review of social divisions and poverty and charts the changing nature of social class. The work of classic (Marx and Weber) and contemporary (Bourdieu and Giddens) social theorists in this area, is introduced. In addition, the idea of globalization is introduced and global inequalities considered.

Chapter 6 moves on to look at the ways in which these disadvantages impact on health and healthcare. Evidence of inequalities in relation to class, gender, 'race' and age are presented and discussed and explanations are considered, particularly recent work on social capital, including Wilkinson's thesis.

PART 2 – HEALTHCARE SYSTEMS AND NURSING

In **Chapter 7**, Gillian Olumide and Hannah Cooke provide the context for this section by examining the *changing* nature of health and social care systems in Britain, linking these changes to shifting political and philosophical viewpoints, economic conditions and technological developments. Thus, a brief history of the British healthcare system and recent healthcare policy is outlined and discussions of social democratic and neo-liberal approaches to health policy are developed and the ideas of the 'Third Way' introduced. The concept of managerialism, introduced in Chapter 4, is further developed in relation to managed healthcare.

In **Chapter 8**, Martin Johnson introduces the concept of power, exploring power and control in relationships between nurses and doctors and between patients and health professionals. By drawing on a number of 'case studies' from nursing practice situations, Johnson illustrates aspects of power in nurse–patient relationships such as social judgement, coercion, authority, humiliation, force, restraint, surveillance and incarceration. Key theorists introduced and/or developed in this chapter are Parsons, Foucault, Steven Lukes and Goffman. Interactionist studies of communications and relationships between professionals and patients are also examined.

In **Chapter 9**, Hannah Cooke develops ideas introduced in Chapter 4 concerning sociological understandings of work and relates them specifically to nursing work. She starts by exploring the origins and developments of modern nursing (including the contributions of Nightingale and Seacole) and also the gendered nature of nursing work. The concept of professionalism is revisited and applied to nursing and linked to changes in nurse education; in addition, the concept of managerialism, this time in relation to nursing, is developed. Cooke also explores the changing boundaries of nursing and changes in the division of labour in healthcare.

In **Chapter 10**, Susan Lambert explores recent policy changes underpinning service developments in community settings for service users with complex care needs, for example older people, people with learning or physical disabilities, people with mental health problems or chronic long-term illness. The contested nature of the term 'community' is explored and boundaries between health and social care are considered further through the classic example of the 'social bath'. The notion of the 'Third Way', introduced in Chapter 8, is developed and described in its application to care in the community. The impact of a 'mixed economy' of care on clients in the community is explored. Studies of informal care are considered in more detail and related to the earlier chapter on families.

PART 3 – THE EXPERIENCE OF ILLNESS

Susan Philpin sets the scene for this section by exploring, in **Chapter 11**, how sociology can contribute to our understanding of the ways in which people, both lay and professional, make sense of health and illness causation. The first part of the chapter compares and contrasts lay and professional understandings of health, illness and risk; key theorists in relation to risk, Beck, Giddens and Douglas, are introduced here. The concept of social constructionism, the idea that interactions between individuals and groups construct what we perceive as reality, is introduced. In addition, and related to this concept, the particular genre of sociology, the 'sociology of the body', is introduced and explored through the analysis of Jocalyn Lawler's study of the ways in which nurses deal with bodies. The work of Foucault and Elias in relation to the body is also considered.

In **Chapter 12**, Lindsay Prior continues to explore differences in lay and professional understandings of health and illness. He starts by charting the change in the status of lay understandings of health and illness noting what he describes as the rise of the 'lay expert'. However, in the second part of the chapter, where Prior contrasts lay and medical knowledge about a specific example – the genetics of breast cancer – he demonstrates the limitations of lay expertise. By contrasting the 'particularity' of lay knowledge (private troubles) with the strengths of sociology to see patterns and structures (public issues) in human misfortune, Prior exemplifies our endeavour in this text to impart the 'sociological imagination'.

In **Chapter 13**, Susan Philpin explores the contribution of sociology to our understanding of the ways in which people experience ill-health. First, Parsons' classic concept of the sick role is introduced and critiqued. Then people's experience of chronic illness is analysed using another classic framework developed by Strauss et al. A number of interpretive studies focusing on the *meaning* of the illness experience for those involved are reviewed, including such methodologies as phenomenology, symbolic interactionism and narrative analysis. Illness is often accompanied by pain and this chapter also explores the ways in which, in addition to the neurophysiological elements of pain, people's experiences of and responses to pain are also influenced by the sociocultural context of that pain.

Illness experience is further explored in **Chapter 14**, where Susan Philpin considers the ways in which this experience is influenced by society's response to people with chronic illness and/or disability. Social reaction to physical and mental illness and disability is explored drawing on insights from sociological studies of the concepts of deviance, labelling and stigma. Classic theorists in this area introduced, or returned to in this chapter include: Goffman, Lemert, Scheff and Rosenhan. Concepts, definitions and models of disability are explained and disabling barriers, both physical and attitudinal, are examined. In addition, anti-discriminatory practice in relation to healthcare is also explored.

Finally, in **Chapter 15**, Hannah Cooke considers sociology's contribution to our understanding of death and dying. She starts by exploring the complex nature of social responses to death, noting changing attitudes, and considers the arguments for and against the proposition that we live in a 'death denying' society and charting the changing attitudes to death and dying. This chapter also considers the growth of hospices and palliative care. It considers communication and awareness in the care of the dying and reviews recent work on the 'disadvantaged dying'.

FURTHER READING

Bauman Z 1990 Thinking sociologically. Blackwell, Oxford.

Gives a good introduction to sociological thought.

Mills C Wright 1959 The sociological imagination. Oxford University Press, New York.

Accessible and readable. You can read more about C Wright Mills at: www.cwrightmills.org You can also read more about the sociological imagination and access resources on social theory at 'A Sociological Tour of Cyberspace' at: www.trinity.edu/mkearl

Porter S 1998 Social theory and nursing practice. Macmillan, London.

Introduces social theory to nurses.

REFERENCES

Bauman Z 1990 Thinking sociologically. Blackwell, Oxford

Berger P 1966 Invitation to sociology. Penguin, Harmondsworth

Cooke H 1993 Why teach sociology? Nurse Education Today 13:210–216

Cooke H 2006 Seagull management and the control of nursing work. Work Employment and Society 20(2):223–243

Cowen H 1994 The human nature debate: social theory, social policy and the caring professions. Pluto, London

Department of Health 1999 Making a difference: Strengthening the nursing, midwifery and health visiting contribution to health and healthcare. Department of Health, London

Department of Health 2002 Liberating the talents: helping primary care trusts and nurses to deliver the NHS plan. Department of Health, London

Department of Health 2006 Modernising nursing careers. Department of Health, London

Giddens A 1976 New rules of sociological method. Hutchinson, London

Giddens A 1986 Sociology: A brief but critical introduction, 2nd edn. Macmillan, London

Giddens A 1995 In defence of sociology. *New Statesman and Society*, 7 April

Giddens A 2001 Sociology. Polity, Cambridge

Goffman E 1983 The interaction order. American Sociological Review 48:1–17

Hart C 2004 Nurses and politics: the impact of power and practice. Palgrave Macmillan, London

Mills C Wright 1959 The sociological imagination. Oxford University Press, New York

Porter S 1995 Sociology and the nursing curriculum: a defence. Journal of Advanced Nursing 21:1130–1135

Porter S 1997 Sociology and the nursing curriculum: a further comment. Journal of Advanced Nursing 26:214–218

Sharp K 1995 Why indeed should we teach sociology? A response to Hannah Cooke. Nurse Education Today 15:52–55

Shields L, Watson R 2007 The demise of nursing in the United Kingdom: a warning for medicine. Journal of the Royal Society of Medicine 100:70–74

Thatcher M 1987 Interview. *Woman's Own*, 31 October

Walsh D 1998 Structure and agency In: Jenks C (ed.) Core sociological dichotomies. Sage, London, p 8–33

Webster C 2002 The National Health Service: A political history. Oxford University Press, Oxford

CHAPTER 2

Thinking sociologically about families and health

Lyn Gardner

KEY CONCEPTS

- Defining families
- Diversity of family forms
- Historical perspectives
- Feminist critiques of families
- Family practices
- Children's perspectives on family life
- Families as care providers
- The anti-family movement

Introduction

'A family is made up of people who support you. Everybody is born with a family. Families are for helping you out'. (Zoe, aged 12, cited in Morrow 1998: 23)

The family is regarded as one of the most important institutions in society; it sits at the centre of both personal and political spheres of life. For individuals, a family can be a 'haven in a heartless world' (Lasch 1995: 6), while others may experience their family as a source of conflict or distress. The myth of the family as either the panacea for all social ills, or the cause of them, permeates through social policy, the models used by health and social care professionals, and the lives of ordinary people (Jones 2002). Therefore, key to understanding the concept of family is to appreciate that it is an *ideological* concept (see Chapter 4). Ideologies about the family shape care provision (which of course includes nursing care), because they shape policy-makers beliefs about what the family is and what it should and should not do. This chapter will consider the development of the contemporary family and its role and function in relation to health and illness.

Nursing and the family

'Nurses working with families of course want to be helpful and reduce or alleviate suffering whenever possible'. Wright & Leahey (2005: 1).

Wright and Leahy offer advice on how to 'avoid or sidestep errors' (2005: 91) in family nursing practice to enable nurses to work with more confidence and competence. The aim of this chapter is to provide nurses with a sound overview of the sociology of the family that may then be *applied to practice* with a sense of confidence.

For nurses, who need to respond thoughtfully and reflexively to people in their care, Nicholson (1999: 77) offers an insightful reminder that:

> *'The categories we have for sorting our world affect how we think about our present situation and possible alternatives'.*

This means understanding differing perspectives on the family and appreciating the wide range of family forms experienced by those in our care. Silva & Smart (1999) emphasize the importance of attending to individual perceptions of family life, rather than simply accepting top-down definitions. Within sociology, the consideration of the individual *subjective* meanings of family follows what classical sociologist Max Weber described as the need for sociologists to achieve a 'subjective understanding of the action of the component individuals' (Weber 1968: 15). Weber believed that sociologists should be concerned with more than offering an explanation of the social world, what he termed *Erklären*, but should seek to achieve understanding or *Verstehen* (we discuss Weber's major ideas in Chapter 4). By accepting this understanding of sociological enquiry, nurses can go on to explore the variety of family arrangements that may more accurately represent the diverse ways that people live in contemporary British society.

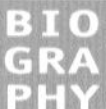

Zygmunt Bauman (1925–present)

Zygmunt Bauman (born 1925, in Poland) was seen as a dissident intellectual in his own country and consequently was forced out of Poland during the late 1960s. He eventually settled in England where he became the first Professor of Sociology at the University of Leeds, until his retirement in 1990. Bauman has been acknowledged as one of the world's greatest social theorists, and is particularly celebrated for his work on modernity and post-modernity (see for example *Modernity and the Holocaust*, 1989; *Globalisation: The Human Consequences*, 1998).

REFLECTION POINT

Consider the various types of family that you have encountered in your practice. How might these differences impact upon care needs?

UNDERSTANDING FAMILIES

Everyday understandings of the family may be taken for granted by nurses and other healthcare professionals, leading to inaccurate assumptions being made about care needs. Thus, it is crucial for nurses to take a step back from their own common-sense understanding of the family and view it from a sociological perspective. By *thinking sociologically* (Bauman 1990), nurses can gain a deeper insight into contemporary family life, and this can enhance the quality of care they provide.

THINKING SOCIOLOGICALLY ABOUT FAMILIES

What is of interest for us in this chapter is Bauman's published work *Thinking Sociologically* (1990). Here he discusses a range of common experiences (family life, for example) and offers examples of thinking sociologically about these experiences. Through these examples, he provides an overview of the discipline of sociology and its related key concepts. Bauman begins his thesis by asserting that sociology is 'first and foremost a *way of thinking* about the human world' (1990: 8, italics as in original), and says that *thinking sociologically* 'helps us to understand other forms of life, inaccessible to our direct experience' (1990: 17). The well-known English writer and actor Alan Bennett makes a similar point in his book *Writing Home* (1994) when he comments:

> *'I go to sociology not for analysis or explications but for access to experiences I do not have and often do not want*

> *(prison, mental illness, birth marks)'. (Bennett 1994: 305)*

Overall, Bauman (and possibly Alan Bennett) believes that the art of thinking sociologically can 'make us more *sensitive*: it may sharpen up our senses, open our eyes wider so that we can explore human conditions which thus far had remained all but invisible' (1990: 16, italics as in original).

Bauman's thesis on *thinking sociologically* illustrates the need for nurses to base their professional judgements about the family upon a broad *evidence base*. Mulhall suggests that:

> *'Knowledge, or evidence, for practice thus comes to us from a wide variety of disciplines, from particular paradigms or ways of 'looking at' the world, and from our own professional and non-professional life experiences'. (Mulhall 1998: 5)*

With this in mind, the chapter will now move on to look at some of the fundamental concepts and issues employed within the sociological study of the family.

What is a family?

Definitions of what a family is, and what it should be, have been debated within political and social discourse for some time. For sociologists, an understanding of what is meant by the term 'family' is essential. Yet it is one of the most intractable issues to be faced within the study of the family. Numerous attempts have been made to define the family in a way that adequately encompasses the diverse family forms that exist, as can be seen in sociology texts which look at the family (Allen & Crow 2001, Bernardes 1997, Featherstone 2004, Silva & Smart 1999). This has led some, for example Gubrium & Holstein (1990), to argue for the rejection of the term 'family' altogether and replace it with 'household'. However, this can be problematic in a number of ways. First, within sociology as well as in everyday life, the terms often merge into one. However, there is an essential distinction to be made between the two (Allen & Crow 2001). A *household* generally refers to a social group, which usually share domestic activities such as eating some meals together, sleeping in the same dwelling, and normally sharing a common domestic budget (Anderson et al 1994, Giddens 2001). Such households may include those who share a kinship link, but there is a growing trend towards single person households and individuals who share a dwelling for economic and situational reasons, such as students.

According to data from the Office for National Statistics (2005), in 2005 there were 7 million people living alone in Britain, which is nearly four times as many as in 1961 (Allen & Crow 2001). Among older people, women over the age of 75 are more likely to live alone than older men to a ratio of 3:5 (Office for National Statistics 2005). Widowhood is a common experience for older women which, not surprisingly, increases statistically with age. Interestingly, a trend in *cohabitation* among older adults has been noted, with the 2001 Census revealing that 5% of men and 4% of women aged between 50–59 lived with a non-marital partner (Office for Population Census and Surveys 2001b). Overall, there continues to be a growing trend in single family households, and as a result, the average household size has decreased from 3.1 to 2.4 during this same time period. In spite of this trend, the majority of people in Britain live in a *family household*: in 2004, 8 out of 10 people lived in a family household compared to 9 out of 10 in 1961 (Office for National Statistics 2005).

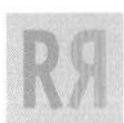

REFLECTION POINT

Think about the ways in which the increasing likelihood for people to be living alone may impact upon their needs for care and support.

According to the 2001 Census, families headed by a person of non-White ethnic background were more likely to have a larger household with dependent children than their White counterparts. For example, almost four out of five Bangladeshi families in Britain had dependent children living at home with them, compared with almost two out of five White families. Bangladeshi and Pakistani families tend to be larger than families from any other ethnic group with 40% having three or more dependent children compared with 28% for Black African families; 20% for Indian families and 17% for White families (Office for Population Census and Surveys 2001b). Nurses should be mindful of the diversity of family forms and family practices, within a range of ethnically diverse groups. By *thinking sociologically*, nurses can avoid stereotyping ethnic groups and be wary of making assumptions about families.

From a sociological perspective, Allen & Crow (2001) add that for clarity it is essential to make a conceptual separation between the two terms 'family' and 'household' despite any overlap. Furthermore, it is essential to appreciate the *perspective of the individuals* who may see themselves as living within a *family*, as opposed to a *household*, which is especially important for nurses who endeavour to build a trusting rapport with those for whom they provide care.

Diversity of family forms

Giddens (2001) suggests that it is more meaningful to talk of *families* rather than *the family*: a term that better represents the diversity of family forms. This apparently slight but significant conceptual move also avoids the problem of idealizing one family form over another, most notably the '*nuclear family*'.

THE UBIQUITOUS NUCLEAR FAMILY

The nuclear family is defined as a small unit of a (usually married) heterosexual couple and their dependent children. Within this arrangement, there are particular expectations and hierarchies that run along gender and age lines. The consequent roles and responsibilities shape the relationships between family members. Despite challenges (which will be explored later in the chapter) the nuclear family form has assumed its dominance within the hearts and minds of wider Western society, and is most commonly held up as the most desirable, and 'normal' family to live in. Yet Bernardes (1997: 3) asserts that 'there is something very strange about this image: it is quite simply unrealistic'. The *idea* of the small and neat nuclear family has considerable potency in that other family forms tend to be defined by reference to it (Muncie & Sapsford 1995).

The idealization of the nuclear family can be problematic for nurses when working with ethnically diverse families who may not conform to the nuclear family stereotype. For example, Pakistani families have developed from a tradition of strong kinship links and extended networks known as *biraderi* and thus may not fit the nuclear family model. Nevertheless, in the West it is widely taken for granted that not only is the nuclear model the best family form, but also the most common in contemporary Western society. Indeed as Bernardes (1997: 2–3) exclaims, 'despite enormous real world variation and diversity', the nuclear family remains the most 'common and popular image' of a family. However, from their research into recent developments in family life, Silva and Smart (1999: 9) reveal the disruption in 'the taken-for-grantedness of primacy of blood and marital relationships', leaving sociologists struggling to provide a vocabulary for new relationships such as step-families or so-called *reconstituted families* (Featherstone 2004).

STEP-FAMILIES

Step-families usually consist of the natural or adopted child (or children) of only one member of the married or cohabiting couple. For the first time, the 2001 Census allowed for the identification of *step-families*, and as a result found that 10% of all families with dependent children in Britain were *step-families*. The Census also highlighted the tendency for children to remain with their mother following any break-up of a partnership or marriage, with over 80% of such families consisting of natural mother and step-father. Not surprisingly, *step-families* were found to be generally larger than non-step-families, with 27% having three or more dependent children compared with 18% of non-step-families. Featherstone (2004), in her book *Family Life and Family Support: a Feminist Analysis*, reminds us that:

> *'Step-families are not the same as nuclear families and they differ from each other in terms of histories and everyday lives. Pre-separation conflict will leave its mark on children' (Featherstone 2004: 132).*

Within the *reconstituted family* (step-family), as Freely (2000) notes, there are ongoing challenges to be faced in terms of relationship building, the re-negotiation of roles, and the creation of a sense of safety and belongingness for all family members, especially children. Nurses need to be mindful of these factors during the planning and delivery of care.

DIVORCE

Britain has witnessed a long-term rise in the rate of divorce particularly since the early 1970s. In 1971 there were 187000 divorced men compared with 1.5 million in 2001, with 296000 divorced women in 1971, rising to 2 million by 2001 (Office for National Statistics 2001). Yet it is important to note here that among certain minority ethnic groups, such as Bangladeshis, rates of marital breakdown and divorce are relatively low. In 2001, almost 70% of divorces in England and Wales were granted to women, most commonly on the grounds of unreasonable behaviour, whereas for men, the most common reason was 2 years separation, with consent (Office for National Statistics 2001).

One explanation for the rise in divorce is offered by Giddens (1992) who argues that women, buoyed up by feminism, are viewing their lives in a different way and are breaking free from traditional models of heterosexual relationships. He argues that women are no longer tied by the force of social customs and beliefs which demanded that they had to marry in order to have children, and needed to live with men to achieve financial security (see Chapter 5 for more about Giddens' major ideas).

In support of Giddens' position, Beck and Beck-Gernsheim (1995) suggest that women appear to be raising their expectations of relationships in terms of intimacy, communication and men's behaviour. In short, 'personal life has become an open project' (Giddens 1992: 8) and women more than men are adopting this stance. Indeed, Stacey (1998) and Ferguson (2001) suggest that men are less well-equipped to face the challenges of a shifting gendered landscape of heterosexual relationships and family life. Yet Jamieson (1997: 40) is less convinced of Giddens' thesis on the transformation of intimate gendered relationships, and argues that he 'seems to underplay the very widespread roots of inequality' within wider society, which impacts upon women's lives and places limits on their life choices. The impact of gender inequality within familial relationships is a recurrent theme within this chapter, and is considered elsewhere in relation to care roles.

CIVIL PARTNERSHIPS

Perhaps one of the most recent examples of the fluidity of the family form is the passing of the Civil Partnership Act that came into force in December 2005, which allowed gay and lesbian couples to formally unify their relationship. According to the Office for National Statistics (2006) within the period 21 December 2005 to 31 January 2006, 3648 civil partnership ceremonies took place, of which 2510 were gay couples and 1138 were lesbian couples. Prior to this formal recognition of same sex partnerships, many lesbian women in particular felt excluded from the privileged heterosexual nuclear family of marriage and children (Bryson 2002).

Historical perspectives

It is useful at this point to offer a brief review of the historical development of the family. This further challenges the notion of the ubiquity of the nuclear family. Silva and Smart (1999: 4) suggest in their work that 'there is both continuity and diversity in family life at the end of the twentieth century'. So, does a look at the past reveal a more consistent picture of family life? Reviews of the historical contributions to the sociological understanding of the British family uncover a range of explanations and perspectives on the growth and development of the family.

First, there appears to be consensus on the view that the effects of the economic expansion of industrial towns resulted in population shifts from rural to urban settings. This meant that the traditional *extended families*, which consisted of a number of people living together (or very close by) in one household all bound by kinship ties and roles such as grandparent, uncle and aunt, brothers and sisters with their spouses and children, were replaced by the economically more mobile nuclear family. Thus the economic and social support of the extended family was being replaced by a smaller family form (*the nuclear family*), seen by many social commentators as a better 'fit' with advancing industrialization and urban living.

Within sociology, the influential American sociologist Talcott Parsons, saw the modern nuclear family as functional to a developing capitalist society. Parsons described nuclear families as 'factories which produce human personalities' (Parsons 1955:16). He described the following functions of the modern nuclear family:

> *'We therefore suggest that the basic and irreducible functions of the family are two: first the primary socialisation of children so that they can truly become members of the society into which they have been born; second, the stabilisation of the adult personalities of the society' (Parsons 1955:16).*

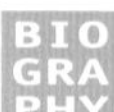

Talcott Parsons (1902–1979)

Talcott Parsons was an American sociologist who originally studied as a biologist. Arguably this influenced the particular brand of functionalism which Parsons developed, which has been criticized for its over emphasis on consensus and equilibrium and its failure to take adequate account of inequality and social conflict. Parsons was a central figure in Harvard University's Department of Sociology and was one of the most influential sociologists of the mid-twentieth century. Parsons was influenced by Weber and Durkheim and also by the Italian economist Vilfredo Pareto. He produced a theory of the social system, which he called structural functionalism. In it, he argued that the crucial feature of social systems like biological organisms was maintaining homeostasis and that all parts of society had to be understood in terms of their functional relationship to the whole system. Like many other sociologists, he attempted to combine human agency and structure in one theory. Major works include:

- *The Structure of Social Action* 1937
- *The Social System* 1951
- *Family, Socialization and Interaction Process* (with R Bales) 1955
- *Economy and Society* (with N Smelser) 1956
- *Politics and Social Structure* 1969

Parsonian functionalism dominated sociological thought about the family throughout the 1950s and 1960s, and thus the extended family and wider kinship roles were largely rendered invisible and 'assumed to have withered away with the rise of modern industrial society' (Twigg & Atkin 1994: 2). However, the now famous study of kinship in the East End of London by Young and Wilmot (1957) served to challenge this position, as it revealed a picture of intergenerational support within families, most significantly delivered by women. Further challenges came from a burgeoning feminist sociology, which challenged the Parsonian assumption that the contemporary nuclear family functioned in the interests of all its members drawing attention in particular to its negative impact on women.

The historical development of British family life cannot be seen as a smooth, linear process, not least because of the presence of ethnically diverse family forms. Within such families, the influence of other traditional or religious practices will go some way in shaping their family life, such as the principles of Islam which place importance and emphasis on family obligations (Hylton 1995). The evidence considered here shows what Simpson (1998) describes as a decline in significance of the nuclear family, and a growth in '*unclear families*'. Whatever form family life takes, it is important to note that nurses should approach with sensitivity, any discussion with people in their care of the experience of family life, and be aware that there are those 'who feel excluded from or damaged by particular families' (Featherstone 2004: 25) or experiences. For example individuals may be damaged by abuse or domestic violence and this can have lasting negative effects on health.

Feminist critiques of the family

A large body of feminist work emerged to challenge the unequal power relationships within the family, with many claiming that the ideology of the nuclear family served to legitimate and perpetuate patriarchal divisions and hierarchies.

THE SEXUAL DIVISION OF LABOUR

There is an expectation that domestic and parenting responsibilities are divided up along gender lines. This is called the *sexual division of labour*, whereby household tasks and parenting/care roles are divided between the man and the woman, with the latter most often taking on the majority share, resulting in men traditionally being seen to hold more power both within the family and the public sphere.

BIOGRAPHY

Ann Oakley (1944–present)

Ann Oakley (born 1944 in London, England) was the only child of Kay Titmuss, a social worker and Richard Titmuss, one of the foremost social policy theorists of his time. She was one of the first students to take sociology at Oxford University. From her first academic book (she also wrote fiction) *Sex, Gender and Society* published in 1972, to her most recent work the *Ann Oakley Reader* (2005), Ann Oakley has focussed her attention on feminism, and the experiences and roles of women in society. Her work has been influential and ground-breaking, for example her thesis on the role of housewife, and the significance of housework in women's lives. She is also credited for bringing attention to the problem of the medicalization of childbirth, and the experience of the transition to motherhood with her books *From Here to Maternity: Becoming a Mother* (1979) and *Women Confined: Towards a Sociology of Childbirth* (1980).

HOUSEWORK

Ann Oakley produced the best known study on housework which revealed the significance of domestic labour within women's lives. She wrote two books: *The Sociology of Housework* and *Housewife*, both published in 1974. It is widely acknowledged that taking responsibility for childcare and housework inevitably results in 'lost opportunities' for those individuals (namely women), especially in the sphere of public life (Chapman 2004: 27). Oakley (1974 Housewife: 222) puts this more forcefully by stating that 'housework is directly opposed to the possibility of human self-actualization' and goes on to assert that 'women's domesticity is a cycle of learnt deprivation and induced subjugation: a circle decisively centred on family life' (1974 Housewife: 233). Oakley firmly locates the subjugation of women at the door of the family. In her book *Taking it Like a Woman* (1984) published a decade later, her critical stance towards the institution of the family remained equally robust. She placed the family at the centre of political forces which served to marginalize women, most specifically the housewife and mother. She was particularly critical of the 'gender-differentiated nuclear family' (1984: 201), along with other feminist writers such as Barrett and McIntosh (1982). Within the confines of the nuclear family, she argued, gendered roles were established and nurtured. Oakley claimed that:

> *'Women mother. Daughters are transformed into mothers. An autonomous sense of self . . . does not need to develop. Women's sense of identity is thus dangerously bound up from early childhood with the identities of others. Not so for men, who as little boys look into their mothers' faces and see what they learn is not a reflection of their own . . . So if it isn't in love that women are lost, it's in the family. The tension between the interests of the family and the interests of women as individuals has been rising for some two centuries. It is not possible for these interests to be reconciled'. (Oakley 1984: 201)*

Earlier, Oakley (1974) had advocated for the abolition of the family as a way of freeing both men and women from the shackles of household and (nuclear) family practices. She believed that:

> *'The family's gift to women is a direct apprenticeship in the housework role. For this reason, the abolition of the housewife role requires the abolition of the family, and the substitution of more open and variable relationships' (Oakley 1974: 236).*

Feminist critiques of the family, and most particularly the nuclear arrangement, have been both vociferous and highly influential within the study of 'the family'. One of the earliest feminist voices to be heard was that of American Betty Friedan who wrote about 'the problem with no name' in her influential book *The Feminine Mystique* (1963). The 'problem' she described was the isolating and self-limiting role of housewife and mother: she wrote of the experience of suburban American women caught up in an unfulfilling cycle which contrasted starkly with their husbands' role as 'breadwinners' in the world of work. In a review of her contribution to feminism, Bryson (2002) points out that Friedan referred to a particular model of family life (the nuclear family), yet this was not necessarily the experience of family life familiar to many working-class and Black women. Indeed, as bell hooks (1984) points out, many Black women at the time worked as domestic help for the disenchanted white middle-class women Friedan spoke of in *The Feminine Mystique*. In a further critique of these early feminist views of the family, Marxist feminists, Barrett and McIntosh (1982) sought to emphasize the significant influence of the state in maintaining the gendered status quo within the nuclear family as part of a wider pattern of inequality which went beyond simply gender.

LONE-PARENT FAMILIES

The supposed ubiquity of the nuclear family form was also being challenged by the increase in lone-parent families (almost exclusively headed by women), particularly evident from the 1970s. In 1971, there were an estimated 570000 lone parent households in Britain; this figure rose to over 1 million by 1986 and climbed to 1.6 million a decade later in 1996 (Haskey 1996). Most recent figures from the 2001/2002 General Household Survey suggest that lone-parent families with dependent children now make up 6% of all households, with the majority headed by mothers (9/10 lone families are headed by women) (Office for Population Census and Surveys 2001a).

It is also important to consider the intersection of ethnicity or 'race' upon the formation of lone-parent families. Somerville (2000) noted from her research that more than one-third of African-Caribbean women were registered heads of household, which perhaps aligns with a sometimes held stereotyped view of Black women. However, Reynolds (2002) suggests that this picture may be misleading as it represents only a transitional stage of family life for many Black women. It is also important to note the negative economic impact of divorce and/or lone-parenthood and the consequent material disadvantage, particularly for women. Somerville (2000) found that economically disadvantaged women were more likely to become lone mothers, and in general, rates of early marriage and divorce or separation are highest among the poorest families. This further compounds the economic disadvantages that lone-parenthood confers.

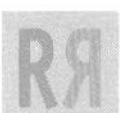

REFLECTION POINT

Consider the potential challenges for parents and children in lone-parent families.

Family practices

A key piece of research by Stacey (1991) revealed the complexity of family life, family forms and family practices. She carried out an ethnographic study of the kinship networks of primarily White working class people in the USA, and revealed a complexity of family arrangements which she called the *post-modern family.* However, Stacey asserted that this description was

> *'Not a new model of family life, not the next stage in an orderly progression of family history but the stage where the belief in a logical progression of family history breaks down ... the post-modern family lurches forward and backward into an uncertain future'. (Stacey 1991: 18)*

Although her research was conducted in the USA, it resonates with the picture here in Britain (Morgan 1996, Silva & Smart 1999). For example Smart et al (2001), look at the fragmentary effects of divorce upon childhood. For clarity and a greater understanding of contemporary family life, we can usefully draw upon Morgan's (1999) conceptualization of *family practices* (originally outlined in Stacey's work), where he emphasizes the interplay between factors such as work, income, culture and policy within families. This shapes the division of labour and consequent power differentials between family members. Put simply, 'family life is often characterized in terms of flux and fluidity' (Morgan 1999: 13) and accordingly, individual families tend to frame domestic practices (such as housework and childcare) in different ways, depending on the prevailing demands and opportunities of the time.

Cultural expectations about family life and the sexual division of labour have altered substantially over the past 30 or 40 years. Most significantly, women's lives have been transformed during the last century with increased demands and opportunities in terms of education, employment, income and relationships. As a result, the assumption of husband as bread-winner and wife as home-maker has been repeatedly challenged over the decades.

It now makes more sense to distinguish between 'caring for' the home and family members, and 'caring about' the family. The former implies undertaking the actual work required, whereas caring *about* your family emphasizes the emotional aspects. This notion of the *emotional labour* expended by parents (most specifically mothers) has been taken up by writers such as Jagger and Wright (1999) and Hochschild (1989), whose earlier work framed the concept more broadly to look at paid 'caring' roles such as airline attendants (Hochschild 1983) (see Chapter 3).

Children's perspectives on family life

Children within the family are expected to accept the more passive role of being cared for and supported by their parents. Morrow's (1998) study on children's perceptions and experience of family life offers some interesting insights into a child's eye-view of familial/ gender roles and relationships. When asked the questions 'what is a family?' and 'what are families for?' the children's answers generally focussed on who was important to them and what those people did for them. For example, Nadia, aged 9 says that:

> *'My mum is important to me because she feeds me and clothes me and loves me very much. My dad is important to me because he pays for the food I eat and the clothes I wear. He cares for me and loves me very much'. (cited in Morrow 1998: 24)*

Morrow (1998: 19) points out that 'gender roles within the household were clearly differentiated', particularly within Pakistani families, as illustrated in the quote from Nadia above. The sexual division of labour is evident in the family of Mark who is 13, when he says that:

> *'My mum is important because she cooks me food and [does the] washing. My dad is important to me because he takes me to work with him so I get to go on roofs at people's houses'. (cited in Morrow 1998: 23)*

Similar studies by Brannen et al (2000) and Smart et al (2001) both point to the importance of the provision of love and care from significant people (especially parents) within the family, and thus echoes the opinions expressed by the children in Morrow's study. From this, it appears that children tend to be less concerned with the shape or structure of their family, and more focussed on the quality of relationships with family members, and are more inclusive in their conception of 'family'. Significantly for nurses working with children it is vital to note that both parents are important to children irrespective of whether they live with them or not.

Families as care providers

The sociologist Ann Oakley (1993) has suggested that *professional* healthcare providers sometimes underestimate the part families and communities play as *providers of care*, and may fail to appreciate the role of families within the broad *experience* of health, illness, care and recovery. The family might easily be described as the 'cornerstone' of the care-giving system. Indeed, a relatively recent government strategy paper, Caring about Carers: a National Strategy for Carers, stated that 'caring forms a vital part of the *fabric and character* of Britain' (DoH 1999a: 5, italics as in original). However, recognition of familial care-giving has not always been quite so evident. Ground-breaking work by sociologists, such as Land (1978), Finch and Groves (1980, 1983), Qureshi and Walker (1989) and more recently, Finch and Mason (1993) revealed new understandings about familial obligations and caring. Indeed, research such as this opened up debate and attracted governmental interest in the significance of informal carers.

During the late 1980s and early 1990s there was a new push for *care in* (and of course *care by*) the community, which was set out in the NHS and Community Care Act, 1990. Subsequently, The Carers (Recognition and Services) Act 1995 was the first piece of legislation to specifically acknowledge the needs and rights of informal carers (see also Chapter 10). It defined carers as 'someone who provides a substantial amount of care on a regular basis to another' and excluded paid carers and voluntary workers. The Act gave informal carers the right to an assessment of their own needs as part of the overall assessment of the cared-for person. Increasingly, the needs of carers are being recognized within governmental policy, including the National Service Framework for Older People (DoH 2001) and The National Service Framework for Mental Health (DoH 1999b).

A further example of the increasing acknowledgement of the significance of carers was that for the first time the 2001 Census contained a question which asked about the provision of unpaid care. From this data it was revealed that in *England and Wales, 5.2 million people identified themselves as unpaid carers* in response to the following question:

> *'Do you look after, or give any help or support to family members, friends, neighbours or others because of long-term physical or mental ill-health or disability, or problems related to old age?' (Office for Population Census and Surveys 2001b)*

From this, the Census also revealed the age and gender demographics of caring. By far the largest group of carers were people over 50, with more than one-in-five people aged 50–59 providing some form of unpaid care. Retired people were more likely than the average to be carers (17%), and those people not in paid work (for example housewives) (24%), were the most likely to provide care. In terms of gender, women outnumbered men in all age groups, and within the 50–59 age group approximately one in four (24.6%) women provided some form of unpaid care compared with 17.9% of men (Office for Population Census and Surveys 2001b).

From the results of her work, Graham (1983) had warned of the consequences of viewing women as a *reserve army of labour* as unpaid informal carers. She highlighted the detrimental effects of this role, which often left women devalued by society. Karp (2001) endorses this view and locates the essence of the problem with society's belief (and hence governmental belief) in the privatized nature of the family. He contends that:

> *'... history has set in motion a process that relegates care-giving to the private domain of family life, sees it as largely the natural moral obligation of women to accomplish, and devalues it as an activity'. (Karp 2001: 251)*

Feminist researchers have looked at the specific contribution women make to care-giving within families – from housework to childcare and care of older relatives. Finch, in an early contribution to the appreciation of the informal care work undertaken by women, coined the phrase 'for community read family, for family read women' (1984: 4). Such challenges served to disrupt the ideological status quo, and the long-held assumptions about the role of women within the family and society as a whole.

However, findings from the 1985 General Household Survey (Green 1988) revealed that a significant minority of informal carers are men. While women continue to outnumber men in care-giving roles, the experience of male carers cannot be marginalized. From his research with carers of a family member with mental illness, Karp (2001) identified that the *perception* of the care role was gendered. Women deeply felt an *obligation* to care, which contrasted with a more pragmatic approach by men. Yet whatever the gender, or other distinctions, it is important to appreciate that 'everyone feels the effect of caring' (DoH 1999a: 11), from the person being cared for by their family, to the professional care providers. It is also important to acknowledge the impact upon other members of the family such as children, perhaps as carers themselves. As we shall see later in the chapter, different families meet the challenges of caring and manage the experience of illness in different ways.

THE IMPACT OF ILLNESS ON THE FAMILY

From their research into the impact of chronic illness, Patterson and Garwick (1994) found that families showed themselves to be resilient and adaptive in response to the challenges of care responsibilities. Nevertheless, the considerable impact upon families faced with the challenge of caring is well documented (see for example Rolland (1994), who looks at the caring role of families with children experiencing chronic illnesses such as Type 1 diabetes). Within such families, there is significant potential for stress and disruption (Patterson & Garwick 1994) and relationships between family members (siblings, parents and extended family) may be altered as a result of the care-giving role. The American sociologist, Arthur Frank, offers a somewhat bleak, yet undoubtedly well observed, perspective on the experience of being the carer of a family member when he says that:

> *'As little we know of illness, we know even less of care. As much as the ill person's experience is denied, the care-giver's experience is denied more completely'. (Frank 1991: 107)*

Frank explores further in his book *The Wounded Storyteller* (1995) the need for people who are ill to tell their stories, or *illness narratives*, as a way of making sense of their experiences. Implicit in Frank's work is the recognition that such narratives are witnessed by others: carers *listen* to the stories of sickness. In this way carers, and perhaps other members of the family, are implicated in the person's sickness and so it becomes a part of their own life experience and life story.

SUPPORT FOR FAMILIES

Recognition of the role of informal carers has become more widespread with the implementation of the Carers' (Recognition and Services) Act in 1995. This piece of legislation was recently developed and updated. The Carers' (Equal Opportunities) Act, 2004 was implemented in April 2005 (see www.direct.gov.uk). In a review of the Act, Lloyd (2000: 7) suggests that the new legislation 'illustrates clearly the intention to raise the social status of unpaid care', through the use of words in the document such as 'unsung heroes', 'value' and 'pride' in relation to the carer role. Yet Lloyd acknowledges that there is still more work to be done in relation to understanding the psychological, and deeply complex, aspects of caring. Nurses are well equipped to take up this challenge both from a research perspective and within their day-to-day practice.

THE FAMILY AND MENTAL ILLNESS

For the family of a person with a mental illness, the role of care giver and supporter can indeed be complex, and accordingly may be fraught with tension and difficulty. Karp explores the experiences of carers of mentally ill family members through in-depth interviews with carers, in his book *The Burden of Sympathy*. He points out that:

> *'Unlike most physical illnesses, caregivers to the mentally ill (especially parents) must often contend with the possibility that they are somehow implicated in the creation of the other's problem'. (Karp 2001: 23)*

Carers may find themselves positioned as the 'enemy by their loved one', suggests Karp (2001: 23). This position is graphically illustrated by a mother interviewed during Karp's research who recounted the distressing experience of initiating the forced hospitalization of her daughter:

> *'She didn't do anything wrong. What has she done wrong to deserve people doing this to her? ... It breaks my heart to see her having to be restrained by four big huge men ... and she's crying and screaming, 'Where's my mother?' 'Why isn't my mother helping me?' It feels like my poor daughter saying, 'Mom, if you love me, how can you let this happen to me?' And yet, I'm doing it out of love ... Getting her help, you know, 'cause that's the only way she's going to get better. I can't take her home and she doesn't understand this .... (Retired secretary, cited in Karp 2001: 79)*

There is a considerable history to the linking of problems with, and problems within, the family to the creation of mental illness. Castel (1988), in his historical overview of the regulation of madness in France, cites the work of Morel in the nineteenth century and his theory of mental illness as a product of degenerate reproduction (that is, children born to mentally ill parents will in turn be vulnerable to such illnesses themselves). Indeed, interest in the possibility of genetic vulnerability to mental illness has endured, with some schools of modern psychiatry still conducting work within this field. However, Rose (1989) identifies the post-war period of the 1940s and 1950s as a time when the professional gaze turned to focus on the internal workings of the family: a distinctly psychological approach. It was around this time that psychoanalyst Frieda Fromm-Reichmann coined the term '*schizophrenogenic mother*' (Fromm-Reichman 1948) to describe an emotionally cold mother who withheld affection from her baby and by doing so supposedly caused the child to develop schizophrenia in later life. These ideas were pursued even further by the so-called 'anti-family' movement in the 1960s and 1970s (Laing & Esterson 1970). In spite of their limited evidence-base, these ideas influenced professional carers and consequently they made the role of family carer even more difficult than it already was. Their legacy has, argues Jones (2002), had a negative impact upon the relationships between family carers and healthcare professionals.

Discussion points

1. How might the changes in family structure impact upon its ability to provide care and support for its members?
2. From your experience in practice, discuss the ways in which a family member's chronic illness impacts upon the rest of the family

CHAPTER SUMMARY

So what is a family? We might all respond differently to that question, with our answers probably based upon our own experiences or expectations of family life. This chapter has highlighted both the diversity of family life and the family as a site of inequality. Inequalities and social diversity are two themes which you will re-visit throughout this book.

Most of us may feel we know what a family is, but if we are required to 'think sociologically' as Bauman (1990) suggests, and respond to the question in a more open-minded way, it is unlikely we would reach a unanimous agreement on what a family actually is. Yet, this apparent lack of certainty over what a family is can be positively re-framed, and seen as the essence of an open and non-judgemental partnership between nurses and the families with whom they work.

REFERENCES

Allen G, Crow G 2001 Families, households and society. Palgrave, Basingstoke

Anderson M, Bechhofer F, Gershuny J (eds) 1994 The social and political economy of the household. Oxford University Press, Oxford

Barrett M, McIntosh M 1982 The anti-social family. Verso, London

Bauman Z 1990 Thinking sociologically. Blackwell, Oxford

Beck U, Beck-Gernsheim E 1995 The normal chaos of love. Polity, Cambridge

bell hooks 1984 From the margin to the centre. South End Press, Boston

Bennett A 1994 Writing home. Faber and Faber, London

Bernardes J 1997 Family studies. Routledge, London

Brannen J, Heptinstall E, Bhopal K 2000 Connecting children: care and family life in later childhood. Routledge Falmer, London

Bryson V 2002 Feminist debates: Issues of theory and political practice. Palgrave Macmillan, Basingstoke

Castel R 1988 The regulation of madness: The origins of incarceration in France. Polity Press, Cambridge

Chapman T 2004 Gender and domestic life. Changing practices in families and households. Palgrave Macmillan, Basingstoke

Department of Health 1999a Caring about carers: A national strategy for carers. DoH, London

Department of Health 1999b The National Service Framework for Mental Health. Stationery Office, London

Department of Health 2001 The National Service Framework for Older People. Stationery Office, London

Featherstone B 2004 Family life and family support. Palgrave Macmillan, Basingstoke

Ferguson H 2001 Social work, individualization and life politics. British Journal of Social Work 31(1):41–55
Finch J 1984 Community care: developing non-sexist alternatives. Critical Social Policy 9:6–18
Finch J, Groves D 1980 Community care and the family: a case for equal opportunities. Journal of Social Policy 9(4):487–514
Finch J, Groves D 1983 A labour of love: Women, work and caring. Routledge & Kegan Paul, London
Finch J, Mason J 1993 Negotiating family responsibilities. Routledge, London
Frank A 1991 At the will of the body. Houghton Mifflin, New York
Frank A 1995 The wounded storyteller. University of Chicago Press, Chicago
Freely M 2000 The parent trap: Children, families and the new morality. Virago, London
Friedan B 1963 The feminine mystique. Penguin, Harmondsworth
Fromm-Reichman F 1948 Notes on the development of treatment of schizophrenics by psychoanalytic psychotherapy. Psychiatry 2:263–273
Giddens A 1992 The transformation of intimacy: Sexuality, love and eroticism in modern societies. Polity, Cambridge
Giddens A 2001 Sociology. Polity, Cambridge
Graham H 1983 Caring: labour of love. In: Finch J, Groves D (eds) A labour of love: Women, work and caring. Routledge & Kegan Paul, London, p 13–30
Green H 1988 General Household Survey 1985: Informal carers. HMSO, London
Gubrium J F, Holstein J A 1990 What is family? Mayfield, Mountain View, California
Haskey J 1996 Population Review: (6) Families and households in Great Britain. Population Trends 85:7–24
Hochschild A 1983 The managed heart: The commercialization of human feeling. University of California Press, Berkeley
Hochschild A 1989 Second shift: Working parents and the revolution at home. Viking Penguin, Harmondsworth
Hylton C 1995 Coping with change. Family transitions in multi-cultural communities. National Stepfamily Association, London
Jagger G, Wright C (eds) 1999 Changing family values. Routledge, London
Jamieson L 1997 Intimacy: Personal relationships in modern societies. Polity, Oxford
Jones D W 2002 Myths, madness and the family the impact of mental illness on families. Palgrave, Basingstoke
Karp DA 2001 The burden of sympathy. How families cope with mental illness. Oxford University Press, Oxford
Laing R D, Esterson A 1970 Sanity, madness and the family. Penguin, Harmondsworth
Land H 1978 Who cares for the family. Journal of Social Policy 7(3):257–284
Lasch C 1995 Haven in a heartless world: The family besieged. Norton, New York
Lloyd L 2000 Caring about carers: only half the picture? Critical Social Policy 20(1):136–357
Morgan D 1996 Family connections: An introduction to family studies. Polity, Cambridge
Morgan D 1999 Risk and family practices. In: Silva E, Smart C (eds) The new family? Sage, London, p 13–30
Morrow V 1998 Understanding families: Children's perspectives. National Children's Bureau, London
Mulhall A 1998 Nursing, research and the evidence. Evidence-based Nursing 1(1):4–6
Muncie J, Sapsford R 1995 Issues in the study of the family. In: Muncie J, Wetherell M, Dallos R et al (eds) Understanding the family. Sage, London, p 7–37
Nicholson L 1999 The play of reason. From the modern to the postmodern. Open University Press, Buckingham
Oakley A 1974 Housewife. Allen Lane, London
Oakley A 1984 Taking it like a woman. Random House, London
Oakley A 1993 Essays on women, medicine and health. Edinburgh University Press, Edinburgh
Office for Population Census and Surveys 2001a General Household Survey 2001/2. Online. Available: www.statistics.gov.uk
Office for Population Census and Surveys 2001b Great Britain 2001 Census. Online. Available: www.statistics.gov.uk
Office for National Statistics 2001 Living arrangements. Online. Available: www.statistics.gov.uk
Office for National Statistics 2005 Living arrangements. Online. Available: www.statistics.gov.uk
Office for National Statistics 2006 Civil partnerships. Online. Available: www.statistics.gov.uk
Parsons T 1955 (with Robert Bales) Family socialisation and interaction process. Free Press, Glencoe
Patterson J, Garwick A 1994 Family meanings and sense of coherence. In: McCubbin H, Thompson E, Thompson A et al (eds) Sense of coherence and resiliency: Stress, coping, and health. University of Wisconsin Press, Madison, p 71–89

Qureshi H, Walker A 1989 The caring relationship: Elderly people and their families. MacMillan, Basingstoke

Reynolds T 2002 Re-analysing the black family. In: Carling A, Duncan S, Edwards R (eds) Analysing families: Morality and rationality in policy and practice. Routledge, London, p 69–76

Rolland J S 1994 Families, illness, and disability: An integrative treatment model. Harper Collins, New York

Rose N 1989 Governing the soul: The shaping of the private self. Routledge, London

Silva E B, Smart C (eds) 1999 The new family? Sage, London

Simpson B 1998 Changing families. Berg, Oxford

Smart C Neale B, Wade A 2001 The changing experiences of childhood: Families and divorce. Polity, Cambridge

Somerville J 2000 Feminism and the family: Politics and society in the UK and USA. Palgrave Macmillan, Basingstoke

Stacey J 1991 Brave new families. Basic Books, New York

Stacey J 1998 Dada-ism in the 1990s: getting past baby talk about fatherlessness. In: Daniels C R (ed.) Lost fathers: The politics of fatherlessness in America. Palgrave Macmillan, London, p 51–83

Twigg J, Atkin K 1994 Carers perceived: policy and practice in informal care. OUP, Buckingham

Weber M 1968 Economy and society: An outline of interpretive sociology. Bedminster Press, New York

Wright L M, Leahey M 2005 The three most common errors in family nursing; how to avoid or sidestep. Journal of Family Nursing 11(2):90–101

Young M, Wilmot P 1957 Family and kinship in East London. Routledge & Kegan Paul, London

CHAPTER

3

Thinking sociologically about religion and health

Hannah Cooke

KEY CONCEPTS

- Secularization
- Theodicy: explaining suffering
- Church, sect and cult
- 'New age' beliefs and fundamentalism
- Religion and health
- Spiritual care

Introduction

Religions are concerned with life's meaning and with explanations of pain, suffering and death. Thus, their importance to sociologists of health and illness might seem obvious. Nevertheless, religion has been strikingly neglected by sociologists of illness. Williams (1993b), has suggested that this has been because both medicine and sociology are highly secular and have therefore regarded religion as unimportant.

When sociologists have turned their attention to religion, it has often been only to predict its death. Meanwhile healthcare has become an increasingly secular domain with only a few remains of its religious foundations. For example, the routine of ward prayers at the start of each shift, which this author remembers from her nurse training, is largely a thing of the past. However, as nurses in particular have come to define their interest in the patient as *holistic*, there has been a new interest in religion and spirituality. This is reflected in a proliferation of books on *spiritual* issues (McSherry 2000, Narayanasamy 2001). These changes reflect both the changing role of nursing and the changing role of religion in contemporary society.

In this chapter, we will look at classical and contemporary sociological studies of religion and their application to healthcare. We will consider how these can help us to understand the complex relationships between religion, society, illness and healthcare in the contemporary world.

Classical sociological accounts of religion

The key theme which has united much sociological writing about religion is that of **secularization**. By secularization, we mean the progressive decline of the importance of religion in the world. Many sociologists of health and illness have assumed that secularization is an inevitable feature of modern society but the empirical evidence to support this assertion is complex and contradictory.

It is important to distinguish between secularization and secularism. Secularization refers to the declining significance of religion; what Max Weber described as the '*disenchantment of the world*' (Gerth & Wright Mills 1970). Secularism refers to a materialist system of thought which rejects religious beliefs as irrational. One of the leading contemporary proponents of secularism is Richard Dawkins (2006). Secular rationalism draws on a philosophical distinction between *reason* and *faith*. Faith is seen as superstitious and backward and thus the decline of religion is seen as a positive and progressive development in the modern world. Secular rationalism can be traced back to the eighteenth century 'Enlightenment' period following the French revolution, when science and rationality became increasingly influential in society. This was an era of massive social, political and economic change heralding the dawn of the industrial revolution. This 'Enlightenment' way of thinking is now often described as *modernism*.

The influence of secular rationalism on sociological theories of religion is obvious. Many of them proceed from an assumption that religion entails a suspension of reason, which requires explanation. Many secularist sociologists therefore seized on evidence of the decline of religion as a reason for optimism. It was evidence of the increasing 'enlightenment' of the world. A pessimistic reading of the evidence for secularization on the other hand, sees it as representing a decline in moral and communal values. Furthermore, in an era of global warming faith in scientific progress has itself been severely curtailed.

Beckford (1989) suggests that it is impossible to disentangle the sociological view of religion from wider social theories and problems. Classical sociologists shaped their theories about religion in response to their attempts to understand the massive social changes brought about by the industrial revolution. They were particularly concerned by the problems of deprivation and disharmony they saw following in its wake. According to Beckford (1989), sociological thinking about religion has failed to keep pace with the changing nature of society and is still rooted in these classical theories. This is particularly true of the theory of secularization which, according to Beckford, has failed to appreciate that the disappearance of nineteenth-century forms of religion does not necessarily imply the disappearance of religion itself. As a starting point therefore, we need to understand how classical nineteenth-century sociologists viewed religion and the way in which their ideas have shaped contemporary debates. We will then consider how our society has changed and the way in which religion has adapted to contemporary social conditions. According to some authors, we now live in a *post-industrial* or *post-modern* age.

MARX'S ACCOUNT OF RELIGION

Marx's view of religion was typical of nineteenth-century secular rationalism in its dismissal of religious beliefs (to read about Marx's major ideas, see Chapter 5). Marx saw religion as a form of *human self alienation*. Marx's ideas drew on the work of the nineteenth-century philosopher Feuerbach (1957), who described the idea of God as an *alienation* of the highest human powers. According to Feuerbach, humans projected their own power onto a deity and thus became estranged from their true nature. Humanity had only to see behind this disguise to grasp that religion was an illusion. Liberation and progress would then result from the establishment of a humanist belief system. Marx agreed with Feuerbach in seeing religion as a form of alienation.

> *'The more the worker expends himself in work the more powerful becomes the world of objects which he creates in face of himself and the poorer he himself becomes in his inner life, the less he belongs to himself. It is just the same in religion. The more of*

himself man attributes to God, the less he has left of himself'. (Marx, cited in Bottomore & Rubel 1973: 178)

Marx took Feuerbach's concept of alienation and applied it in a new way. For Marx, the source of alienation was not religion itself but the economic relations of society. Workers were not oppressed by their beliefs but by the new relations of industrial capitalism which exploited them. For Marx, religion was problematic because of the role it played in reconciling working people to that oppression. Religion expressed fundamental values of compassion, freedom and justice but it encouraged the exploited to accept the status quo and aspire to salvation in an after-life rather than realizing these values on earth.

> *'Religious suffering is at the same time an expression of real suffering and a protest against real suffering. Religion is the sigh of the oppressed creature, the sentiment of a heartless world and the soul of soulless conditions. It is the opium of the people. The abolition of religion, as the illusory happiness of men is a demand for their real happiness. The call to abandon their illusions about their condition is a call to abandon a condition which requires illusion'. (Marx, cited in Bottomore & Rubel 1973: 41).*

Thus Marx looked forward to a society rid of oppression in which justice would be realized on earth and religion would become unnecessary.

REFLECTION POINT

We have seen that Marx was concerned with the ways in which industrial society produced *alienation* – a sense of powerlessness. How do you think that a sense of alienation might affect a person's health? How did Marx think that religion contributed to a sense of alienation? Do you think that he was right to criticize religion in this way?

DURKHEIM AND RELIGION

If Marx was concerned with the inequality and oppression created by industrial capitalism, then the sociologist Emile Durkheim was concerned above all with the breakdown of communal values and the social order. Marx has given us the concept of *alienation* – a sense of self estrangement engendered by the oppression of capitalist social relations. By contrast, Durkheim saw contemporary humanity as threatened by the condition of **anomie**. *Anomie* refers to a sense of normlessness (from the Greek anomia absence of law) – the individual's estrangement from societal rules and values. Durkheim believed that anomie led to suicide, crime and social breakdown.

BIOGRAPHY Emile Durkheim (1858–1917)

Emile Durkheim was a French sociologist from a Jewish background. He is credited along with Herbert Spencer with being the founder of sociology as an academic discipline and with changing forever the way we would think about and study society. Durkheim was a socialist and his work addressed the problems of social deprivation and disharmony that followed in the wake of the industrial revolution. He believed that religion had played an important part in promoting social cohesion and that professions would play an important part in promoting civic morals in industrial societies.

Durkheim was concerned to establish the social origins of social problems, such as crime and suicide. Durkheim presented a critique of individualistic explanations of social behaviour. He said that social phenomena were 'social facts' which could not be explained simply by reference to the motivations or propensities of individual actors (methodological individualism). Social facts had, according to Durkheim, their own logic which was not reducible to explanations at the biological or psychological level. Social facts are external to any particular individual considered as a biological entity and act as an external constraint on individual choices and actions. They are 'endowed with coercive power, by ... which they impose themselves upon him, independent of his individual will'. A social fact can hence be defined as 'every way of acting, fixed or not, capable of exercising on the individual an external constraint' (Rules of the Sociological Method 1895).

Durkheim's major works include:

- *Division of Labour in Society* 1893
- *Rules of the Sociological Method* 1895
- *Suicide* 1897
- *Elementary Forms of the Religious Lifestyles* 1912
- *Professional Ethics and Civic Morals* (published in 1955)

For Durkheim, some form of religion was necessary to society if anomie was to be contained. Religion was the means, whereby society collectively expressed its central values and identity through ceremonials and rituals. In his major study of religion, The Elementary Forms of Religious Life ([1912] 1976), he tried to outline the different forms that these rituals took and the functions that they performed. Durkheim believed that *there was something eternal in religion* although the dynamic nature of society meant that religious forms and beliefs would change. Religion promoted social cohesion and acted as a 'social cement'. Durkheim was preoccupied with the way in which industrialization both threatened and changed the basis of social cohesion. However, religion would survive because:

> *'There can be no society which does not feel the need of upholding and reaffirming at regular intervals the collective sentiments and the collective ideas which make up its unity and its personality'. (Durkheim [1912] 1976: 427)*

Durkheim predicted that while religious *institutions* might decline, the functions of religion would persist. Whereas, in pre-industrial society, religious worship was largely collective, in modern society, religion would become individualized. Religion would express the sacredness inherent in each individual as an expression of a moral community. Durkheim's ideas have found expression in the work of contemporary sociologists who have argued that religious beliefs have persisted but have become increasingly individualistic and privatized. Thus, Luckmann (1967) described this new private form of religion as 'invisible religion'.

RR REFLECTION POINT

We have seen that Durkheim believed that religion was like an invisible glue that helped to hold society together. Durkheim believed that this was because it helped people to express shared social values. What values do you think that people share within contemporary society? How are these expressed? How important are shared values in healthcare? What part do you think that religion plays in this?

WEBER'S VIEW OF RELIGION

Max Weber was concerned both with the way in which society shaped religious ideas and also with the way in which religious ideas influenced society (Weber's major ideas are discussed in Chapter 4). Weber's ideas about the interplay of religion and society are expressed in particular in his best known study on the influence of Protestant ideas on the rise of capitalism (Weber 1974). Thus, Weber was interested in the social psychology of religion and he has a lot to say that is of relevance to healthcare. He paid particular attention to the ways in which religions construct explanations of suffering and death. Such justifications and explanations of suffering are described as *theodicies*.

The idea of suffering as a form of punishment is of profound importance in almost all religious traditions. Weber says that the fortunate are not content with good fortune alone, but need to believe that they have a right to be fortunate. Thus, wealth, power and good health are legitimated by the *theory of good fortune*, and suffering is treated as a sign of *odiousness in the eyes of the Gods*. The possessor of good fortune needs to console his conscience with the belief that he deserves to be favoured as much as the unfortunate deserve their misery.

The poor and suffering still have to make sense of their lot and can find small comfort in the idea that they deserve to suffer. The persistence of injustice and undeserved suffering therefore led to the idea of a saviour or redeemer who will right all wrongs by either '*the return of good fortune in this world or the security of happiness in the next world*' (Weber 1920, reprinted in Gerth & Wright Mills 1970). Thus, new theodicies periodically emerge which promise to right the wrongs of the world and offer salvation to the poor and suffering. Examples include the Christian Messiah and the Cult of Krishna in Hinduism.

Weber saw the modern world as characterized by increasing rationalization. The spread of rationality pushed the need for explanations of suffering to the margins of our consciousness. Rationality had *demystified* the world. Science, however, can explain how events such as sickness occur, but it is limited in its explanations of why such events occur. Weber's discussion of theodicies reminds us that these questions remain central to how people make sense of the world. According to Clark:

> *'How and why questions seem therefore to keep alive the distinction between science and religion. When related to some conditions of human misfortune – say sickness – they may be posed as the opposition between two problems 'how is my condition caused' and 'why is this happening to me.' Where does the individual find answers to these "why" questions?' (Clark 1982: 7)*

How individuals find meaning in suffering is key to understanding a person's response to illness. Weber's ideas suggest that these 'why' questions are marginalized by secular rationalism. The rise of modern medicine is one instance of the increasing rationalization of the world with its central focus on how illness is caused and its location of the source of illness in the physiology of the individual. However, for Weber in contrast to some of his more recent followers the disenchantment of the world was 'more of a tendency than an accomplished fact' (Beckford 1989).

There would always be counter tendencies and areas of social life which resisted the process of rationalization. Weber utilized the concept of charisma to explain the rise of new religious and social movements not based on rational or traditional authority.

Charismatic authority is wielded by an individual or social group who are able to achieve power through ideas, revelations, magical power or simply force of personality. Charismatic authority implies the breakdown of existing systems of authority whether rational or traditional and therefore, entails the creation of new and revolutionary social, political or religious movements. By its very nature, charismatic authority is short-lived and charisma becomes 'routinized' as the movement settles down and becomes institutionalized. James and Field (1992) analysed the 'routinization of charisma' in the growing bureaucratization of the hospice movement and we return to this in the final chapter.

Weber's concept of charisma implied that religions would not decline inexorably. New religions would arise with charismatic leaders and existing religions would experience periods of charismatic revival. The significance of the concept of charisma has been variously interpreted. For some charismatic religions are mere punctuation points in the irreversible 'disenchantment of the world', whereas, for others, they show the continuing social significance of religion and the potential of religious movements to overthrow the existing social order.

RЯ REFLECTION POINT

We have seen that Weber believed that religion was important in helping people to make sense of suffering and misfortune. What ideas do you think help people make sense of suffering today? How important is religion to this sense-making process?

Religion: declining or changing?

We can still see the influence of these classical theorists when we look at studies of contemporary religion. However, in the twenty-first century we are arguably facing a different set of social conditions. How different is a matter of debate with some authors seeing the present simply as a continuation of the past; for these authors we continue to live in a largely industrialized modern age in which society will continue to become progressively more secular. For other writers however, we have moved into a new era where we are now disenchanted with science and rationality and new interests in religion and spirituality may develop. These latter authors describe the present as a postmodern or post industrial era (Heelas 1993a). These different schools of thought look at changes in religion in different ways. Three types of evidence have been put forward when examining the changing fortunes of religion in contemporary society:

1. Patterns of religious membership and affiliation
2. Patterns of religious belief
3. The influence of religion on major social institutions.

DECLINING RELIGIOUS AFFILIATION?

When considering changes in religious institutions and their membership we are going to look first of all at the situation in the UK. Later, we will consider whether the UK is typical or exceptional in its attitudes to religion.

Changing patterns of religious affiliation have to be considered in relation to the different types of religious organizations which exist in contemporary UK society. Sociologists have developed a number of typologies of religious organizations. Four main types are generally recognized:

1. Churches
2. Sects
3. Denominations
4. Cults.

Churches are large-scale, formal organizations with professional clergy, which are often highly bureaucratic. They may be closely allied to the state as in the case of the Church of England or the Catholic Church in Eire. The Church of England has suffered a dramatic decline in attendance with only 1.8 million attending regularly in 1992 (Davie 1994a), yet it is still the Church to which the majority (25.5 million of the population) claim allegiance. More recently, Brierley (2005) has suggested that only 6.8% of the population attended church regularly in 2005, yet surveys have shown that the majority of the population continue to claim to be nominally Christian. Most only attend church for significant events such as baptisms, weddings, funerals and Christmas.

In spite of a general decline in active church membership, there remain significant local and regional differences. Congregations still thrive in some areas, particularly rural areas and provinces, such as Northern Ireland. Furthermore, many ethnic minority communities show no signs of adopting the rather lukewarm attitude to religion characteristic of the majority of the UK population. Bruce (1996) argues that religion has an important role in expressing ethnic and cultural identity and that in many of these situations, it is used as a 'cultural defence'. An alternative argument is that these groups retain the more enthusiastic attitudes to religion typical of their country of origin and that it is the UK population which is unusual in its indifference to religion.

The rather dramatic evidence of a decline in active church membership has fuelled arguments in favour of the secularization thesis. The evidence is visible to all as, throughout our towns and cities redundant churches and chapels are converted into shops, warehouses, flats and bingo halls. However, non-Christian places of worship have fared better with many new mosques being built. The rather more buoyant fortunes of other Christian groups have also sometimes gone unnoticed yet few towns of a significant size have not seen the erection of a Kingdom Hall by their local Jehovah's Witnesses and new evangelical churches are also increasing in number.

Sects represent an increasingly important feature of the contemporary religious scene. Sectarian groups such as the Jehovah's Witnesses have usually arisen in radical protest against existing religions often through a charismatic leader. They are highly organized groups which see themselves as true believers and draw strong boundaries between 'them' and 'us'. Many are *millenarian* groups who believe that the end of the world is imminent and only *they* will be saved. Some modern sects have been remarkably successful in exploiting mass communications and marketing techniques to spread their message (Schmalz 1994). Some of the larger sects, such as the Mormons and Jehovah's Witnesses owe much of their success to their use of the techniques of successful business corporations, which is ironic given their ostensible rejection of secular rationalism. Recently, many have added the internet to their armoury of recruitment techniques.

Niebuhr (1929) argued that after a period of time, sects would 'cool down' and become more established and tolerant of other religions. He described these groups as *denominations*.

Denominational groups, such as the Methodists, have suffered very serious declines in membership. It may be that newer sects are learning this lesson and instituting mechanisms for maintaining a sectarian identity and boundaries between members and outsiders. A good example of this strategy of boundary maintenance is the decision of the Jehovah's Witnesses to institute a taboo on blood transfusions in the post-war period (Singelenberg 1990). A more recent example is the strong hostility to psychiatry promoted by the Church of Scientology. The rising fortunes of sectarian groups can be related in part to their successful methods of discipline and boundary maintenance in maintaining their membership. However, other more loose knit new religious groups have also multiplied in recent years.

Cults have been considered a fourth major form of religious organization (Bruce 1996) and one that has received considerable negative media attention (Barker 1989). *Cults* are small loose knit groups with unorthodox religious beliefs. Barker has made a considerable study of these groups and prefers the term *New Religious Movements* as more accurate and less pejorative. Although these new religious movements (or *cults*) have attracted negative media attention in recent years due to their supposed ability to 'brainwash' their members, research suggests that membership is usually short-lived and individuals attracted to these movements can be described as 'seekers' who pursue a variety of unorthodox religious beliefs and practices often simultaneously (Barker 1989). There are however risks that *cults* may pose a threat to the welfare of their members when leaders claim divine authority or when cult members allow important decisions about their lives to be made by others (Barker 1989).

The growth of sectarian groups and *cults* can be related to two competing trends in religious affiliation and belief. First, the growth of fundamentalism and second, the growth of 'new age' religious ideas and beliefs.

Fundamentalism was a term originally applied to the defence of Protestant orthodoxy against modern scientific thought, particularly the theory of evolution. The term has come to be applied more generally to religious movements which defend religious orthodoxy against the encroachments of contemporary culture (Marty & Scott Appleby 1993). Although Islamic fundamentalism has received the most media attention, fundamentalist movements have arisen in all parts of the world and in all religious traditions. For example, Christian fundamentalism is an increasingly important political force in the USA. Key features of fundamentalist movements include:

> *'A general hostility towards a rationalist post-Enlightenment view of the world; an emphasis on supernatural intervention in daily mundane affairs; a restored patriarchy under a charismatic leader who draws his legitimacy from God ... initial intransigence, born of millennial expectations followed (when the millennium fails to materialize) by some form of accommodation or bargaining with the larger world; a tendency to 'fight back' against the current of the times while appropriating those aspects of contemporary culture that seem necessary or desirable'. (Ruthuen 1993)*

The globalization of social life brings us into increasing contact with other religious traditions. The fundamentalist response to making sense of increasingly fragmented world views is to choose one all-encompassing view of the world and stick with it. Fundamentalists also see themselves as fighting back against the encroachments of secular rationalism and may become increasingly interested in obtaining secular power to achieve their ends. Robertson (1989) saw globalization as leading to the politicization of religion and the 'religionization' of politics. Davie (1994b) predicted a growth of intransigent and competing fundamentalisms. The Al Quaida attack on the world trade centre and the subsequent 'war on terror' have made their words seem prophetic. It would be difficult in the light of recent events to continue to maintain that religion is of no political significance in the modern world.

New age religion has been an alternative response to contemporary conditions. While for some the response to changing times has been found in fundamentalism or the fierce allegiance of sectarianism, another response to the variety of religious ideas and beliefs on offer in a global society is to select your own personal package. New age beliefs have imported market ideas into religion and Davie (1994a) has described this phenomenon as 'supermarket religion'. Our spiritual beliefs no longer reflect a deeply rooted sense of life's meaning and become instead a 'lifestyle' choice. Many authors have described the rise of a loose network of religious or quasi-religious organizations, practices and products, which Heelas (1993b) has described as the '*new age movement*'. This movement encourages us to 'shop around' for our spiritual beliefs and practices. These 'spiritual shoppers' are often described as 'seekers'. 'Seekers' may have shifting allegiances to cult groups or may pursue a more individualistic spiritual path.

New age beliefs have a number of shared features. The first is their eclecticism, 'new age' groups draw on a wide variety of religious ideas and symbols without worrying very much about their logical connections or contradictions. Berger (2001) describes this assembling of bits and pieces as 'patchwork religion'. Loose connections are made through the use of metaphors or umbrella terms, such as 'energy' and 'holism' (Bruce 1996).

For Heelas (1996), the central theme of the new age is the 'sacralization of the self'. This echoes Durkheim's earlier view that religion would come to symbolize the sacredness of the individual. The new age has been linked to a highly individualistic culture which Walter (1993) has described as '*expressivism*', in which self expression and self realization become the highest achievements. This culture (also described negatively by Lasch 1979 as '*narcissism*') finds its secular expression in humanistic psychology and many contemporary forms of therapy. Some of these therapies incorporate some supernatural beliefs so that the line between therapies and cults is sometimes blurred. In these self religions, these ideas are extended; we should not only seek to 'find ourselves', but to find God within ourselves.

Bruce (1996) sees the new age as the apotheosis of a consumerist and individualistic society. The 'new age' places little value on community, self sacrifice or on service to others or a higher power. Bruce argues that it is a 'grand irony' that such groups regard themselves as 'alternative', since they are the perfect product of their time. Bruce says that the 'new age' is the 'acme of consumerism', it is 'individualism raised to a new plane' leading individuals to suppose that 'by knowing oneself, we can know everything'.

New age movements take different forms and encompass religious groups and communities as well as individual therapists and practitioners. Many of the beliefs and practices of the 'new age' have entered the mass market and this is particularly true of 'self-help' manuals and 'alternative' therapies, such as aromatherapy which have spawned an enormous range of consumer products.

BELIEVING WITHOUT BELONGING?

We have painted a picture of declining church membership in the UK coupled with some growth areas, in particular, sectarian and fundamentalist movements and 'new age' movements. Empirical studies have consistently reported high levels of religious belief in spite of declining church membership. Survey results vary depending on how the question is asked but seem to indicate that although belief has declined, the majority of the population continue to believe in God. Surveys in the 1990s found that 68% of the UK population believed in God compared with 79% in the 1960s (Davie 2000). More unorthodox spiritual beliefs also persist and have sometimes increased with 31% claiming to believe in ghosts (compared with 19% in the 1970s); 26% believing in reincarnation; 23% believing in horoscopes and 47% believing in fortune telling (Davie 2000). According to Knoblauch (2003), 60% of the European population have reported in surveys that they have had supernatural experiences.

Three themes can be identified in sociological explanations of 'believing without belonging'. First, the theme of 'self religions' identified with earlier Durkheimian ideas and described in Luckmann's (1967) work as 'invisible' or 'privatized' systems of religion. This would explain the persistence and growth of unorthodox religious ideas and supernatural experiences. The 'new age' movement can be seen as the creation of a cultural milieu for these privatized religious systems. Linked to this sociologists have identified a general decline in membership of communal organizations (otherwise described as a decline in social capital; see Chapters 5 and 6). Declining church membership can be seen as a reflection of declining communal values rather than declining religious values and no different from the decline of football clubs, trade unions etc. (Davie 1994a).

Finally, some social historians have talked of 'common' or 'folk' religion instead of 'private' religion. The existence of high levels of belief alongside low levels of practice are seen as a recurrence of the characteristics of religion before the industrial revolution (Davie 1994a). Recent reports that the majority of the population rate religion as of low importance to their everyday lives (Voas & Crockett 2005) may reflect a long-term UK tradition. Folk traditions and informal practices existing outside formal structures are fairly persistent (Clark 1982, Davie 1994a, 2000). These 'unofficial' religious practices draw on shared meanings and are not entirely personal. Such beliefs may not be prominent in everyday life, but may be drawn on at times of transition or crisis, such as childbirth, illness and death. The recent examples of mass mourning following for example the death of Princess Diana fit in with the idea of religious folk traditions. (Davie 2000). Some authors have likened this folk tradition to a *God of the gaps*. God is only appealed to or consulted when everyday coping mechanisms have failed, such as in times of personal crisis, bereavement or illness (Abercrombie 1970).

DECLINING RELIGIOUS INFLUENCE?

If most areas of our life are controlled by secular institutions and our God is a *God of the gaps*, then religion may have little influence in our lives whatever the faith we profess. Thus, Voas and Crockett (2005) suggest that recent British polls have charted a decline in the numbers of people stating that religion was important in their lives. This is the argument made by Bruce (1996); religion is an increasingly marginalized and moribund force in contemporary society. Thus, one of the theories of secularization concerns the decline of religious influence in the world.

Public religion refers to the active participation of religious groups in public affairs (Casanova 1994). Casanova suggests that this involves engagement at a variety of different levels and that while the privileged position of religion within the state may have declined, this does not mean that religious groups cannot engage successfully with politics and civil society. In the USA, for example we have seen many examples of faith groups engaging very successfully in public life often wielding enormous influence. Faith groups have become increasingly vociferous on matters concerned with human rights, morality and ethics. Mainstream religious groups as well as fundamentalist movements have engaged in political debate and public affairs. Casanova (1994) has argued that religious groups have become more differentiated: that is they have become more separate from state institutions such as the healthcare and education systems. However, the state has increasingly withdrawn from the provision of services with the introduction of 'market' approaches to welfare provision and we have moved towards a 'mixed economy' of services. The scope for faith groups to engage in public life may substantially increase as political developments in the USA have recently indicated.

A final point about the influence of religion in the modern world concerns the role of religion globally. Much of the debate focuses on data from Britain and Western Europe. Yet these countries may be exceptional; across much of the globe, there is little evidence of secularization and religious affiliation and influence may actually be increasing (Berger 2001). This is not just the difference between 'modern' Western societies and less industrialized nations. Polls of the American public suggest that 96% believe in God and 67% believe that religion is 'very important' in their lives (Powell et al 2003).

In summing up, we can say that sociological studies of contemporary religion have produced a complex picture of competing trends. While there is evidence of declining church membership in the UK, there is also evidence of a high level of religious belief independent of church organizations. For some, this represents the active pursuit of *self realization*, through *new age* religion. For others, religion is a more marginal part of existence, more properly described as a *God of the gaps*. At the same time, there is a definite backlash against secularization with an increase in groups offering a fundamentalist outlook on life. The public influence of religion is changing. Religion may play a smaller part in many state institutions such as state schools but faith groups continue to play an important part in public life and it is possible that this will increase as the state withdraws from welfare provision and we move towards a 'mixed economy' of welfare.

Clearly, this complex pattern of contemporary religious life has an impact on the responses of individuals to illness, suffering and death, which is worthy of our attention. In addition, we may wish to consider the effect of these cultural influences on nursing.

REFLECTION POINT

We have seen that lots of different forms of religious belief exist. There are also diverse religious groups and variations in people's relationships to religious groups. Reflect on your own religious beliefs and practice. What impact do you think that they have on your attitudes to your own health?

Religion, illness and health

A number of authors have considered the influence of religion on health and illness. Much of this research has occurred in the USA where faith groups have considerable public influence as we have discussed. One factor, which has interested a number of sociologists, is the apparent relationship between religious affiliation and health. Put simply, it has been suggested that the religious tend to live longer and be healthier (Hummer et al 2004, Jarvis & Northcott 1987, Levin 1994, Miller & Thoresen 2003). Explanations have focused on the way in which religions offer social support and promote a healthy lifestyle. The beneficial effects of religious practices such as prayer, meditation and yoga have also been studied (Seeman et al 2003). Finally, religious belief has been posited as providing beneficial psychological effects such as 'inner peace' and a sense of life's meaning (Miller & Thoresen 2003). This brings us back to our earlier discussion of theodicy and the role of religion in beliefs about health, illness and suffering.

In spite of the detailed attention, which has been paid to lay concepts of health in recent years, very little attention has been paid within this literature to the impact of spiritual beliefs on health beliefs. Williams (1993b) has suggested that the moral and religious components of health beliefs are easily overlooked by the researcher particularly as religious beliefs have become more private. Williams (1990) described a '*Protestant legacy*' in the accounts of health given by his Scottish respondents. Popular moral conceptions of health reflected Protestant theological debates. His respondents expressed views of health and illness, which were close to Weber's '*theodicy of good fortune*'.

The healthy owed their good fortune to a hard-working and virtuous existence, whereas the sick had '*brought it on themselves*'. Blaxter (1993) noted similar moral views of illness and a sense of guilt among respondents who 'gave in' to sickness. In Blaxter's respondents, good health was so clearly synonymous with virtue that respondents claimed to be healthy even when this flew in the face of all the available evidence. One respondent recounting the early death of most of her close relatives concluded '*We were a healthy family*'. Williams (1993a) has described the career of the chronically sick in terms of the pursuit of virtue as they strive to assert themselves as morally blameless in spite of the stigma of their condition.

The Judaeo-Christian tradition contains a legacy of religious ideas, which place responsibility for health on the individual and see good health as a reward for a virtuous life. These ideas lead to a deep-rooted resistance to accepting the social causes of ill health (Blaxter 1990). Similar beliefs may exist in other religious traditions and affect the individual response to illness (Agrawal & Dalal 1993). There is clearly much more to be learned about the effect of various religious traditions on beliefs about health and illness and research in this area is needed.

As regards the recent changes in religions in our own society summarized earlier, we can draw out a number of implications for healthcare. First, there are increasing numbers of people who are only nominally religious and whose beliefs are informal and privatized. Such individuals may only turn to religion in times of personal crisis, but their beliefs about health and illness may be influenced by religious traditions with which they have only a tenuous connection. In studies by Williams and others of health beliefs, a Protestant version of the '*theodicy of good fortune*' seems to be common and may have the potential to create unnecessary guilt.

Second, the growth of fundamentalist and sectarian groups, presents new challenges for healthcare workers. Fundamentalism is by its nature, in opposition to secular rationalism. Medicine is an area of secular rationalism most likely to conflict with fundamentalist groups through its involvement in issues of life, death and sexual morality.

Fundamentalist groups have become increasingly involved in debates about contraception, abortion and genetic medicine and conflicts on these areas seem bound to increase. Additionally, some sectarian groups prohibit specific medical practices such as the Jehovah's Witness ban on blood transfusions. These groups pose some serious legal, political and ethical challenges to liberal democracies. The sociological and psychological literature on sectarian groups and new religious movements is polarized between psychologists and psychiatrists who claim that these groups exercise techniques of brainwashing and 'mind control' (West 1993) and a more liberal view that individuals generally enter and leave these groups of their own free will (Barker 1989). An intermediate position is taken by some authors suggesting that the social pressures of sect membership affect the validity of an individual's judgement. This applies particularly to informed consent and refusal of treatment (Young & Griffith 1992). If as Davie (1994b) suggests, we may become a world of '*competing fundamentalisms*', current medical ethical guidelines based on assumptions of religious toleration and individual freedom may be put under increasing strain and may struggle to adapt to the pressures of this changing social context.

Finally, we live in a multicultural and multiethnic society. Thus, nurses must deal with patients from diverse religious backgrounds and must understand and make provision for diverse religious beliefs and practices. As we noted earlier many ethnic minority communities have remained much more steadfast in their religious practices than the UK population generally.

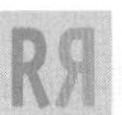
REFLECTION POINT

We have discussed the diverse religious backgrounds that people may come from and the ways in which religion can impact on health. How can you use this understanding to improve your assessment of patients?

Religion, spirituality and nursing

In this final section, we will briefly consider the influence of changing religious ideas and practices on nursing. Nursing has traditionally had strong associations with religion. According to Rafferty (1997) 'religious enthusiasm' was an important motivation for nineteenth-century nursing reform with religious sisterhoods playing an important role. The tradition of service and vocation which was fostered by early nursing reformers is still an important influence for many nurses. However, some nursing writers have lamented the way in which nursing has moved from this earlier religious tradition of 'service' and 'vocation' towards the 'self religions' that we discussed earlier (Bradshaw 1994).

The recent popularity of 'new age' ideas in nursing, which we will explore in this section, may reflect a contemporary version of the traditional link between nursing and religion. 'New age' ideas are linked to a particular discourse about health and illness which has found recent expression in nursing through its interest in 'holism' and the subjective world of the patient. The influence of 'new age' ideas and the 'self religions' is particularly apparent in nurses' contemporary ideas about 'spiritual care'. There is also an enormous popular interest in complementary therapies in nursing many of which derive their philosophical bases from new age religions (Bruce 1996).

The contemporary nursing literature on spiritual care contains considerable debate about the nature of spirituality. The emerging consensus in the literature is that spirituality is separate from religion (Dyson et al 1997, McSherry & Draper 1998). The literature asserts that spiritual care is a cornerstone of 'holistic' nursing practice. The particular conception of holism expressed in this literature is of the individual as a 'bio-psychological-spiritual being' (Narayanasamy & Owens 2001). Thus, the literature on spiritual care routinely erases the social context of the individual. This includes the cultural and religious context of an individual's 'spiritual' beliefs with spirituality conceived in individualistic terms. Thus, a widely cited definition of spirituality in the literature is that provided by Murray and Zenter (1989:16).

> *'A quality that goes beyond religious affiliations, that strives for inspiration, reverence, awe, meaning and purpose, even in those who do not believe in any god. The spiritual dimension tries to be in harmony with the universe, strives for answers about the infinite and comes into focus when the person faces emotional stress, physical illness or death'.*

It is common therefore for this literature to repudiate the connection between spirituality and a belief in God or to redefine God as a 'higher power' or 'life principle'. Thus, according to Dyson et al (1997) 'whatever the person takes to be the highest value in life' can be defined as their 'God' and this can include 'work, money, personal gain'. The connection therefore between the nursing literature on spirituality and 'new age' beliefs or the 'self religions' seems self evident. Indeed Dyson et al (1997) identify spirituality with 'healthy self love'. This is a far cry from the ideas of self sacrifice and vocation which inspired nineteenth century nurse reformers. This view of spirituality may be an unsympathetic one for patients who continue to associate spirituality with traditional religious values. Ironically nurses' attempts firstly to lay claim to their own definition of spirituality and secondly to detach spirituality from religion could represent yet another attempt to both secularize and m-edicalize the sacred.

Discussion points

1. How much influence do you think that religion should have in society?
2. What are your own spiritual beliefs? How do they influence you as a nurse?
3. What part do you think that religion should play in healthcare?
4. How much information about their religious beliefs do you think that nurses should ask for from patients?
5. How much right do you think that patients should have to demand or refuse treatment on religious grounds?

CHAPTER SUMMARY

This chapter has introduced you to sociological thinking about religion. We have used this chapter to introduce you to the three 'classical' social theorists: Karl Marx, Emile Durkheim and Max Weber, by discussing the different ways in which they thought about religion. We have seen that Karl Marx was particularly concerned about the ways in which ordinary working people were exploited by industrial capitalism and saw religion as excusing that exploitation. Emile Durkheim was preoccupied with the ways in which religion undermined a sense of community and the shared values and rituals that held society together. Max Weber examined the different ways that we make sense of suffering. He also discussed the ways in which the industrial society had changed the way we see the world. Rationality had 'disenchanted' the world and marginalized questions about the meaning of suffering. This is very relevant to healthcare. According to Clark, science and rationality can answer the question of how we become ill but cannot ask the question: 'why did this happen to me?

This discussion has led us on to look at the question of whether religion is actually declining in modern society or just changing. This is something that sociologists have argued about for many years. The debate about this question draws on three kinds of evidence: first, whether people belong to religious organizations; second, whether people believe in God or the supernatural and finally, whether religion has any influence in the world. The evidence is very mixed. While religion is declining in some places, it is also developing new forms and new areas of influence. Two important (but very different) new movements are 'new age' religion and religious 'fundamentalism'.

Changes in the place of religion in society have an important impact on the ways in which people cope with and make sense of illness, suffering and death. This can have an impact on people's health. Recent changes in religions, such as the growth of fundamentalism offer new challenges to nurse when they are helping patients to make sense of the experience of illness. Nurses have become increasingly interested in spirituality but need to be careful not to detach their understanding of spirituality from a broader understanding of religion and its place in society.

FURTHER READING

Davie G 1994 Religion in Britain since 1945: Believing without belonging. Blackwell, Oxford.

Davie provides a good introduction to the sociology of religion.

Williams R 1993 Religion and illness. In: Radley A (ed.) Worlds of illness: Biographical and cultural perspectives on health and disease. Routledge, London, p 71–91.

Williams provides a valuable sociological discussion of religion and health.

McSherry W 2000 Making sense of spirituality in nursing practice. Churchill Livingstone, Edinburgh.

Narayanasamy A 2001 Spiritual care: A practical guide for nurses and healthcare practitioners. Quay Publishing, Wiltshire.

McSherry and Narayanasamy introduce spiritual care to nurses.

REFERENCES

Abercrombie N, Baker J, Brett S 1970 Superstition and religion: the God of the gaps. In: Martin D, Hill M (eds) A sociological yearbook of religion. SCM, London, p 93–129

Agrawal M, Dalal A 1993 Beliefs about the world and recovery from myocardial infarction. Journal of Social Psychology 133(3):385–394

Barker E 1989 New religious movements: A practical introduction. HMSO, London

Beckford J 1989 Religion and advanced industrial society. Unwin Hyman, London

Berger P 2001 Reflections on the sociology of religion today. Sociology of Religion 62(4):443–445

Blaxter M 1990 Health and lifestyles. Routledge, London

Blaxter M 1993 Why do the victims blame themselves? In: Radley A (ed.) Worlds of illness: Biographical and cultural perspectives on health and disease. Routledge, London, p 124–142

Bottomore TB, Rubel M 1973 Karl Marx: Selected writings in sociology and social philosophy. Penguin, Harmondsworth

Bradshaw A 1994 Lighting the lamp: The spiritual dimension of nursing care. Scutari, London

Brierley P (ed.) 2005 The UK Christian handbook: Religious trends No. 5: The future of the church. Christian Research, London

Bruce S 1996 Religion in the modern world: from cathedrals to Cults. Oxford University Press, Oxford

Casanova J 1994 Public religions in the modern world. Chicago University Press, Chicago

Clark D 1982 Between pulpit and pew: Folk religion in a North Yorkshire fishing village. Cambridge University Press, Cambridge

Davie G 1994a Religion in Britain since 1945: Believing without belonging. Blackwell, Oxford

Davie, G 1994b Religion in post-war Britain: a sociological view. In: Obelkevich J, Catterall P (eds) Understanding post-war British society. Routledge, New York, p 165–178

Davie G 2000 Religion in modern Britain: Changing Sociological Assumptions. Sociology 34(1): 113–128

Dawkins R 2006 The God delusion. Bantam Books, London

Durkheim E [1897] 1970 Suicide. Routledge, London

Durkheim E [1912] 1976 The elementary forms of religious life. Allen and Unwin, London

Dyson J, Cobb M, Forman D 1997 The meaning of spirituality: A literature review. Journal of Advanced Nursing 26(1):1183–1188
Feuerbach L 1957 Essences of Christianity. Harper, New York
Gerth HH, Wright Mills C 1970 (eds) Max Weber: Essays in sociology. Routledge, London
Heelas P 1993a The new age in cultural context: the pre-modern, the modern and the post-modern. Religion 23:103–111
Heelas P 1993b The sacralization of the self and new age capitalism. In: Abercrombie N, Ward A (eds) Social change in contemporary society. Polity, Cambridge, p 139–166
Heelas P 1996 The new age movement: Celebrating the self and the sacralization of modernity. Blackwell, Cambridge, MA
Hummer R, Ellison C, Rogers R 2004 Religious involvement and adult mortality in the United States: Review and perspective. Southern Medical Journal 97(12):1223–1230
James N, Field D 1992 The routinization of hospice: Charisma and bureaucratization. Social Science and Medicine 34:1363–1375
Jarvis GK, Northcott HD 1987 Religion and differences in morbidity and mortality. Social Science and Medicine 25(7):813–824
Knoblauch H 2003 Europe and invisible religion. Social Compass 50(3):267–274
Lasch C 1979 The culture of narcissism. Abacus, London
Levin J 1994 Religion and health: Is there an association? Social Science and Medicine 38(11): 1475–1482
Luckmann T 1967 The invisible religion. Macmillan, New York
Marty ME, Scott Appleby R 1993 Fundamentalism observed. Chicago University Press, Chicago
McSherry W 2000 Making sense of spirituality in nursing practice. Churchill Livingstone, Edinburgh
McSherry W, Draper P 1998 The debates emerging from the literature surrounding the concept of spirituality as applied to nursing. Journal of Advanced Nursing 27:683–691
Miller W, Thoresen C 2003 Spirituality, religion and health: An Emerging research field. American Psychologist 58(1):24–35
Murray R, Zenter FB 1989 Nursing concepts for health promotion. Prentice Hall, New york
Narayanasamy A 2001 Spiritual care: A practical guide for nurses and healthcare practitioners. Quay Publishing, Wiltshire
Narayanasamy A, Owens J 2001 A critical incident study of nurses' responses to the spiritual needs of their patients. Journal of Advanced Nursing 33(4): 446–455
Niebuhr HR 1929 The social sources of denominationalism. Henry Holt, New York
Powell L, Shahabi L, Thoresen C 2003 Religion and spirituality: Linkages to physical health. American Psychologist 58(1):36–52
Rafferty A 1997 Nursing history and the politics of welfare. Routledge, London
Robertson R 1989 Globalization, politics and religion. In: Beckford J, Luckmann T (eds) The changing face of religion. Sage, London, p 10–23
Ruthuen M 1993 The audio-vision of God. *The Guardian* 1 May
Schmalz MN 1994 When Festinger fails: Prophecy and the Watch Tower. Religion 24:293–308
Seeman T, Dubin L, Seeman M 2003 Religiosity/ spirituality and health: A critical review of the evidence for biological pathways. American Psychologist 58(1):53–63
Singelenberg R 1990 The blood transfusion taboo of Jehovah's Witnesses: Origin, development and function of a controversial doctrine. Social Science and Medicine 31(4):515–523
Voas D, Crockett A 2005 Religion in Britain: Neither believing nor belonging. Sociology 39(1):11–28
Walter T 1993 Death in the new age. Religion 23:127–145
Weber M 1974 The Protestant ethic and the spirit of capitalism. Unwin, London
Williams G 1993a Chronic illness and the pursuit of virtue in everyday life. In: Radley A (ed.) Worlds of illness: Biographical and cultural perspectives on health and disease. Routledge, London, p 92–108
Williams R 1990 A Protestant legacy: Attitudes to death and illness among older Aberdonians. Oxford University Press, Oxford
Williams R 1993b Religion and illness. In: Radley A (ed.) Worlds of illness: Biographical and cultural perspectives on health and disease. Routledge, London, p 71–91
West LJ 1993 A psychiatric overview of cult related phenomena. Journal of the American Academy of Psychoanalysis 21(1):1–19
Young JL, Griffith EH 1992. A critical evaluation of coercive persuasion as used in the assessment of cults. Behavioural Sciences and the Law 10:89–101

CHAPTER 4

Work, professionalism and organizational life

Hannah Cooke

KEY CONCEPTS

- The changing division of labour
- Bureaucracies and markets.
- Total institutions
- Taylorism and Fordism
- Professionalism
- Emotional labour
- Managerialism
- McDonaldization

What is work?

According to Williams (1983: 334–335)

> *'Work is the modern English form of the noun* weorc *(Old English) and the verb* wyrcan *(Old English). As our most general word for doing something, and for something done, its range of applications has of course been enormous. What is now most interesting is its predominant specialisation to regular paid employment'.*

According to Nicholls (2005: 374–376)

> *'Thirty years later, what is most interesting is that "work" does not automatically suggest regular, full-time or even paid employment. Part of the reason for this is that work has itself become a contested concept'.*

We spend much of our lives working and much work goes on outside paid employment; housework and voluntary work, for example. As Nicholls indicates, there have been debates over the recognition of non-paid work, such as housework, which have changed our perceptions of work. However, paid work is still central to most people's lives. A central feature of contemporary society is its complex division of labour. Whereas in pre-industrial societies, households often produced most of their own goods and services, in contemporary British society, vast areas of work are organized into specialized jobs for which individuals receive wages. The structured inequalities in society which we examine in Chapters 5 and 6 largely centre around a person's status in paid work. Paid work in contemporary society has come to serve many functions beyond the provision of goods and services. It provides us with a sense of status and identity, and a place in society. We live in a society that places enormous value on paid work and which often demeans other forms of work. Such a society may leave us less and less time and space for unpaid work. Instead of baking our child a birthday cake, we are encouraged to buy one from the supermarket (Hochschild 2001). Instead of caring for our children, under schemes such as 'welfare to work', we are expected to *buy* childcare while we go out to work (Mooney 2004).

BOUNDARIES OF WORK AND EMPLOYMENT

The centrality of this economic model of work should not blind us to the fact that many goods and services are still produced outside formal employment. It has been estimated for example that if unpaid domestic work was paid for at the same average rate as paid employment, then the value of this work to Britain could be calculated as 122% of gross domestic production (*Guardian* 1997). Most of this unpaid work takes place in families the majority of it is carried out by women as we discussed in Chapter 2.

Our role as nurses alerts us to the fragile boundary between paid employment and unpaid work, particularly where women's work is concerned. Nurses produce a human service, but the fact that most of the tasks which we carry out in our daily employment are being carried out somewhere by an unpaid carer causes difficulties when we wish to claim special expertise and professional status. The increased throughput of hospital patients and renewed emphasis on 'community care' has intensified the pressures to move patients from paid to unpaid care. Ironically this is happening at a time when people often have less time to provide such care due to increased working hours. Britain has the longest working hours in Western Europe and recent surveys have shown that one-fifth of the population work more than 48 h/week (Office of National Statistics 2006). The move to informal care has been driven by the continuing pressure to contain health spending. Boundaries between unpaid work and paid employment are constantly shifting and we look in more detail at unpaid (informal) care in Chapters 2 and 10.

THE DIVISION OF LABOUR

Much of our understanding of the division of labour is founded on Durkheim's major work; 'The Division of Labour in Society' (Durkheim [1893] 1984). According to Durkheim, in pre-industrial societies, the division of labour is simple, most people are involved in similar occupations and people are bound together by shared experiences and beliefs. Work is often organized through kinship ties. Durkheim describes these close knit traditional societies as bound together by *'mechanical solidarity'*. With industrialization and urbanization comes a breakdown of traditional forms of solidarity. Modern industrial society has an extremely complex division of labour with a huge number of different work roles. This leads to a more individualistic society with many different ways of life, values and beliefs. The danger for modern society is that individualism will lead to a breakdown of social ties. Durkheim says that the problem of how to keep order in industrial societies is solved by the creation of *organic solidarity. Organic solidarity* is based on the acceptance of difference through a recognition of mutual interdependence. The development of highly specialized roles which are interdependent is a key feature of organic solidarity. However, the risk of a breakdown of community values (a condition that Durkheim called anomie) is always present. Durkheim saw the professions as playing a key role in maintaining a moral community in conditions of organic solidarity (Durkheim [1950] 1992). Professions are carriers of important ideals such as altruism and public service. Durkheim's ideas about the division of labour have informed many attempts to understand role changes in contemporary healthcare (Allen & Hughes 2002).

Work and organizations

Most contemporary work takes place within organizations; we are born in an organization, we are educated in an organization, we will spend our working lives and much of our leisure time in organizations. Most of us will die in an organization (Giddens 2001). Our ideas about organizations have changed over time. The two key ideas that shape contemporary organizations are those of bureaucracy and market.

THE IDEA OF BUREAUCRACY

The word bureaucracy comes from a French word referring to a kind of baize cloth used to cover desks. It means, literally, the rule of those who sit behind desks. The term bureaucracy has always had negative connotations. The most important classical sociological study of bureaucracy was by Max Weber. Weber produced a balanced account of bureaucracy highlighting both its strengths and weaknesses.

Weber thought the rise of bureaucracy was inevitable. He saw it as the form of rational administration most suited to large scale social systems. Weber saw bureaucracies as governed by instrumental rationality (rather than traditions, values or feelings) and believed that this had both strengths and weaknesses. Weber identified the following characteristics as typical of bureaucratic systems (see Gerth and Mills 1970).

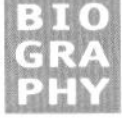

Max Weber (1864–1920)

Max Weber was born in Erfurt in Germany in 1864. His father was a prominent German politician. Weber was an important German sociologist and political theorist and is best known for his thesis of the 'Protestant Ethic,' relating Protestantism to capitalism (see Chapter 5), and for his ideas on bureaucracy. He also carried out a major study of world religions, which we considered in Chapter 3. He is considered to be one of the founders of modern sociology.

Weber argued for an objective and value-free approach to social research. Like Durkheim he highlighted the importance of social structure yet he also stressed the importance of meaning and consciousness in understanding social action.

Weber has been described as an 'action theorist'. He believed that human societies were the cumulative outcome of people's actions. He was interested therefore in the ideas that shape human choices. However, he also recognized that the circumstances that people find themselves in constrain their actions. Understanding human actions means trying to place ourselves in other's shoes and appreciate their circumstances – Weber called this kind of understanding *verstehen*. According to Weber we can classify actions by their motivations (rationalities). There are four types of rationality:

1. Traditional rationality – 'I did it because it's always been done that way'
2. Affective rationality – 'I did it because I care'
3. Value rationality – 'I did it because it was the right thing to do'
4. Instrumental rationality – 'I did it because it was profitable/cost-effective'

Weber believed that contemporary society was increasingly dominated by instrumental (technocratic) rationality at the expense of other motivations and values. He called this process the 'disenchantment' of the world and saw it as having both positive and negative consequences.

Weber's key works include:

- *The Protestant Ethic and the Spirit of Capitalism* 1904
- *Economy and Society* 1914
- *Sociology of Religion* 1916

THE CHARACTERISTICS OF A BUREAUCRACY

- There are fixed rules governing all areas of activity. Rules are more or less exhaustive and can be learned
- There is a clear cut hierarchy with clears lines of accountability
- The management of the modern organization is based upon written documents
- Officials are full time and salaried and their work is governed by formal training and examinations
- There is a clear separation between the individual's private life and working life.

Weber believed that bureaucratic organizations had advantages in terms of fairness and efficiency because they were governed by strict and impartial rules and procedures. This prevented individuals from using the organization to promote their own personal interests by, for example, promoting their family and friends into positions of power regardless of their ability. In theory at least, in bureaucracies, open competition and formal rules of employment mean the appointment of the best person for the job. Cronyism and favouritism should not be part of a properly run bureaucracy.

Weber recognized that bureaucracies could have unintended negative consequences such as inflexibility and dehumanization and he talked pessimistically about the 'iron cage' of instrumental rationality. To appreciate the potentially dehumanizing effects of bureaucratic systems we have only to turn to sociological studies of institutional life such as Goffman's work on total institutions (see *Asylums*).

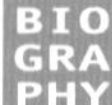

Erving Goffman (1922–1982)

Erving Goffman was an interactionist sociologist. He was therefore, like Weber, an action theorist. Interactionists however, see action as a two-way process and are interested in the meanings which people give to the world around them and how they interpret the behaviour of others. Goffman often used the metaphor of the stage (described as a 'dramaturgical perspective') to describe the ways in which people act in everyday life – hence we talk about people 'acting' social 'roles'. Goffman completed a large number of qualitative studies of social interaction. His study of asylums was influential in changing the way we care for people with mental health problems. His major works include:

- *The Presentation of Self in Everyday Life* 1959
- *Asylums* 1961
- *Stigma* 1963

TOTAL INSTITUTIONS

Total institutions are those institutions which regulate the entire existence of those who reside in them. Residents are often cut off from the outside world. Examples of total institutions described by Goffman include asylums, prisons, monasteries, boarding schools and army barracks. Institutions for the sick are of particular interest to us as health professionals and Goffman's own study was of the life of inmates of a mental hospital (Goffman 1968). He describes the attributes of a total institution as follows:

> *'First all aspects of life are conducted in the same place and under the same single authority. Second, each phase of the member's daily activity is carried on in the immediate company of a large batch of others, all of whom are treated alike and required to do the same thing together. Third all phases of the day's activities are tightly scheduled, with one activity leading at a prearranged time into the next ... Finally the various enforced activities are brought together into a single rational plan purportedly designed to fulfil the official aims of the institution'. (Goffman 1968: 17)*

Goffman was particularly concerned with the ways in which these institutions stripped the individual of their identity; a process he described as the 'mortification of the self'. Standardized treatment and rigid routines enforce conformity and refuse to recognize individuality. Inmates have to find ways of 'making out' in order to survive institutional life and retain a sense of self; some acquiesce in the system and become 'colonized', others withdraw or distance themselves by 'playing it cool'. For many, total institutions can have damaging effects.

Goffman's depiction of total institutions gives us a bleak picture of the bureaucratic control of the everyday lives of individuals. His work helped to speed up the closures of large healthcare institutions such as mental hospitals. His work also influenced the attacks on state bureaucracies that have been fashionable since the 1960s. The impersonality of bureaucracy has led critics to describe it as fundamentally inhuman. These criticisms have also driven the demands to 'modernize' public organizations such as the NHS. Central to the process of 'modernization' is the demand to expose public bureaux to business values and the disciplines of the 'market'. We must remember however that the market is also governed by instrumental rationality (the profit motive) so that markets do not necessarily rescue us from the worst features of bureaucracy. These attacks on bureaucracy ignore what Weber called the 'ethic' of bureaucracy; its impartiality and clear cut rules of conduct. This 'ethic' offers protection from cronyism, corruption and the arbitrary exercise of power (Du Gay 2000). The much criticized 'one size fits all' model of standardized welfare services at least offered a minimum level of equity which may be lost if 'choice' becomes a dominant value. Du Gay suggests that these ethical ideals of bureaucracy such as fairness, impartiality and playing by the rules are essential to democracy. We will consider next what the idea of the market has to offer.

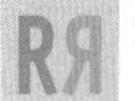

REFLECTION POINT

We have seen that 'total institutions' organize inmates' everyday lives bureaucratically. Goffman used the concept of the 'total institution' to describe the ways in which institutions can undermine our autonomy and sense of self. You may find yourself working with patients who have to spend a long time in hospital or other types of institutional care such as a nursing home. What do you think that you can do to help people who are being cared for to preserve their sense of autonomy and individuality?

THE IDEA OF THE MARKET

> *'I want no gold and I want no silver. I have enough to eat and I have a good and beautiful wife and a son whom I love and who is strong and well formed. What is gold to me? The earth brings a blessing and the fruits of it and my herds of cattle bring blessings. Gold brings no blessing and silver brings no blessing. They are only good to look at. I can't put them in my belly when I am hungry so they have no value. They are only beautiful like a flower that blooms or a bird that sings. But if you put the flower in your belly it is no longer beautiful, and if you cook the bird it sings no longer' (Traven,* The Treasure of the Sierra Madre, *cited in Kahn 1997: 69).*

Kahn quotes Traven's popular novel about Mexican peasants to illustrate a critique of markets, which sees them as based on a culture of greed and a worship of money in which people have lost sight of the true value of the world around them. The ideas expressed here echo Marx's distinction between the 'use value' of an object, i.e. its value to human health and happiness and its 'exchange value', i.e. its monetary price. These critical ideas offer us a way into thinking about what the idea of the market actually stands for.

According to Clarke (2005a) the word 'market' originally referred to a place where people met to trade goods. This view of a market as a place has given way to a more abstract idea of the market as the fundamental way of organizing human society (Carrier 1997). Our modern conception of the market owes much to the ideas of the classical economist, Adam Smith, who described society as regulated by the 'hidden hand of the market'. This means that market societies are composed of millions of individual transactions, which combine to produce equilibrium if the market is left alone to regulate itself (Carrier 1997). Thus according to pro-market economists (often described as economic liberals because of their desire to 'liberate' the market) if everyone is free to engage in the pursuit of private profit then over time the 'hidden hand' of the market will achieve prosperity for all. The greatest good for the greatest number is better achieved by self-interest than by altruism (Lubasz 1992). Thus a goal of society should be to remove any obstacles to a 'free market' and to open as many areas of social life as possible to market mechanisms.

This idea of the market is based on two key assumptions which are contested by critics. First, the idea of the market is based on a particular idea of human nature. This is often described as the idea of 'economic man'. This is the idea that buying and selling is a universal human activity and that the instrumental pursuit of profit ('calculating avarice') is a fundamental human characteristic. This is a matter of some dispute particularly amongst anthropologists who study pre-industrial societies. Thus Douglas (1992) says that market societies were relative latecomers as types of human organization. It is their dominance in the industrial West, which has led to a rewriting of our ideas about 'human nature'. Both bureaucracies and markets are dominated by instrumental rationality in different ways (to put it simply bureaucracies are concerned with rules and hierarchies and markets with money and profits). Weber's ideas about different types of rationality alert us to the possibility that other motivations (traditions, values, beliefs, feelings) may govern human behaviour. Traven's depiction of the Mexican peasant at the start of this section illustrates the view that these other motivations are more desirable and authentic, and if we abandon these we become a people who 'know the price of everything and the value of nothing' (Oscar Wilde 1892). These issues are pertinent to an occupation such as nursing where altruism and 'vocation' remain important but contested ideals.

Second, the idea of the market is based on the idea that in a 'free' market everyone can participate on an equal footing. Our discussions of inequality in Chapters 5 and 6 will question this idea. Opponents of the market argue that markets are always shaped by structured inequalities and thus reward the rich and powerful (Carrier 1997, Clarke 2005a). This view of markets argues that the extension of markets leads not to prosperity but to deepening inequality.

Strong ideas about the market as *the* fundamental form of human social life have led to a social programme which extends market mechanisms into all areas of life. The alternative view, which is that markets are just one way of organizing social life, leads to suggestions that there are some areas of social life which should be governed by other values and motivations (our personal and family life for example). Healthcare is one area where public service and altruism have been important ideals and where the role of markets has been contested (Pollock 2004). However, recent healthcare reforms in many countries have introduced market mechanisms into public healthcare systems.

Thus, the idea of the market now underpins many contemporary, taken for granted ideas in healthcare. Market ideas encourage us to see health as a commodity which we can buy and ourselves as 'healthcare consumers' rather than patients. It is market ideas that encourage us to believe that greater 'competition' and 'choice' will produce greater 'efficiency' and higher standards. These ideas assume that market motives (profit, self interest) govern the behaviours of both healthcare workers and patients. We will return to these ideas in Chapters 7 and 9.

RR REFLECTION POINT

We have seen that the idea of the market has become a very influential way of organizing contemporary social life. This has led to an increase of 'business methods' in healthcare and increased consumerism amongst patients. Putting the market at the centre of social life reflects a particular set of beliefs about human nature. In particular it reflects the idea that people are normally motivated by the self interested pursuit of profit. Think about the factors that motivated you to become a nurse. What values underpinned your decision? How well do you think that market ideas explain your own motivations and values?

Work in the industrial age

We have noted that a key feature of contemporary society is the industrial division of labour. Individuals work in highly specialized employment often in large scale organizations such as the NHS. The popular picture of the industrial revolution is of a time of technological change when great inventions such as the steam engine and the Spinning Jenny revolutionized the production of goods and services. More revolutionary was the change in the social organization of work affected by the introduction of the factory system (Thompson 1968). Prior to the creation of mills and factories the worker followed the production process from start to finish. The weaver, for example, produced a piece of cloth for sale in the local Piece Hall. Following industrialization, the production process was divided into a series of tasks completed by different workers under the control of the factory manager.

Early exponents of the industrial division of labour such as Adam Smith noted the increase in productivity that could be achieved by breaking a job down into its simplest components and dividing these up between different workers. It was Charles Babbage in 1832 who pointed out that industrial production was also more profitable because it could employ less-skilled, cheaper labour. In purchasing a 'whole' task the employer must pay the rate for the most skilled part of that task, whereas if a task is broken up, many parts of the task may be more cheaply obtained (Watson 2003). This 'Babbage principle' continues to exert an influence, for instance on whether nurses are allowed to deliver 'whole person' care in nursing. Nursing skill mix is still often determined by the 'Babbage principle' and this can undermine nurses' attempts to provide holistic care. We will look at this again in Chapter 9.

The aim of the factory manager was to exert discipline over the worker to ensure maximum productivity. There was considerable opposition to the deskilling of the industrial system. Initially industrial discipline was draconian and was resisted by the populace with early mills employing mainly women and children. According to Hammond and Hammond (1949: 33):

> *'In the modern world most people have to adapt themselves to some kind of discipline, and to observe other people's timetables, to do other people's sums, or to work under other people's orders, but we have to remember that the population that was flung into the brutal rhythm of the factory had earned its living in relative freedom, and that the discipline of the early factory was particularly savage ... No economist of the day, in estimating the gains and the losses of factory employment ever allowed for the strain and violence a man suffered in his feelings when*

he passed from a life in which he could smoke or eat, or dig or sleep as he pleased to one in which somebody turned the key on him and for fourteen hours a day he had not even the right to whistle'.

This was a period in which techniques of social control proliferated. One of the instruments that helped to impose factory discipline on the populace was the New Poor Law (1834). The New Poor Law was the first systematic attempt to link welfare to work (Mooney 2004). The Act was based on the principle of 'less eligibility', which said that those in receipt of welfare should have a harsher life than the worst paid worker. The Poor Law led to the widespread development of workhouses, (whose conditions were graphically depicted by Charles Dickens in *Oliver Twist*) and ushered in an era of incarceration (Scull 1977) in which the socially deviant and indigent were subject to the disciplines of a whole array of new total institutions, such as sanatoria, orphanages, workhouses and asylums. The inmates of such institutions were expected to learn new habits of order and discipline and nurses played a major role in the creation of these institutions.

TAYLORISM

The most developed expression of the industrial division of labour can be found in the work of Frederick Winslow Taylor. Taylor's system of 'scientific management' involved breaking tasks down to their smallest components; these could then be measured to establish the quickest and most efficient means to complete that task which Taylor described as the 'one best way' (Taylor 1947). Taylorist systems produce tasks that are small and fragmented and the worker has no control over his/her work. Taylor wanted to separate the planning of work tasks from their execution in order to minimize the costs of both labour and job training. He also favoured an arms length 'minimum interaction' model of relations between managers and workers. Watson (2003) suggests that he regarded workers as 'economic animals' who 'would allow managers to do their thinking for them'. Braverman (1974) has argued that the influence of Taylorism has led to attempts to de-skill and routinize work across the entire labour force leading to work intensification. Taylorism can be seen in nursing where tasks are fragmented and nurses are required to adhere to rigid protocols and routines. Work intensification can be seen in efforts to get 'more for less' out of the nursing workforce (see Chapter 9).

In 1832, Charles Babbage had recognized the potential to weaken the bargaining power of workers by fragmenting work tasks. Taylor took this a step further believing that it was possible to treat each worker as an individual economic unit. Taylor wanted a different rate for every worker in order to eliminate any 'community of interest' between workers. We can see his continuing influence on healthcare in recent innovations, such as Agenda for Change.

FORDISM

Taylorism coincided with the development of the moving assembly line and that system of production that has come to be known as Fordism. Henry Ford apparently adopted the moving assembly line after watching workers in his local abattoir in the process of disassembling cattle. Fordism combined Taylorist management practices with the intensification of production through increased automation. The goal of Fordism was the large scale mass production of goods in order to achieve economies of scale. We can see the influence of Fordism in the 'modernization' of healthcare where small hospitals and GP practices are seen as inefficient and where services are centralized to achieve economies of scale. Fordism also recognized that mass produced goods required mass markets. The higher wages offered to workers as an incentive to work in the car industry were also a recognition that factory workers were to become important consumers of mass produced goods (Watson 2003). The need for stable mass markets also underpinned the commitment to the welfare state during this era and thus the models of welfare professionalism that went with it.

RR REFLECTION POINT

In the next section we are going to think about professionalism and what it means to different people. Before beginning this section, think about your own views about professionalism. Do you believe that nursing is a profession? What does 'being professional' involve? Write a list of behaviours that indicate professionalism. What are the advantages of professionalism? What are the disadvantages?

PROFESSIONALISM

Watson (2003: 252) describes professions as:

> *'Occupations which have been relatively successful in gaining high status and autonomy in certain societies on the basis of a claimed specialist expertise over which they have gained a degree of monopoly control'.*

This particular view of professions stresses the privileges that professionals gain from their professional status and has something in common with George Bernard Shaw's ([1911] 1971) assertion that 'all professions are a conspiracy against the laity'. This view sees professions as characterized above all by autonomy and a monopoly over the practices of the professional. The profession maintains this monopoly through strategies of 'occupational closure' such as restricting training places and allowing only members of the profession to perform certain functions. Thus for example, medicine has delegated some tasks to nursing but has largely maintained control over matters of clinical judgement such as diagnosis (Allen & Hughes 2002).

This way of looking at professions became particularly common in the 1970s and 1980s. In particular, Eliot Freidson's (1975) influential work on professions laid particular stress on professional autonomy and professional 'closure' as the defining features of a profession.

Freidson's analysis of professions was in sharp contrast to earlier studies of professions which emphasized the traits to which they aspired. One influential list of traits was Greenwood's (1957) 'attributes of a profession'. This was elaborated by Millerson (1964) to give the following list:

- Skill based on theoretical knowledge
- The provision of education and training
- The testing of member competence
- The existence of a professional body
- Adherence to a code of conduct
- Emphasis on altruistic service

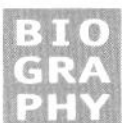

Eliot Freidson (1923–2005)

Eliot Freidson was a New York professor of sociology. He began his academic career at the University of Chicago and was influenced by the 'Chicago school' of sociologists. He also worked for British intelligence during the Second World War. He was a leading figure in the sociology of medicine and his book *Profession of Medicine* was considered a landmark in the study of professions. His work contained both a critique of, and an attempt to reform and defend the professions. His *Professionalism: The Third Logic* attempted to establish professionalism as a third model for the organization of work alongside Adam Smith's free market and Max Weber's bureaucracy. Major works include:

- *Profession of Medicine* 1970
- *Doctoring Together* 1976
- *Professionalism Reborn* 1995
- *Professionalism: The Third Logic* 2001

The trait approach was criticized as being simply a 'wish list' in which professionals elaborated their aspirations rather than a description of what professions were actually like. Certainly, lists of traits became 'shopping lists' for occupations that were aspiring to professional status. Thus for example nursing leaders actively pursued some of the items on the list such as nursing theories, nursing degrees and a code of conduct in order to raise the status of the occupation.

Since the 1970s the idea that the superior expertise of professionals and their ethic of service entitles them to a degree of autonomy has come under sustained attack. 'Medical dominance' has been an important target. For example, Ivan Illich (1976) (a former priest) attacked medicine from a particular moral and religious stance. He accused doctors of being 'iatrogenic' – literally 'sickening'. Doctors undermined health through 'clinical iatrogenesis'; this referred to adverse incidents in medicine such as medical errors and the side effects of drugs. Illich also accused doctors of 'cultural' and 'social' iatrogenesis. Doctors, he said, undermined health by eroding individual responsibility. Illich believed that medicine created dependence and undermined our capacity for personal growth through suffering.

A further attack on medicine came from the lawyer Ian Kennedy (1983) who claimed to have 'unmasked' medicine and who accused doctors of a lack of accountability. Kennedy wanted to develop a new, less paternalistic relationship between doctors and patients which emphasized individual responsibility. The critiques of both authors were in tune with the growing trend towards market approaches to welfare.

These challenges to professionalism have led the welfare professions' claims to altruism, vocation and special expertise to be treated with considerable cynicism. As we have become a more consumerist society our contemporary attitude to professionals has been described as being characterized by a 'decline of deference'. This means that the profession's claims to exercise discretion and 'professional judgement' have come under attack. Professionals have found themselves subject to increased scrutiny and control. Professional autonomy rests on the claim that professional knowledge is indeterminate; in other words it contains a high level of variability and uncertainty. Thus doctors have claimed that clinical judgement requires a high level of personal expertise to adapt treatment regimens to the unique needs of each individual patient.

Jamous and Pellouille (1970) have argued that all professions employ both indeterminate and technical knowledge. Technical knowledge can be codified in procedures which can be regulated externally and which offer a uniform set of procedures for standard types of case. Indeterminate knowledge is exercised through the skill and judgement of the individual professional who is able to treat each individual case as unique. Jamous and Pellouille suggest that recognition of professional indeterminacy has to be granted by those in power. When this recognition is revoked the autonomy of a professional group is eroded and professionals are forced to engage increasingly in technical work. What this means in practice is that professionals are increasingly forced to follow procedures and protocols and given less opportunity to exercise professional judgement and deliver individualized care. We then see professionals being subjected to Taylorist controls with tighter work specifications (protocols, service frameworks, targets, etc.), intensification of work and greater managerial scrutiny (audits, performance reviews etc). In particular, there has been increased pressure on the professions to produce marketable outcomes and competitive working practices (Warhurst & Thompson 1998).

Krause (1996) suggested that the professions were the 'last guilds'. Guilds were associations of skilled craftsmen who offered mutual aid and support. According to Krause capitalism and the state have 'finally caught up' with the last guilds and professional autonomy is 'slowly fading'. The professions are losing control over the workplaces, their associations, their markets and their relationship to the state; a process which McKinley and Arches (1985) have called 'proletarianisation'.

Critiques of medical dominance found a sympathetic hearing with nurses who used attacks on the 'medical model' to advance their own occupational position. Nurses have been slow to realize the potential costs to nursing of medicine's loss of professional autonomy. The voice of the cynics has been ascendant for so long that we have forgotten that the service ideals of the professions could actually protect the weak as well as the strong. Durkheim (1992) saw the professions as playing an important role in promoting civic morals in industrial societies which the contemporary consumerist and market based models of service may not easily replace. Crompton (1990) suggests that the professions are neither purely idealistic nor purely self seeking. Professions embody the contradictions underlying the division of labour in modern society. While protecting their own interests they can also embody 'institutionalized altruism' and can 'moderate the excesses of the market' (Watson 2003).

Changes in the professional status of doctors have been presented optimistically as indicative of greater consumer power and a decline in paternalism. The pessimistic view suggests that the decline of professional autonomy entails a loss of public service ideals and the creation of 'assembly line' medicine which serves corporate interests rather than patients (McKinley & Marceau 2002). These contradictory accounts of changes in the status of professionals mirror similar debates about changes in the workplace which we will consider next.

RЯ REFLECTION POINT

We have reviewed the idea that professional autonomy is declining. Some authors have been optimistic about this seeing it as a positive outcome of increased consumer power. Other writers have been pessimistic and have seen this as an indication of the increased power of big business and the state. From your own experience jot down evidence for and against the proposition that the professional status of nurses is declining. How would you conclude that the professional status of nurses has changed?

Work in the 'post-industrial' age

CHANGING WORKPLACES

In the post-war period there has been a marked change in the economic structure of the UK and thus a change in employment patterns. Industries, such as coal, steel and shipbuilding have declined leading to economic depression and unemployment in areas such as the North East of England and South Wales. This has been in part due to the creation of 'global' markets leading multi-national companies to move labour intensive industries to countries where labour costs are cheaper such as South-east Asia. Thus changes in work are often explained with reference to the process of 'globalization'.

Globalization refers to the process whereby different nations, regions and people's of the world become economically, politically and culturally interdependent.

At the same time, automation and the growth of information technology have allowed industries to shed workers in a process of 'industrial shakeout' encouraged particularly through the 1980s to increase efficiency and competitiveness.

During this period the service (or tertiary) sector has increased in size and importance with the growth of services such as banking, retailing, leisure industries and to some extent healthcare. The growth in the size and importance of the service sector has been referred to as the 'tertiarization' of the economy and it has a number of implications. First, it implies a growth in white collar jobs and a corresponding decline in manual work. Second, many jobs in service industries such as shop work and office work involve interaction with customers and thus employ a different set of skills. Physical skills become less important than interpersonal skills. Thus the growth in service industries had produced a corresponding increase in job opportunities for women and is in part responsible for their increased participation in the labour market. There are implications for nursing since women now have greater choice of employment leading to greater recruitment and retention problems in nursing. This has led to attempts to recruit nurses from a wider range of backgrounds and from overseas.

The debate about the implications of this change in the workplace has been polarized into those who see post industrial society as offering better jobs to all and those who are much more pessimistic. The research evidence tends to suggest that there are winners and losers in the new economy. The change from manufacturing jobs to service jobs does not necessarily mean a change to better jobs. While some service jobs are well paid and rewarding others are insecure and badly paid. Beynon (1997) cites Reich (1992) suggesting that there are a 'privileged fifth' mainly in the media and communications industries (lecturers, journalists, public relations consultants, advertising executives, web designers, etc.). Beynon describes this group as 'symbolic analysts' (or 'spin doctors') and suggests that we live 'their interpretive world', which may be why we may have an unrealistically optimistic view of changes at work. The reality for most is very different to that for the privileged fifth who dominate print and the airwaves. Many service jobs involve the delivery of mundane services (cleaners, care assistants, waiters, supermarket cashiers) for low wages. There has been a steady decline in full time, stable employment and Beynon (1997) describes the rise of the 'hyphenated worker' – those in part-time, casual or temporary work. This is a much more negative image of changes at work than that of authors who describe the rise of the 'portfolio career' leading to a new world of opportunities (Handy 1989).

Handy's ideas influenced the introduction of 'professional portfolios' in nursing, which offered 'flexible' careers as a positive opportunity for nurses (Davies 1990). However, flexible work for nurses has often meant bank and agency work with poor conditions and prospects. An important reason for the growth of casual labour in the care sector has been privatization. According to Beynon et al (2002), 2 million public sector jobs were lost between 1981 and 1999.

A less positive account of labour flexibility than Handy's has been given by two authors who took low paid jobs in the service sector and wrote about their experiences (Ehrenreich 2002, Toynbee 2002). Both authors vividly describe not only the low wages and back breaking work but also the disrespect with which mundane service workers were treated by both 'customers' and employers. This was not the 'portfolio career' but 'one dead end job after another' (Watson 2003).

EMOTIONAL LABOUR

The growth in personal service industries has led to a growing interest in the different set of skills which such industries require. Hochschild (1983) has described the interpersonal aspects of service work as 'emotional labour'.

Emotional labour involves work activity in which the worker is required to display particular emotions in the course of providing a service. What is interesting about emotional labour is that it is managed. Hochschild has studied the management practices which have developed to attempt to manipulate workers' emotions to fit to the needs of the organization.

BIOGRAPHY

Arlie Hochschild (1940–present)

Arlie Hochschild is professor of sociology at the University of California, Berkeley, USA. She is the author of several books including: *The Managed Heart: Commercialisation of Human Feeling* (1983), *The Time Bind: When Work Becomes Home and Home Becomes Work* (1997) and *The Second Shift* (1990). Hochschild's coined the term 'emotional labour' and her work is concerned with the place of women within the labour market and within the household. She is also concerned with the impact of the market on human life particularly the commercialization of personal and emotional life. Her work has had considerable influence on the analysis of nursing work.

In her study of Delta airlines, hostesses were exhorted by trainers not only to smile but to 'really mean it'. Hochschild employs a distinction between deep and surface acting to describe what is expected when emotional labour is required. In surface acting we try to change our outward appearance such as gestures and tone of voice. The other way to act is deep acting as propounded by the Russian director, Constantin Stanislavski. Stanislavski encouraged actors to conjure up the appropriate feelings by training their imagination; to get into the shoes of the character. Similarly airline hostesses were required not merely to put on a smile but to work on their inner feelings in order to summon 'genuine' friendly and sympathetic service for the customer.

Managers do not always want to encourage positive feelings in their employees. Hochschild's study also encompassed the rather different emotional repertoire of Delta's debt collectors.

> *'The corporate world has a toe and a heel, and each performs a different function; one delivers a service, the other collects payment for it. When an organization seeks to create demand for a service and then deliver it, it uses the smile and the soft questioning voice. Behind this delivery display, the organization's worker is asked to feel sympathy, trust and good will. On the other hand, when the organization seeks to collect money for what it has sold, its workers may be asked to use a grimace and the raised voice of command. Behind this collection display the worker is asked to feel distrust and sometimes positive bad will'. (Hochschild 1983: 137)*

Thus, the emotions we feel at work have come to be subject to the control and scrutiny of managers. To some extent this marks the extension of Taylorist management practices to new areas of work. Sometimes this can involve the management of surface acting. The scripted interactions of the staff of fast food chains who ask us to go 'supersize' and tell us to 'have a nice day' come into this category. In service industries where interaction with the customer is more prolonged however management may try to achieve a more penetrating control of workers' emotional display by attempting to manipulate the inner feelings of their workforce. The critical question to reflect on is the extent to which nurses control their own emotional labour. The issue of the growth of managerial control and its extension into new areas is one to which we turn next.

REFLECTION POINT

We have seen that the term emotional labour has been used to describe the ways in which we have to work on our feeling in the workplace. It also describes the ways in which our feelings may be exploited and controlled by employers. How useful is the idea of emotional labour in nursing? Think about

Continued

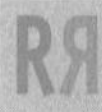

REFLECTION POINT—cont'd

aspects of nursing which involve emotional labour? How much scrutiny and control do managers exercise over nurses' emotion work? To what extent do you think that nurses exercise professional autonomy when undertaking emotion work?

MANAGERIALISM

The term 'management' according to Williams (1983) came from the verb *maneggiare*, which referred to the training of horses, literally meaning 'to take in hand'. Today the term 'management' refers to the practice of directing and organizing an activity, enterprise or group (Clarke 2005b).

In 1945 Burnham argued that a 'managerial revolution' was taking place in which a new class of salaried managers was taking over control of enterprises (Burnham 1945). This marked a move from personal control of organizations (the family firm) to impersonal control (the limited company owned by banks, insurance companies, etc.). In the post-war period, the managerial class made successful efforts to establish it self as a professional group in its own right with the establishment of business schools, management theory and professional associations of managers in various industries. There has been considerable debate as to whether the managerial class continue to serve the interests of those who employ them (states, corporations, etc.) or whether as a class it has come to serve its own interests (becoming the 'fat cats' described in the tabloid press). According to Clarke (2005b) the USA led the way in developing the managerial class and has been instrumental in exporting managerialism worldwide. Management models developed quite rapidly in the latter part of the twentieth century. Many have been short lived and have had a very limited evidence base ('re-engineering', 'transformational leadership', 'the one minute manager', etc.) but they have generated considerable publicity and drama and have exerted considerable influence (Clarke 2005b).

Just as we have been encouraged to let market ideas govern more areas of our lives, so too have we been encouraged to see 'management' as an activity that should direct more and more of our lives. Self-help books encourage us to 'manage' our homes, relationships and children according to business principles. More recently, the growth of the managerial class has been documented most extensively in the growth of managerial power within public services. Managerialism in public services (also described as 'new public management') is associated with the claim that public services should become more 'business like' and with the extension of market ideas into public services (Clarke & Newman 1997, Cutler & Waine 1994).

Traynor (1999) suggests that we can regard managerialism as an ideology. Traynor thus casts doubt on managerial claims as to the 'scientific' basis of managerialism and asks us to view it as a social practice serving particular interests.

The term ***ideology*** refers to an abstract set of (often political) ideas often with the additional sense that these ideas serve the interests of a powerful group and justify their power. In this sense, ideology is often seen as a set of ideas which excuse injustice and inequality.

The political case for managerialism in the public sector was laid out in an influential work by the management consultants Osborne and Gaebler (1992). They wanted to 'reinvent government' in the image of private corporations. Their agenda for public sector reform was as follows:

- Competition between service providers
- Empowering citizens by pushing control out of bureaucracies into communities
- Focusing on outcomes rather than inputs
- Organizations and persons driven by missions and visions not by rules and regulations
- Re-defining clients as customers

- Preventing problems before they emerge rather than simply treating them once they have arisen
- Earning money not just spending it
- Decentralizing authority and encouraging participative management. Using market type mechanisms rather than bureaucratic techniques and practices
- Catalysing partnerships between public, private and voluntary sectors.

Essentially Osborne and Gaebler wanted to break up public services and introduce private sector competition and their ideas can be clearly seen to have influenced recent reforms in the NHS (see Chapter 7). They thought that bureaucratic rules and procedures should be replaced by the discipline of a competitive market. A number of recent authors have pointed out some of the contradictions in the managerialist agenda (Clarke & Newman 1997, Du Gay 2000, Pollitt & Bouckaert 2000, Traynor 1999).

These can be summarized as follows:

- Increase central control but free local managers to manage
- Save money but raise standards
- Motivate and empower staff but intensify work and downsize
- Empower consumers but ration and standardize services
- Reduce bureaucracy but increase regulation, inspection and audit.

These contradictions mirror contradictory discourses in the management literature. On the one hand, managers see themselves as imposing Taylorist controls in order to get 'more for less' from their workforce – this is the 'scientific management' strand of managerial discourse. On the other hand, managers see themselves as 'winning hearts and minds', empowering staff, promoting teamwork and shaping corporate culture-this is the 'human relations' strand of management discourse. According to Traynor (1999), both strands aim for the same thing-greater control over the workforce. We turn next to the work of George Ritzer who has extended the critical analysis of managerialism further in the concept of 'McDonaldization'.

McDONALDIZATION?

There are two visions of the future and the present. One conjures up a world of work in which we are all progressively de-skilled as managerial controls tighten and more of our work becomes prescribed and routinized (Braverman 1974). The other envisages the creation of a post-industrial knowledge-based society in which many more people will have rewarding jobs in the information and service sectors. A large 'core' of highly trained staff will be valued for their knowledge and skills and will be 'empowered' by 'transformational' managers. Similar contradictory visions are apparent in recent efforts to 'modernize' nurses careers (DoH 2006).

Ritzer (1996) has argued that far from entering an era in which workers and consumers are 'empowered', we are entering an age of 'McDonaldization'. McDonaldism has extended assembly line techniques to the service sector. McDonalds is the success story of our time emulated by countless corporations both public and private. McDonaldism has four basic dimensions: efficiency (cost-cutting), calculability (quantification), predictability and increased control through the substitution of non-human for human technology (robots, computer programs). Another important element of McDonaldization is its ability to shift labour and service costs onto the consumer. McDonalds reduces its own costs by 'putting customers to work', filling their own cups with drinks, clearing their own tables just as Ikea puts its customers to work transporting and building their own furniture. As with all rationalized systems McDonaldization produces negative by-products such as the dehumanization of customers and employees and unintended inefficiency and waste.

As a counter to the argument that post-industrial society has seen a breakdown of Fordist and Taylorist regimes of work, Ritzer argues that such regimes have extended enormously. For Ritzer the idea that we have entered an era of consumer choice and flexibility is an illusion.

> *'First, homogenous products dominate a McDonaldized world. The Big Mac, The Egg McMuffin and Chicken McNuggets are identical from one time and place to another. Second, technologies such as Burger King's conveyor system, as well as the French fry and soft drinks machines throughout the fast food industry are as rigid as many of the technologies of Henry Ford's assembly line system. Further, the work routines in the fast food restaurant are highly standardized. Even what the workers say to customers is routinized. The jobs in a fast food restaurant are deskilled; they take little or no ability. The workers are homogenous and the actions of the customers are homogenized by the demands of the fast food restaurant (for example, don't dare ask for a rare burger). The workers at fast food restaurants are interchangeable. Finally, what is consumed is homogenized by McDonaldization. Thus in these and other ways Fordism is alive and well in the world although it has been transformed into McDonaldism'. (Ritzer 1996: 152)*

According to Ritzer, McDonaldization has entered healthcare with increased managerialism. The McDonaldization of medicine has irrational consequences. It takes control away from frontline healthcare work, standardizes professional work and makes healthcare professionals feel increasingly alienated. From the patient's point of view it is apt to make patients feel like just a number in the system. It shifts the costs of care back on to the patient demanding more and more self treatment and care. Masked by a rhetoric of 'empowerment' this actually marks the creation of a 'flat-packed' model of care (Cooke 2002). Despite a rhetoric of consumerism, according to Ritzer, McDonaldization is dehumanizing and depersonalizing healthcare.

RR REFLECTION POINT

We have seen that Ritzer believes that the principles of fast food service delivery are being applied to more and more areas of life. These involve standardization, cost cutting, quantification (making numbers the most important way of evaluating the service) and increased use of non-human labour such as computers. They also involve a self service model that makes the customer do more of the work. Can you think of examples of these changes in healthcare? To what extent do you think that healthcare is becoming McDonaldized?

Discussion points

1. To what extent can we regard the health service as a bureaucracy? What are the good and bad points about the bureaucratic organization of healthcare?
2. To what extent do you think that healthcare should be organized according to the principles of the market? What are the advantages and disadvantages of a market approach to healthcare?
3. Discuss the values that you believe should underpin the organization of healthcare.
4. To what extent do you think that we can regard nursing as a profession?

CHAPTER SUMMARY

This chapter asked you to think about what work is and to reflect on the boundary between paid and unpaid work. It introduced you to Durkheim's theories about the division of labour which help us to understand how work is organized in society. The chapter also looked at how work has changed in contemporary 'postindustrial' society. The growth in service industries has led to a growing recognition of the importance of 'emotional labour' and you are asked to reflect on the implications of this for nursing. We also looked at the changing role of the professions and considered the ways in which a growth in managerialism is subjecting professionals to increased controls. In particular we considered Ritzer's concept of McDonaldization and the possibility that we are moving to a 'fast-food' model of healthcare.

This chapter also introduced you to different ideas about organizations, in particular the ideas of bureaucracy and market. It discussed the arguments for and against bureaucracies and markets as ways of organizing important social functions such as healthcare. Debates about changes in organizations, the kind of work we do, and the kind of work we value, reflect some fundamental differences in ideas, both about the kind of society we live in now, and the kind of society we ought to live in. Behind these debates are differences in values and beliefs which are not simply reducible to technical questions of 'what works'. These debates will recur throughout our discussions of healthcare and nursing in this book.

FURTHER READING

Watson T 2003 Sociology, work and industry. Routledge, London.

Gives a comprehensive review of the recent sociology of work.

Mooney G, ed. 2004 Work: Personal lives and social policy. Open University Press, Buckingham.

Gives a review of relationships between work and welfare

Ehrenreich B 2002 Nickel and dimed. Granta Books, London.

Toynbee P 2002 Hard work. Bloomsbury, London.

Both Ehrenreich and Toynbee give enlightening personal accounts of service work in the 'new' economy.

REFERENCES

Allen D, Hughes D 2002 The division of labour in healthcare. Palgrave Macmillan, Basingstoke

Beynon H 1997 Changes at work: Working paper 19. Manchester International Centre for Labour Studies, University of Manchester, Manchester

Beynon H, Grimshaw, DP, Rubery J et al 2002 Managing employment change: The new realities of work. Oxford University Press, Oxford

Braverman H 1974 Labour and monopoly capital. Monthly Review Press, New York

Burnham J 1945 The managerial revolution. Penguin, Harmondsworth

Carrier J 1997 The meanings of the market. Berg, Oxford

Clarke J 2005a Market. In: Bennet T, Grossberg L and Morris M (eds) New Keywords. Blackwell, Oxford

Clarke J 2005b 'Management' In: Bennet T, Grossberg L and Morris M (eds) New keywords. Blackwell, Oxford

Clarke J, Newman J 1997 The managerial state. Sage, London

Cooke H 2002 Empowerment. In: Blakely G, Bryson V (eds) Contemporary political concepts. Pluto, London, Ch 9

Crompton R 1990 Professions in the current context. Work, Employment and Society 5(4):147–166

Cutler T, Waine B 1994 Managing the welfare state. Berg, London

Davies C 1990 The collapse of the conventional career: The future of work and its relevance for post registration education in nursing, midwifery and health visiting. English National Board for Nursing, Midwifery and Health Visiting, London

Department of Health (2006) Modernising nursing careers. Department of Health, London

Douglas M 1992 Risk and blame: Essays in cultural theory. Routledge, London

Du Gay P 2000 In praise of bureaucracy. Sage, London

Durkheim E [1893] 1984 The division of labour in society. Macmillan, London

Durkheim E 1992 Professional ethics and civic morals (Routledge Sociology Classics). Routledge, London

Ehrenreich B 2002 Nickel and dimed. Granta Books, London

Freidson E 1975 Profession of medicine. Dodd, Mead, New York

Gerth H H, Mills, C W 1970 From Max Weber. Routledge and Kegan Paul, London

Giddens A 2001 Sociology. Polity, Cambridge

Goffman E 1968 Asylums: Essays on the social situation of mental patients. Penguin, Harmondsworth

Greenwood E 1957 Attributes of a profession. Social Work 2:45–55

Guardian 1997 £739 – the hidden earning power in your home that gets swept under the carpet. 7 October

Hammond J L, Hammond B 1949 The town labourer (1760–1832) Vol I. British Publishers Guild, London

Handy C 1989 The Age of Unreason. Business Books, London

Hochschild A 1983 The managed heart: Commercialisation of HUMAN Feeling. University of California Press, Berkeley

Hochschild A 2001 The time bind: when work becomes home and home becomes work. Owl Books, New York

Illich I 1976 Limits to medicine. Marion Boyars, London

Jamous H, Pellouille B 1970 Changes in the French Hospital System. In: Jackson J (ed.) Professions and professionalism. Cambridge University Press, Cambridge, p 111–152

Kahn J 1997 Demons, commodities and the history of anthropology. In: Carrier J (ed.) The meanings of the market. Berg, Oxford, p 69–98

Kennedy I 1983 The unmasking of medicine. Granada, London

Lubasz H 1992 Adam Smith and the invisible hand of the market. In: Dilley R (ed.) Contesting markets: Analyses of ideology, discourse and practice. Edinburgh University Press, Edinburgh, p 37–56

Millerson G 1964 The qualifying associations. Routledge and Kegan Paul, London

Mooney G (ed.) 2004 Work: Personal lives and social policy. Open University Press, Buckingham

Krause E 1996 The death of the guilds: Professions, states and the advance of capitalism, 1930 to the present. Yale University Press, New Haven

McKinley J, Arches J 1985 Towards the proletarianisation of physicians. International Journal of Health Services 15(2):161–195

McKinley J, Marceau L 2002 The end of the golden age of doctoring. International Journal of Health Services 32(2):379–416

Nicholls T 2005 Work. In: Bennet T, Grossberg L, Morris M (eds) New keywords. A revised vocabulary of culture and society. Blackwell, Oxford, p 374–376

Office of National Statistics 2006 Social Trends No 36 Palgrave, Macmillan, Basingstoke

Osborne D, Gaebler T 1992 Reinventing government. Addison-Wesley, Reading, MA

Pollitt C, Bouckaert G 2000 Public management reform: A comparative analysis. Oxford University Press, Oxford

Pollock A 2004 NHS plc. Verso, London

Ritzer G 1996 The McDonaldization of society. Pine Forge Press, Thousand Oaks, CA

Scull A 1977 Decarceration. Prentice Hall, NJ

Shaw G B 1971 (first published 1911) The doctor's dilemma. Penguin, Harmondsworth

Taylor F W 1947 Scientific management. Harper and Row, New York

Thompson EP 1968 The making of the English working class. Penguin Books, Harmondsworth

Toynbee P 2002 Hard work. Bloomsbury, London

Traynor M 1999 Managerialism and nursing. Routledge, London

Warhurst C, Thompson P, eds. 1998 Hands hearts and minds: Changing work and workers at the end of the century. In: Workplaces of the future. Macmillan, London, p 1–24

Watson T 2003 Sociology, work and industry. London, Routledge

Williams R 1983 Keywords: A vocabulary of society and culture (revised edn). Fontana, London

Social class, poverty and health

Ronnie Moore

KEY CONCEPTS

- An historical review of social divisions
- Poverty and definitions of poverty
- The changing nature of social class
- Contemporary debates about classical sociological theories of class
- Globalization and its impact on poverty and health inequalities

Social differences and social strata

A Vaudeville comedian once declared, 'I don't care to belong to a club that accepts people like me as members'. Behind this comical one-liner is a subtle recognition of important and pervasive issues of social differentiation and social status. When we talk of social differences, we often refer to various physical characteristics, ideas or behaviour which set us apart from others. Ethnic identity, for example, separates us. Other characteristics may also divide us. We may align ourselves to, or be aligned by others to, a particular group or groups. We talk of local, regional and national identities such as Northerners, Southerners, Scots, Irish or English, or of religious identities such as Jews, Catholics, Muslims or Protestants. In contemporary society, popular culture has also introduced new identities that signify a preference for particular interests or lifestyle choices such as that of Goths (see Hodkinson 2002).

These are important markers and such labels carry a particular currency in terms of identity and belonging. This is not a local phenomenon either. If we look at other cultures in different parts of the world, we also see a tendency to differentiate people. The caste system in India provides a particularly good example of a complex and highly structured social system where a person's caste position assigns their social position. This emphasizes strict social boundaries and is tied to religious practice and to how daily life is organized. The caste system not only stresses differences but importantly illustrates another phenomenon, that of social stratification (the dividing of a society into grades, levels or classes). This implies a layering in terms of hierarchy and status assigned at birth until death, where the person cannot chose to enter or leave their caste. The caste system is thus an extremely rigid form of social stratification.

When we look at Britain, we see that historically social stratification rested on a feudal system and on the ownership of land. The ruling elite (the nobility), were able to command power, status, privilege and wealth. This was maintained and socially reproduced through grace and favour and through the legal right of inheritance. The rise of industrialization however, meant that the basis of social stratification in Britain changed dramatically. The shift from an agrarian based economy to the modern, cash nexus (capitalist) economy comprehensively altered the nature of the social structure and the ancient order in Britain, and consequently people's lives.

Within a developing and expanding industrial labour market, the basis of social stratification also came to rest increasingly on a social position in the workforce and on a market position in an economy based on exchanging labour for money. Much of the old ruling elite (hereditary aristocracy) still remained at the apex but important changes were occurring. The aristocracy had traditionally looked down on people who were in 'trade' but increasingly the new rich such as industrial or business entrepreneurs become part of the ruling elite. Inheritance however remained an important factor socially reproducing the elite. At the same time, the enclosure movement was forcing rural workers off the land into towns and cities to form the new industrial working class.

The initial phases of industrialization brought extremely harsh economic and social conditions. With virtually no regulation, the industrial workforce was vulnerable to unscrupulous employers and often forced to work long hours in very dangerous conditions (see Chapter 4). The very young, the infirm and the old did not escape these hardships; they worked in factories, mills and mines in a wretched industrializing world. Unrestricted (free market) commercial freedom meant that employment did not make people immune to suffering and poverty. Poor employment conditions meant that the majority of the industrial workforce was condemned to a life of misery and poverty. The labouring class lived in pitiable conditions, with overcrowding, poor nutrition and poor sanitation.

The growth of the middle classes

The industrial revolution in Britain and the development and expansion of an economically powerful British Empire were to have major social and economic consequences locally (and later globally). As industrialization attracted people to the large urban areas in search of work, it brought with it geographical and social mobility and cultural contact within and between nations. It constituted a reshaping of the geographical spread of the population of Britain and changed the way that the population was stratified. This changed the nature of family and social life (see Chapter 2) and gave rise to a more complex social order with a variety of different social groups or classes. The basis of one's station or class was now linked to employment and position in the labour market.

As industrialization gathered momentum throughout the nineteenth century, jobs diversified. In the labour market, some skills were able to command higher levels of income and better conditions. Industrialization meant that new professions formed to organize and manage a developing capitalist economy, i.e. engineers, accountants. The expansion of the British Empire also fuelled the demand for new administrative occupations which expanded throughout the Victorian period including government officials, teachers, lawyers, doctors and clerks. Out of this emerged a very broad category of people who made up 'the middling' or middle class. Over the past century, this professional sector has expanded dramatically (Routh 1980).

The ethos driving the Victorian middle classes was the idea of individualism, independence, thrift and a moral and spiritual belief in hard work and merit. These virtues are embodied in what Max Weber (see Chapter 4) has described as the 'Protestant Ethic'. Weber believed this ethic was a necessary condition for the growth of capitalism in certain parts of Europe (Bendix 1966, Hamilton 2001). Underlying this ethos was the belief that the individual was responsible for his or her own actions and condition. Industrialization was believed to have created the possibility for upward social mobility into the middle and upper classes and this was seen as positive proof that a fair meritocratic system had replaced an inherently unfair system of nepotism and aristocratic privilege (Gunn and Bell 2003, Saunders 1990). The focus was on the moral attitude of the individual and on their responsibility for their social class and economic condition. This ideology was not new. The 'deserving' and 'undeserving' were survivals of an older ethos.

Poverty

THE POOR IN HISTORY

In great monarchies, and in early parliamentary democracies, the poor were regarded as an enduring problem. Historically, they were categorized into different groups including vagrants, paupers, migrants, the sick, the old and the able bodied poor. An important distinction arose between the 'deserving' and the 'undeserving' poor. As early as 1531, an Act of Parliament officially differentiated between the 'able-bodied' vagrant and those vagrants that could not help being in the position that they were in because of disability or sickness (Kumar 1984). This coincided with the expansion of towns and cities in which an earlier form of capitalism (described as mercantile capitalism) expanded from the sixteenth century onwards. The able-bodied poor were identified as 'sturdy beggars' and were seen as not wanting to work for a living. They were regarded as being a threat to the moral, religious and political order of the day. Begging for example, was considered a threat to public order and legislation made slothfulness a crime punishable by flogging. Ill-health was regarded suspiciously and seen as an excuse for laziness. Sir Thomas More for example, condemned the work-less as 'Sturdy and valiaunte beggars cloaking their idle lyfe under the colours of some disease or sickness' (Garraty 1978: 28). There was however, some recognition that, in certain circumstances, the able bodied might not be in a position to work because no work was available. Thus, for example, another Act was passed in 1572 recognizing some groups, such as redundant soldiers, as being genuinely unemployed, thus exempting them from the penalties of the extreme vagrancy laws.

Since the Elizabethan Poor Laws of 1597, official attitudes to the poor in Britain have been embodied in a series of Acts. Legislation reflected the general reluctance of government to take responsibility for the poor and infirm. It was widely held that official actions to help the poor would simply encourage idleness and thus make matters worse. Historically, relief from poverty was regarded as a matter for the family, sometimes with the assistance of the church. Rather than being seen as socially caused, poverty was seen as an individual matter, due to personal misfortune, or to character or moral defect.

Although the poor law provided basic relief from hardship and deprivation, its primary function was not charitable; rather it ensured that the poor were effectively managed. The legislation provided for a harsh system of public provision for the poor and destitute. The New Poor Law Amendment Act of 1837 marked a new approach to poverty coinciding with the growth of industrial capitalism (see Chapter 4). The aim now was to exert greater discipline on the able bodied poor by forcing them into workhouses if they wished to obtain relief.

It was these Acts that guided official attitudes towards the poor for the rest of the nineteenth century and arguably up to the present day 'welfare to work' policies (see Chapter 4). By the middle of the nineteenth century, workhouses were common throughout Britain. One of the effects of the harshness of this legislation was that it encouraged workers and their families to become geographically mobile in search of work. Official attitudes to the poor continued to link poverty to a pathology of the poor person; a moral defect rather than a defect in the social, political and economic environment in which that person lived. In other words, the focus was on the individual rather than the way society was organized and it was individual failings that were perceived as the cause of poverty.

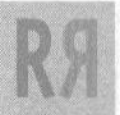

REFLECTION POINT

We have seen that historically attitudes to the poor have often been harsh and unsympathetic. Help for the poor in places such as workhouses was often little more than punishment and the poor were blamed for their poverty. Think about recent coverage of the issue of poverty that you may have seen in the media. Are people more sympathetic to poverty today? To what extent do you think that the poor are still blamed for their condition?

DEFINITIONS OF POVERTY

Concerned figures such as Charles Dickens provided a literary window to this world in novels such as *Oliver Twist*. For social commentators such as Friedrich Engels and Karl Marx, the problem lay in the social and economic circumstances that the working poor, unemployed and infirm found themselves in. This presented a challenge for Engels:

> *'I have now to prove that society in England daily and hourly commits ... social murder ... and so hurries them into the grave before their time. I have further to prove that society knows how injurious such conditions are to the health and the life of the workers, and yet does nothing to improve these conditions'. (Engels 1892: 96)*

Marx believed that these circumstances were the result of exploitation and uncontrolled capitalism where the poor were tied into cycles of poverty. Thus, poverty reproduced itself with successive generations. Marx and Engels viewed social class in terms of a theory of social change and also believed that it was important to understand society in order to change it.

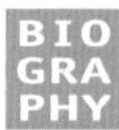

Karl Marx (1818–1883)

Karl Marx was a German philosopher, economist and political theorist. He studied philosophy at the University of Berlin and became part of a group of radical philosophers called the young Hegelians who were influenced by the work of G W F Hegel. Marx began his career as an editor of a liberal newspaper in Cologne but his political views brought him into conflict with the authorities and after a brief exile in Paris and Brussels he settled in Britain. Much of his work was produced in collaboration with Friedrich Engels, who was the son of a wealthy manufacturer and who supported Marx for much of his life. Marx struggled with poverty and ill health for most of his life. He died in 1883 and is buried in Highgate cemetery. To read more about Marx's life, see Francis Wheen's (1999) excellent biography.

One of Marx's central ideas was the concept of *alienation*. In his earliest work, *Economic and Philosophical Manuscripts* (1844) Marx described the alienated nature of labour under capitalism and contrasted it with the idea of a communist society in which freedom and cooperation would prevail. He said of alienation: 'Money is the alienated essence of man's work and existence; the essence dominates him and he worships it'.

In the German Ideology (1845), he and Engels developed the idea of *historical materialism*. They believed that history could be understood by reference to material conditions rather than ideas and personalities. In particular, they believed that conflict and struggle between opposing forces was the motive force of history. They said 'Life is not determined by consciousness but consciousness is determined by life'.

Marx joined the Communist League in Paris in the 1840s and he and Engels were invited to produce a succinct statement of Communist philosophy. They published the Communist Manifesto in 1848. It began 'the history of all hitherto existing societies is the history of class struggle' and concluded 'Workers of the world unite. You have nothing to lose but your chains'.

Marx spent much of the rest of his life analysing the capitalist production process. He produced two major works *Das Capital* in which he developed the *theory of surplus value* and the *Grundrisse*, which was published after his death.

Marx developed many influential ideas and his ideas have extended beyond the Communist movement. His writings about economics and sociology have influenced many thinkers who do not share his political views.

Other important observers at the time also exposed the effects of urban life on the industrial poor. One of the most influential reformers of the period was the founder of the Salvation Army, Charles Booth, whose *Life and Labour of the Peoples of London* (1889) provided a bleak historical account of what the life of the poor was like. Booth showed that poverty, bad working conditions, low income and bad health were related. He defined poverty existing when income was not large enough to sustain physical health, otherwise known as the subsistence level. For Booth, poverty meant being in a constant state of want and struggling for the basic essentials to survive.

Thus, social reformers tried to identify a fixed point of income, beneath which it would be impossible for a person to live and work. This became known as the absolute definition of poverty. It regarded poverty as relating solely to the amount of income necessary for maintaining a person's health and ability to function. This was an extreme distinction in that it defined a level of subsistence which was the absolute minimum for maintaining health. Those who had the bare essentials to survive were not categorized as being in poverty. Booth demonstrated that, even according to this minimal definition, large numbers of people in Britain were living in poverty. The sociological importance of this work was that it provided an important starting point for the subsequent debate on social conditions, poverty and health. By establishing measurable (albeit crude) levels of poverty and devising means whereby it could be defined and understood, Booth stimulated public and academic debate which would inform research into poverty and health.

An important contribution to this debate is the work of Peter Townsend. Townsend's concept of 'relative poverty' argues that absolute definitions of poverty do not take account of the fact that people's requirements do not stay the same as society changes. In *Poverty in the United Kingdom* (1979), Townsend argues that absolute definitions of poverty are inappropriate and poverty rather than being defined in absolute terms should be defined in relation to the general living standards in society at a given point in time. In other words, a person should be regarded as being in poverty if they cannot afford those things which are regarded as basic to everyday life by most people. This approach suggests that in modern society poverty is regarded as not having what are deemed to be basic necessities. More recently, Mack and Lansley (1985) have used public opinion surveys to show that there is actually public consensus as to what are regarded as necessities.

REFLECTION POINT

We have seen that in Victorian times, people tried to define a level of 'absolute poverty'. This was the minimum that people needed just to stay alive; in other words just above starvation level. There has more recently been an attempt to replace this with the concept of 'relative poverty'. This tries to define the level of income required to participate in society. It therefore involves an effort to establish what most people think are basic essentials for that society at the time. More than twenty years ago Mack and Lansley (1985) showed that there was public consensus about what were regarded as necessities at that time. Make a list of the things that you think are the necessaries of life today to which everyone should have access? Do you believe that this should include just the basics we need to survive such as food, clothing and shelter? Alternatively, do you think that this should also include things that enable people to participate in society and its customs (for example, the ability to buy family Christmas presents)?

Social class

DEFINING SOCIAL CLASS

Our discussion so far has illustrated the fact that social differentiation has existed throughout history but has been dynamic and changing. With the rise of modern capitalism, societies stratified into a hierarchical system, based primarily on economic status and social prestige. The consequences of such a dramatic reordering of British and other industrial societies intensified the harsh conditions of the poor, especially the 'labouring poor'. Marx in particular was concerned with early industrialization and with its effects on social structure and social class.

Marx was particularly interested in the mechanisms that produced and reproduced class inequality and what he called 'class consciousness'. He argued that a person's chances of living, surviving and providing for themselves and their family were linked to the relationship to what he termed 'the means of production'. Capitalists and industrialists appeared to profit under capitalism since they owned and controlled the means of production (i.e. the factories and mills that the workers laboured in, and the raw materials of production such as cotton and steel).

However, the working poor (who had only their labour to sell to survive) were exploited. For Marx the distinction was clear. There existed two social classes – those who own the means of production (the wealthy bourgeoisie), and those who must sell their labour to survive (the proletariat). His outlook was critical. He argued that the nature of the relationship was antagonistic and based on exploitation. For Marx, wealth determined life and health chances and an economic definition was therefore crucial as a measure of social position or class.

Marx believed that the rich would accrue more and more wealth since they not only owned finance but also controlled the mechanisms of finance. Marx predicted that this would eventually lead to a concentration of capital among the rich. This would ultimately lead to a class revolution since capitalism was based on exploitation and thus the interests of the bourgeoisie and the proletariat were diametrically opposed. The theory behind this was the idea of a dialectic (after the German Philosopher, Hegel). This was the idea that the struggle of opposites will eventually lead to progress and the creation of new conditions.

Central to Marx's ideas was his theory of alienation (see also Chapter 3). Workers perceived themselves being subjected to market forces of supply and demand, i.e. constrained by the market which was beyond their control.

The net result of this was that workers became alienated and estranged from what they produced. This is the sense of loss of control of one's life and one's destiny. Marx believed that only with the end of capitalism would humans be free to fulfil their truly social nature.

THE CHANGING NATURE OF SOCIAL CLASS

Marx believed his ideas to be central to a general understanding of social and class inequality and not bound by national borders. He believed that capitalism would only be overthrown by international revolution. In some ways, his vision foresaw the importance of international capitalism and what we now understand as globalization. For some, though, Marx's theory was over-deterministic. It appeared to overplay the influence of structural mechanisms such as capitalism and underplay human 'agency'. That is, the extent to which people are able to exercise personal choice as opposed to being subject to social forces beyond their control. For example, Marx talked of 'economic capital' but failed to recognize other forms of capital which later theorists suggest are important to life and social living. For example, more recently Pierre Bourdieu developed the notion of social or cultural capital (which is discussed later in this chapter).

Social stratification thus appeared to develop in a more complex way than Marx has predicted particularly through the expansion of the middle classes. Class conflict rather than increasing as Marx suggested, appears to have been contained, via trade union collective bargaining and the development of the welfare state. Marx's prediction of a unified (and international) class consciousness 'a class for itself' did not emerge; rather, local and national identities and cultures continued to exert an important influence. The working class as defined by Marx have not developed a unified international consciousness.

Historical accounts of industrialization identify various stages of development. While Marxists talk about early and late phases of capitalism, non-Marxists have talked of early, mature, late and post-industrial phases and of modernity and post-modernity. The historical significance here is that the nature of work and the nature of our society has changed and is still changing. The social significance is that working and living practices are influenced by this and these epochs appear to mark distinct stages in the development of human society. Social classes appear to be more fluid and therefore more complex than Marx suggested. Rather than classes polarizing, the class structure in advanced industrial societies appeared to become more complex and differentiated.

Writing shortly after Marx, Max Weber agreed with Marx that economics produced class differences, but for Weber a definition social class based solely on economic factors was of limited use. While Marx emphasized social structure, Weber stressed human action. Weber suggested that power or political influence and prestige also helped to determine a person's social status. Weber's ideas on social stratification suggested three important connected elements.

1. *Class:* the economic relationship to the market
2. *Status:* honour, prestige and social standing
3. *Party:* political power and affiliation

All three elements interact and are important for what Weber called 'life chances'. Wealthy industrialists for example, may own the means of production, but managers, because of their position or expertise might have the power to make important business decisions. Similarly religious leaders may have social status and cultural influence but little economic or political power. For Weber, social strata reflected the distribution of power (Gerth & Mills 1946). Weber's focus on status and occupation was an important sociological shift and provided a more nuanced discussion of social class issues which dealt with dynamic changes in the occupational structure and appeared to be more able to explain the complexity of the twentieth-century class system.

Following Weber, John Goldthorpe and colleagues allocated seven separate class categories taking account not only of wealth but also power and social status. This became highly influential and paved the way for practical working definitions of social class based on occupational status (see Leete and Fox 1977, Szreter 1984). This helps sociologists and other academics and professionals observe demographic, social, political, economic and health trends. The neo-Weberian approach to measuring social class structure is further developed by Lockwood, Goldthorpe and colleagues (see Goldthorpe 1980).

Applying social class criteria to different social groups was a commanding feature of British sociology up to the 1980s. This linked economic position, social identity and political preference. Class was defined using the Registrar General's scale of social class was commonly applied. This defined five broad strata, based on occupation.

THE REGISTRAR GENERAL'S CLASSIFICATION OF SOCIAL CLASS

I. Professional
II. Managerial/Technical
IIIa. Skilled (non-manual)
IIIb. Skilled (manual)
IV. Partly skilled
V. Unskilled
VI. Other

Since 2000, this has been refined into the UK National Statistics Socioeconomic Classification (NS-SEC), which is now used in all official surveys.

THE NATIONAL STATISTICS SOCIOECONOMIC CLASSIFICATION OF ANALYTIC CLASSES

1. Higher managerial and professional occupations
2. Lower managerial and professional occupations
3. Intermediate occupations
4. Small employers and own account workers
5. Lower supervisory and technical occupations
6. Semi-routine occupations
7. Routine occupations
8. Never worked and long-term unemployed.

While Goldthorpe and colleagues refined practical ways to measure social class, other important neo-Weberians produced theories to account for changes in social class (see Giddens 1981). In the 1980s, Giddens developed Weberian ideas on class structure and described what he calls '*structuration*' (or duality of structure). Structuration theory suggests that social structures determine people's action but human action also has an impact on these structures. Giddens was thus interested in the nature of agency and structure and the relationship between the two (Giddens 1984).

In recent years, it has been suggested that traditional perceptions of social status are becoming blurred. Care assistants are now on the Queen's Honours list as well as business gurus. In addition, we now see iconic figures of our time such as rock/pop or sporting stars juxtaposed with former nobility, landed gentry, financiers and industrialists. Such changes reflect social transformation (arguably the

BIOGRAPHY Anthony Giddens (1938–present)

Anthony Giddens was born in London and studied sociology at Hull, Cambridge and the London School of Economics. He was a professor of sociology at Kings College Cambridge and from 1998–2003 was Director of the London School of Economics. Giddens was closely associated with the New Labour project and was an architect of the political ideas of the 'Third Way' and an advisor to Tony Blair. He received a peerage in 2004. Giddens has written widely on a variety of topics and of particular influence are his ideas about structuration, reflexivity, globalization and the Third Way.

'tertiarization' of the economy discussed in Chapter 4), just as they did in the industrial revolution and are evidence of the dynamic nature of social stratification.

REFLECTION POINT

We have seen that since the industrial revolution, the concept of class has been the most important way of describing the way in which social inequality has structured people's life chances. Sociologists have disagreed over the exact nature of class. Particularly important have been arguments about whether class just involves economic differences or whether it also involves cultural and political differences. We have also seen that the class structure has changed particularly through the growth of the middle class. Although social inequality has persisted, we have noted that cultural ideas about class have changed dramatically. Think about what the idea of social class means to you. What class would you describe yourself as belonging to? What image do the terms middle class, working class and upper class conjure up? Do you think that these stereotypes accurately portray individual members of these groups?

Critical theories of social class

In spite of the challenges to the Marxist theories outlined above, when considering social class some theorists argued that Marxist interpretations of class should not be dismissed. These authors believed that exploitation and inequality were still important features of contemporary society which should be critically challenged. One particular group of German theorists known as the Frankfurt School was interested in the idea of a 'critical' theory rather than 'traditional' theory. These included Adorno, Marcuse, Horkheimer and Habermas and their ideas have continued to be developed by other theorists. Following Marx, the stated aims of critical theory are not simply to seek to understand the world, but to effect emancipatory change within it. Anti-racist and feminist theories have also developed a critical stance towards contemporary society and are included in modern understanding of critical theory.

Scambler and Higgs (1999) for example, are sympathetic to the Marxist position and suggest that class has not diminished its sociological potency as a means of understanding the social world. They reject the postmodern approach which sees class as just an idea rather than something that has real material effects and consequences. They argue that while we have seen important economic and political changes this has not meant the end of social class. An inspection of recent literature on inequalities and health serves to illustrate this point. Much of the literature points to clear relationships between social class, illness and life expectancy (Chandola (1998, 2000), Moore & Harrisson 1996).

Thus many Marxist and non-Marxist sociologists argue for the continued importance of social class as a concept (Erikson & Goldthorpe 1992, Scambler & Higgs 1999, Wright 1997). One sociologist who has done much to refine and develop contemporary conceptions of social class is the French sociologist, Pierre Bourdieu.

Bourdieu was concerned with how inequalities are produced and persist and the practices that reproduce inequality (for example of class and gender). Key ideas in Bourdieu's work include habitus, field and capital. According to Bourdieu, all human action takes place in social fields. The term '*field*' describes the objective social and economic circumstances in which a struggle for resources takes place. The field then is concerned with what Bourdieu calls 'economic and political profit' (Jenkins 1992). Fields are distinguished by the resources that are at stake, for example employment status, fame, artistic or intellectual prestige or political power. A field can be seen as a

BIOGRAPHY Pierre Bourdieu (1930–2002)

Pierre Bourdieu was born in the south of France and studied philosophy in Pau and Paris. He then became a lecturer in Algiers in 1985 at the time of the Algerian struggle for independence from the French colonial administration. He wrote a seminal study of the Algerian situation and went on to write a further 30 books and 300 papers during his lifetime. Bourdieu was an anthropologist, sociologist and philosopher who wrote on a wide range of topics including colonialism, class, education, language, art and television. His best known work was *Distinction* in which he developed his ideas about social and cultural capital. Bourdieu was also a political activist who campaigned against neo-liberalism and globalization for example by supporting small French farmers in their campaign against McDonalds. He said of the impact of neo-liberalism, 'ours is a Darwinian world of insecurity and stress'.

forcefield within which an individual is subject to particular social pressures. It can also be seen as a battlefield within which the battle for status and position is constantly waged (Wacquant 1998). An example of field would be the division of labour within healthcare. For example, a student entering nurse training is subject to a variety of social pressures and the dispositions that he or she bring into this situation will determine how well he or she succeeds in his/her career.

How an individual, such as our student nurse, gets on in a particular field depends on their mastery of the practices of the field, which Bourdieu calls the 'feel for the game' According to Bourdieu, individuals enter the field with a particular habitus. Bourdieu derived the term *habitus* from the Greek word *hexis,* which relates to deportment, manner and style (May 1996). A habitus is a set of acquired dispositions involving things such as lifestyle, dress, manner of speaking, body language and personal taste as well as beliefs. Bourdieu sees these dispositions as learnt and socially acquired – they are neither natural nor innate. However, because these dispositions are acquired from early childhood they become second nature so that we are unselfconscious in our practice and thus they appear to be natural. Further because they are bodily-practices, they profoundly affect our whole relationship to the world. For example, Bourdieu gives the example of traditional societies in which women must walk behind men with their eyes lowered (Jenkins 1992). It does not take much imagination to see that such practices would over time have profound physical effects as well as altering our outlook (literally) on the world. Thus, our student nurse brings certain dispositions with them and these are learnt not innate. This may be one reason why, for example, men occupy a disproportionately large number of senior positions in nursing (see Chapter 9).

Different groups or classes in society develop a different habitus. *Habitus* therefore constitutes the mechanism whereby we internalize external constraints such as inequalities of race, gender and class. The dispositions that people acquire thus depend on their position in society. Bourdieu is also concerned with the social value of a particular habitus. He says that individuals are endowed with different amounts of capital dependent on their social position. For Bourdieu capital is any resource that is effective in bringing success in a particular social field. He distinguishes three principal types of capital: economic (wealth), cultural and social.

Cultural capital focuses on the different cultural resources of individuals from different classes. Of central importance are the different educational resources of school children from different social classes. This includes high expectations of parents and teachers and echoes earlier work of British and American educationalists. Parents from more privileged classes provide children with cultural capital, the attitudes and knowledge that make the educational system a comfortable familiar place in which they can succeed easily. Bourdieu is critical of the view that educational success or failure is solely down to natural ability. Further, Bourdieu and Passeron (1973), discuss cultural reproduction suggesting that social institutions such as schools and hospitals reproduce advantage and disadvantage. Capitalist societies depend on a stratified social system, where the working class has an education suited for manual labour: levelling out such inequalities would threaten the social order.

REFLECTION POINT

We have seen that Bourdieu used the term *habitus* to describe the way in which very fundamental aspects of our persona such as ways of walking and talking can be shaped by social inequality. Thus for example, women may have been taught from an early age to be submissive and the working class to 'know their place'. Our own society has changed rapidly and we have been encouraged to see it as a society in which everyone who wants to can succeed. However, the reality is that social mobility remains very limited and Bourdieu's ideas have been seen as a useful way of understanding why it is still very difficult to move out of the class into which we are born. We have seen that Bourdieu used the term *cultural capital* to describe the subtle ways in which privilege and disadvantage are passed down the generations. Bourdieu showed for example, that middle class children feel more comfortable in educational settings. Now think about healthcare settings? What 'cultural capital' do you think that patients need to negotiate a visit to a GP or outpatient clinic?

Bourdieu has also defined *social capital,* which refers to valued social networks which are regarded as resources. We find common sense understandings of *social capital* referred to in expressions such as 'it's not what you know but who you know'. Bourdieu defines *social capital* as, 'the aggregate of the actual or potential resources which are linked to possession of a durable network of more or less institutionalized relationships of mutual acquaintance and recognition' (Bourdieu 1984). Social capital is the collective value of all available social networks and their social, political, economic and other (health) advantages. Thus social advantage and disadvantage depend not just on wealth but also on the possession of cultural and social capital. Bourdieu's recognition of multiple forms of capital recognizes the possibility of human agency and choice. Individuals can rise above their circumstances but Bourdieu also recognizes the subtle ways in which privilege and disadvantage are passed down the generations.

Bourdieu also describes a fourth type of capital which he calls *symbolic capital. Symbolic capital* refers to the ability of a particular class or group to impose its world view on others particularly when this conceals or obfuscates objective reality. This results in what Bourdieu calls *symbolic violence.* Bourdieu uses the term *symbolic violence* to refer to the ideological basis of domination. 'Every power to exert symbolic violence, i.e. every power which manages to impose meanings and to impose them as legitimate by concealing the power relations which are the basis of its force, adds its own specifically symbolic force to those power relations' (Bourdieu & Passeron 1977: 4).

Bourdieu saw *symbolic violence* as leading to social suffering (and consequently negative effects on health and welfare) and attempted to document this suffering in a series of case studies (Bourdieu 1999). One of his examples is the treatment of a sick person as an object. He quotes one woman in hospital who says 'you really are just a piece of straw'. Bourdieu says that the logic of the hospital makes sick persons with their suffering seem 'like one more obstacle to the smooth operation of the institution'. Symbolic violence is committed when sick and disabled individuals internalize the sense of worthlessness that the institution conveys to them (see also Chapter 8). Similarly, symbolic violence occurs when the poor or members of ethnic minorities internalize negative views of themselves and their class. Thus not only does symbolic violence help to perpetuate inequality it also has deleterious effects on the health and welfare of the disadvantaged such as stress and low self-esteem. We will explore this more in Chapter 6.

REFLECTION POINT

We have seen that Bourdieu used the term 'symbolic violence' to describe the ways in which inequality is justified and reproduced. He was particularly concerned with the ways in which the disadvantaged were forced to internalize a negative self image. To what extent do you think that the healthcare system reproduces inequality? Think about your own experience of dealing with disadvantaged healthcare users such as the poor, elderly, disabled or homeless. Is symbolic violence a useful concept for describing some of the experiences of these users? Can you think of examples of 'symbolic violence' from your own experience?

These various forms of capital relate to resources based on group membership, relationships, networks of influence and support. For Bourdieu these different types or forms of capital interact and influence each other. Bourdieu suggests that the social structure is defined by the distribution of capital. The working class have less **economic capital** (income and wealth) but also less **cultural capital** (valued dispositions, valued cultural goods, educational credentials and skills), less **social capital** (valued network and social resources) and less **symbolic capital** (ability to shape the dominant world view in society).

GENDER, ETHNICITY AND SOCIAL CLASS

Gender and ethnicity are also important in class positioning but placing these within a social class framework has been problematic. As Anthias (2001) suggests dividing people into permanent class and status groupings has limited explanatory power if gender and ethnicity are not taken into account. This is because class groups are cross cut by gender and ethnicity (Anthias 2001). In other words, gender and ethnicity can have an impact on life chances independent of social class. For example in Chapter 2, we looked at the impact of family practices on women's life chances. In addition, ethnicity can affect life chances through for example racial stereotyping. If we simply allocate a 'status' category to gender and ethnicity we fail to understand their important characteristics and differences, both from each other, as well as other status groupings such as occupational or consumption based groups (Anthias 2001: 841). Anthias is critical of traditional approaches which have sought to measure and incorporate gender and ethnic groupings simply in terms of social class. She argues that this is less meaningful and is of limited use. She does however suggest that it is possible to incorporate gender and ethnic divisions into stratification analysis by using Bourdieu's (1987) ideas.

SOCIAL COHESION, SOCIAL CAPITAL, HEALTH AND WELL-BEING

The concept of social capital has become a popular one in recent times (Kawachi et al 1979, Portes 1998). The political scientist Robert Putnam has develops the idea of social capital from a different perspective to Bourdieu. On the basis of his fieldwork in both Italy and the USA, Putnam argues that social capital is a key component to building and maintaining democracy. He uses the term 'social capital' to refer to involvement in civil society through institutions such as churches and voluntary organizations that allow people to build up social networks as well as building a sense of community. He points up the benefits of social capital suggesting that high levels of social capital were associated with lower crime rates, higher levels of prosperity and better health and happiness: '... the haves engage in much more civic activity than the have-nots ... social inequalities may be embedded in social capital' (Putnam 2000: 358).

This however is a complex area since shared ties and identities, in addition to these positive aspects, can also impose constraints on individuals and groups and may not always be beneficial (Putnam 2000). Putnam distinguishes between two types of social capital:

1. *Bridging*, i.e. the value assigned to social networks and connections that reach (horizontally) across socially homogenous groups. These are civic networks that enhance community social cohesion.
2. *Bonding*, the second type of social capital (emphasizing a hierarchical patronage system) where there are exclusive ties which bind people who share a similar identity and which shut other groups out. Criminal gangs and some elite groups, for example, are exclusive and self-serving and are said to emphasize bonding social capital, while church groups and clubs create bridging social capital (see also Chapter 3).

Putnam suggests that bridging social capital provides major benefits for societies, governments, individuals, and communities and thus the decline of churches, clubs and societies has important consequences for the individual and society (see Putnam 2000). The potential health consequences of social capital are highlighted in several recent studies (see Klinenberg 2002, Moore 2004). Although the ideas surrounding social capital have been influenced by Emile Durkheim he is rarely acknowledged (Turner 2003). We will explore the influence of social capital on health further in Chapter 6.

POVERTY AND SOCIAL EXCLUSION: GLOBALIZATION AND THE 'FREE MARKET'

From the 1970s, major industrial nations such as the USA, Britain and the European Union have generally tried to adopt a centralist economic policy. The philosophy which underpins this is a throwback to an earlier historical epoch. It is the idea of the free market and a *laissez-faire* approach. This is one which limits government intervention and places few or limited restrictions on business growth and economic development (see also Chapters 4 and 7). This approach celebrates competition, individualism and economic self-sufficiency 'while actively fostering the "inclusion" of the poor and marginalized into the labour market, on the market's terms' (Carpenter 2000). The general philosophy behind this so-called neo-liberal approach was the belief in a trickle down theory where wealth would eventually filter down through the social classes. The evidence below suggests that the reality has been deepening global inequality.

Neo-liberal philosophy and governance is the cornerstone in terms of trade, cooperation and understanding between the major Western capitalist economies. This has become an important ideology in modern democracies (Carpenter 2000). Despite an apparent commitment to 'free' markets, critics see it as involving political and economic domination by large multinational companies as small enterprises are squeezed out since they cannot compete against the major conglomerates. Behind neo-liberalism is the notion of optimistic progression and universality. We witness now a collision of a new global (corporate) world order and competing cultures and identities, where the local market place has given way to an international or world market. Technology has also had an impact. Electronic mass media has collapsed space and time barriers in human communication, enabling people to interact and live on a global scale. In this sense, the globe has been turned into a village by the electronic mass media and virtually instant communication (McLuhan 1962). Mobile phones, home and laptop computers are symbolic representations of this global age. In addition, the unprecedented availability and affordability of air travel has facilitated globalization. Indeed, Albrow (1996) suggests that it marks the creation of a new epoch where communication and exchange is truly global. Globalization means that we can reach beyond old horizons to a worldwide network or web and this has meant an intensification of social relations between people in distant places. Events happening in one part of the globe have consequences for other parts of the globe. Modern high-speed communication means that information, and resources (such as money) can travel around the world in an instant.

Globalization may be viewed as primarily an economic phenomenon involving increased (in terms of volume and speed) interaction, integration of national economic systems through growing international trade capital and investment. Social and cultural and technological exchange and trade increases and borders are losing their relevance. Critics see globalization as a worldwide trend towards a globalized economic system controlled by supranational corporate trade and international banks which are not accountable to democratic processes or national governments. The recent Action Aid Report (2005) provides examples of how power in the world food industry has become concentrated in a few hands. The report suggests that global food companies are dominating markets by buying up seed firms and forcing down prices for staple goods including tea, coffee, milk, bananas and wheat resulting in increased poverty in developing countries. The report suggests that 30 companies now account for a third of the world's processed food; five companies control 75% of the international grain trade; and six companies manage 75% of the global pesticide market. It finds that two companies dominate sales of half the world's bananas, three trade 85% of the world's tea, and one, Walmart, now controls 40% of Mexico's retail food sector. It also found that Monsanto controls 91% of the global GM seed market. Nestlé, Monsanto, Unilever, Tesco, Walmart, Bayer and Cargill are all said to have expanded hugely in size, power and influence in the past decade, directly because of the trade liberalization policies being advanced by the USA, Britain and other G8 nations. The Action Aid report argues that these companies are wealthier than the countries which they deal with. Nestlé, it says, recorded profits greater than Ghana's GDP in 2002, Unilever profits were a third larger than the national income of Mozambique and Walmart profits are bigger than the economies of both countries combined.

Critics have expressed concern about the negative health effects of trade liberalization. The report suggests that 50000 dairy farmers have been forced out of business, after a series of takeovers by Nestlé and Parmalat. In India, an estimated 12000 children worked last year on cotton-seed farms supplying subsidiaries of Bayer, Monsanto, Syngenta and Unilever. Many children were also exposed to dangerous pesticides. In the Indian tea sector – where two big companies control more than half the market – thousands of small-scale tea growers and plantation workers are struggling to earn enough to feed their families. Similar concerns have been expressed about the global labour market. For example, the recruitment of overseas nurses by rich Western countries has deprived some poor African countries of their trained nursing workforce.

While there appears to be a consensus that globalization and neo-liberal policies have meant economic growth, for developed and developing nations the health consequences of Western political policies appear to be coming into sharp relief as individuals in developing countries struggle to survive. Others face the dual problem of dealing with longer life expectancy (in poverty) and fending off traditional killer diseases long since eradicated or controlled in the West. Simultaneously, disadvantaged social groups in developed nations are experiencing an unprecedented growth in obesity (particularly childhood obesity).

Discussion points

1. What are the different ways in which policy-makers have defined poverty? How might these different definitions affect policies to help people in poverty?
2. What are the different ways that people have defined social class? How might different definitions of social class affect our understanding of the ways that social inequalities affect health?
3. What do you understand by the terms 'cultural capital' and 'social capital'? How do you think that these terms could help us to understand the impact of social inequality on health?

CHAPTER SUMMARY

Social class is about differentiating and ranking. But it is also about exploitation and inequality and about relations between different social groups. The concept however has, as we have seen, is a problematic one. The concept is not static, but is influenced by social and technological change and by how it is perceived. Classes and ideas of high and low status differ temporally (through time) and spatially (between different places). If we compare status and job rankings between England and the USA for example, we see that these are not easily matched. Yet, sociologists are aware that some individuals and groups in society fare better, and some fare worse in terms of wealth and socioeconomic status and this appears to influence health and health chances (Moore & Harrisson 1996). While some sociologists have spent a good portion of their working lives trying to understand, define and defend the idea of social class others have questioned the usefulness of the concept in contemporary society.

The classic approaches to social class are outlined and a major debate has been about the issue of 'structure' and 'agency' and the interplay between both of these influences. Giddens' work has become extremely influential here (not least in the political domain in Britain), while Bourdieu's notion of habitus has become a useful analytical device which has helped in terms of accounting for the position of women and ethnic groups within a wider concept of social class. While social class will continue to be debated, the effects of poverty and inequality will continue to impact on the health of the population. We will look more at the impact of inequality on health in the next chapter.

REFERENCES

Action Aid Report 2005 Power hungry: Six reasons to regulate global food corporations. Online. Available: www.actionaid.org.uk/doc_lib/13_1_power_hungry.pdf 31 Jan 2007

Albrow M 1996 The global age: State and society beyond modernity. Polity, Cambridge

Anthias F 2001 The concept of 'social division' and theorising social stratification: Looking at ethnicity and class. Sociology 35(4):835–854

Bendix R 1966 Max Weber: An intellectual portrait. Methuen, London

Booth W 1889 Life and labour of the people of London. Williams and Norgate, London

Bourdieu P 1984 Distinctions. Routledge, London

Bourdieu P 1987 What makes a social class? On the theoretical and practical existence of groups. Berkeley Journal of Sociology 32:1–18

Bourdieu P 1999 The weight of the world: Social suffering in contemporary society. Polity, Cambridge

Bourdieu P, Passeron J C 1973 Cultural reproduction and social reproduction. In: Brown R (ed.) Knowledge, education and social change. Tavistock, London

Bourdieu P, Passeron JC 1977 Reproduction in education, culture and society. Sage, London

Carpenter M 2000 Health for some: Global health and economic development since Alma Ata. Community Development Journal 35:336–351

Chandola T 1998 Social inequality in coronary heart disease: A comparison of occupational classifications. Social Science and Medicine 47:525–533

Chandola T 2000 Social class differences in mortality using the new UK National Statistics Socioeconomic Classification. Social Science and Medicine 50 (1):641–649

Erikson R, Goldthorpe J H 1992 The constant flux. Clarendon, Oxford

Engels F 1892 The condition of the working class in England. Oxford University Press, Oxford

Garraty J 1978 Unemployment in history: Economic thought and public policy. Harper and Row, London

Gerth H H, Mills C W 1946 (eds) From Max Weber: Essays in sociology. Oxford University Press, New York

Giddens A 1981 The class structure of the advanced societies. Hutchinson, London

Giddens A 1984 Constitution of society: Outline of theory of structuration. Polity, Cambridge

Goldthorpe JH 1980 Social mobility and class structure in modern Britain. Clarendon, Oxford

Gunn S, Bell R 2003 Middle classes: their rise and sprawl. Phoenix, London

Hamilton M 2001 The sociology of religion. Routledge, London

Hodkinson P 2002 Goth: identity, style and subculture. Berg, London

Jenkins R 1992 Pierre Bourdieu. Routledge, London

Kawachi I, Kennedy BP, Lochner K, et al 1979 Social capital, income equality and mortality. American Journal of Public Health 87(9):1491–1498

Klinenberg E 2002 Heat wave: Social autopsy of disaster in Chicago. University of Chicago Press, Chicago

Kumar K 1984 Unemployment as a problem in the development of industrial societies: The English experience. Sociological Review 32(2):187–208

Leete R, Fox J 1977 Registrar General's Social Classes: Origins and uses. Population Trends 8:1–7

Mack J, Lansley S 1985 Poor Britain. Allen and Unwin, London

McLuhan M 1962 The Gutenberg Galaxy: The making of typographic man. University of Toronto Press, Toronto

May T 1996 Situating social theory. Open University Press, Buckingham

Moore RG 2004 Religion, identity and health. In: Kelleher D, Leavy G (eds) Identity and health. Palgrave, London, p 123–148

Moore RG, Harrisson S 1996 In poor health: Socioeconomic status and health chances. A review of the literature. Social Sciences in Health 1(4):221–235

Portes A 1998 Social capital: Its origins and applications in modern sociology. Annual Review of Sociology 24:1–24.

Putnam R 2000 Bowling alone: The collapse and revival of American community. Simon and Schuster, New York

Routh R 1980 Occupations and pay in Great Britain. Macmillan, London

Saunders P 1990 Social class and stratification. Routledge, London

Scambler G, Higgs P 1999 Stratification class and health: Class relations and health inequalities in high modernity. Sociology 33(2):275–296

Szreter SRS 1984 The genesis of the Registrar General's social classification of occupations. British Journal of Sociology 35(4):523–546

Townsend P 1979 Poverty in the United Kingdom. Penguin, London

Turner B 2003 Social capital, inequality and health: The Durkheimian revival. Social Theory & Health 1(1):4–20

Wacquant L 1998 Pierre Bourdieu. In: Stones R (ed.) Key sociological thinkers. Palgrave Macmillan, Basingstoke, p 215–229

Wheen F 1999 Karl Marx. Fourth estate, London

Wright E O 1997 Class counts: Comparative studies in class analysis. Cambridge University Press, Cambridge

CHAPTER

6

Inequalities and health disadvantage

Ronnie Moore

KEY CONCEPTS

- Linking poverty and health
- Linking inequality and health
- Behavioural and materialist explanations for health inequalities
- Social capital and health inequalities
- Gender poverty and health
- Ethnicity, racism and healthcare
- Older people and the experience of poverty and ageism

Introduction

> *'There is no more serious inequality than knowing you'll die sooner because you're badly off'. (Frank Dobson, cited in Shaw et al 2000: 1)*

Britain is one of a number of advanced industrial nations which has experienced major improvements in the health of its population over the last 150 years. The most virulent infectious diseases which characterized the early part of the century are now effectively managed or have gone altogether. Mortality rates have greatly declined and life expectancy has increased significantly. This is a remarkable achievement and is often held as a triumph for medical innovation and science. However, the reasons overall for health gain are, as McKeown (1979) demonstrated, more accurately attributed to factors such as cleaner water, better sanitation, education and contraception. A major consequence of these changes however is that fewer people are born and on average people are living much longer.

This increased longevity has had profound consequences. The nature of common sickness has changed from infectious to chronic degenerative ailments; this has been described as the '*epidemiological transition*'. This transition has presented major social and healthcare challenges. As the overall population stock in the older age categories has increased, there has been increased demand on healthcare services for treatment for degenerative diseases and assistance in coping with the consequences of these.

The statistical trends tell us of overall improvements in the health of the population. However, sociologists and epidemiologists have noted that there are important differences in health chances. This means there are differences in the chances of becoming ill (morbidity) and dying earlier (mortality) between different groups in society. The previous chapter suggested an association between health and social class or wealth. For example, good health generally appears to be linked to wealth, while illness appears to be connected to poverty and deprivation. Not only are the differences glaring but there is concern that inequalities in health in Britain are actually getting worse.

Linking, poverty social class and health

The debate surrounding the link between social class and health is controversial, and has been rehearsed in various historical accounts (see Chadwick [1842] 1965). During the nineteenth century, the pioneer of public health, William Farr, was the first to make use of standardized mortality ratios to show up differences in death rates between people living in rich and poor districts. As a result, Farr estimated that almost 65 000 child deaths per year among the poor were avoidable (Whitehead 2000). Throughout the twentieth century, a developing body of research demonstrated serious inequalities in health and healthcare. In particular, research using standardized mortality ratios showed clear and widening inequalities in death rates between the social classes. Townsend's (1979) research in the 1970s for example, noted that those in social class V were two and a half times more likely to die before reaching the age of retirement.

Not only did the research show health inequalities, but it also pointed to a widening of the health gap between the rich and poor. This stimulated intense academic and political debate and the Government eventually commissioned a report to look at the issue. The Black Research Working Group on Inequalities in Health (1980) produced a report confirming significant and widespread class difference in health. The 'Black Report' (1980) concluded that the lower social classes experienced poorer health at all stages of their life in spite of welfare reforms. It also demonstrated a 'social gradient' in health throughout the social strata. Thus according to the Acheson (1998) report the costs of health inequalities are not only borne by the people at the bottom. The report estimated that if the mortality rate of social classes III, IV and V were brought down to that of social classes I and II then 17 000 deaths would be prevented among men under 65 every year. The Whitehall I study of civil servants showed that even junior office staff had worse health and earlier deaths than senior staff (Marmot et al 1984).

A number of socioeconomic factors including environment, unemployment, education, transport and housing (all of which are linked by income), profoundly influence health chances. Although the report highlighted the serious nature of the problem, little was done to implement the measures suggested in the Black report. It did however act as a major catalyst prompting widespread cross national research. The later Acheson Report (1998) commissioned by the Blair government presents a number of recommendations for reducing health inequalities, but implementation remains a problem.

THE WIDENING GAP

Recent research into inequality and ill health tend to support the general findings of the Black Report and point in particular to a widening of the health gap between the rich and the poor. Inequalities in health are found at virtually every stage of the life cycle. Morbidity and mortality rates have been shown to be consistently higher among more disadvantaged economic groups and in socially deprived areas (Marmot & McDowall 1986). Whitehead's (1987) review of inequalities in health came up with new and international findings and further corroborated evidence of class variations in health. Her findings suggested a serious widening of inequalities in health throughout the 1980s. Phillimore et al (1994) further illustrate this. During the period 1981–1991 a widening of mortality differentials was observed for all age categories under 75 years, between the most affluent and the most deprived areas. Other evidence has pointed to socioeconomic status as a major factor influencing morbidity as well as mortality. Yuen et al (1990) inspected acute and chronic self reported illness using data from the

General Household Survey (1981–84) and found an inverse relationship between reported levels of illness and socioeconomic status.

Cross-cultural research shows that health inequalities are an international problem. Pappas et al (1993) compared mortality between socio-economic groups between 1960 and 1986 in the USA. They confirmed that the poor die earlier and have more health problems. They also showed that the disparity was increasing. Health inequalities in the USA are even starker than in the UK. Navarro (2004) suggested that a member of the poorest class in the USA can now expect to die 14 years earlier than a member of the most affluent class.

In 2000, an important study showed that inequalities continued to widen at the start of the new millennium. Some key facts and figures from this study are illustrated below.

BIOGRAPHY

The Widening Gap: Health Inequalities and Policy in Britain

In this study by Shaw et al (2000), 1 million people living in the constituencies with the worst health were compared with a million people living in constituencies with the best health. The 'worst million' lived in deprived areas such as Glasgow and Salford. The 'best million' lived in affluent areas such as Kensington and East Dorset. Living in one of the 'worst million' areas was associated with higher levels of poverty, unemployment, poor housing and poor education.

- The life expectancy gap between men in the 'best million' and 'worst million' was almost 10 years
- Infant mortality in the 'worst million' was almost double that in the 'best million'
- People in the 'worst million' were almost three times more likely to have a long-standing illness
- When compared with the 'best million', 62% of deaths under 65 years in the 'worst million' were avoidable.

The Shaw et al (2000) study was one of a number of recent studies that linked social class inequalities to geographical inequalities. There has been a steady North to South shift in terms of the focus of economic activity in the UK since the end of the 1970s. Smith (1989) demonstrated how different regions of the UK are increasingly acting like magnets either for wealth or social deprivation. As there are geographical distributions of poverty and wealth, so too are there similar patterns for health. There is now a geography of health and wealth in which social deprivation and high morbidity and mortality rates go hand-in-hand.

Extreme morbidity and mortality variations between the Northern and Southern regions of the UK are difficult to ignore. The research illustrates a geographical mapping of poverty and of health and illness (Carstairs & Morris 1989, Phillimore 1989). These patterns may be local as well as regional. For example, life expectancy decreases by 1 year for each of six stops on the London Underground that one travels from Tower Hill into the East End (Shaw 2005). These trends have become more obvious in recent years. We are concerned here with inequalities within the UK but international inequalities have also worsened as our discussion of globalization in Chapter 5 indicated. For example, life expectancy is an astonishing 48 years more in Japan than in Sierra Leone (Marmot 2005).

Explanations for health inequalities

There are several theoretical explanations for health inequalities. These vary and are disputed. The cultural/behavioural characteristics of the poor are said to influence ill-health. It has been argued that the poor are responsible for their own destiny, and that the causes of ill health are personal and/or cultural (which infers choice).

Another explanation postulated is that a type of social Darwinism (natural or social selection) influences or decides health chances. The central tenets of this approach are that social mobility is dependent on health. Poor health leads to poor social and economic status and good health promotes upward mobility. Researchers favouring materialist/structuralist interpretations however, believe that health is dictated by conditions brought about directly by the lack of money and resources.

Theoretical explanations for health disparities have sometimes been presented as being mutually exclusive rather than interdependent. In assessing each of these interpretations, the Black Report underscored the materialist/structuralist explanation as being the most influential. The report identified economic factors, such as income, environment, education, housing and transport as having the most important bearing on health. Disagreements centre on the choice of a master indicator of health and illness; that is, the explanation that is most important. Arguments between theorists and policy makers highlight ideological and political disputes. We will consider the major explanations next.

CULTURAL/BEHAVIOURAL

The lifestyle of the lower socioeconomic classes has been viewed as an important cause of health inequality (DoH 1991). The government's philosophical approach is sympathetic to the view that people are ultimately responsible for their own health. This allows the government to see their role as facilitators and educators, rather than providers of benefits and services. While cultural differences between social classes may explain some of the variation in health, as a single explanation culture/lifestyle is highly problematic and should be treated with caution. It would be misleading to separate lifestyle and behaviour from their social context since these relate to such things as availability of choice (Wilkinson & Marmot 2003). The 'Health and Lifestyles' (Blaxter 1990) survey showed that most people were aware of healthy messages such as those regarding diet, smoking and exercise. However, making healthy choices was a complex matter. Few people had wholly healthy or unhealthy lifestyles; most engaged in a mixture of more or less healthy behaviours, and their choices were subject to a variety of influences including beliefs and material and social circumstances. This survey also showed that people in disadvantaged circumstances were less likely to experience health improvement as a result of lifestyle change owing to the health damaging effects of their material circumstances (see Chapter 11). Graham's (1993) research has also showed the ways in which hardship influences health choices. For some people, life is so difficult now that it seems impossible to worry about the future. She showed, for example, how women in difficult circumstances used smoking to cope with the stresses and strains of everyday life, even though they were aware of its damaging effects.

If we take food as an example of lifestyle, we can see a social gradient in diet quality. The major dietary difference between the social classes is that the poor substitute cheaper, processed foods for fresh foodstuffs. Processed foods are still heavily promoted by the food industry which has an enormously powerful influence on food standards (Wilkinson & Marmot 2003). Nutritional status thus continues to reflect socioeconomic status. Blaxter (1990) found that, among the more disadvantaged, meeting energy demands was an important consideration. While middle class women were preoccupied with providing a 'well balanced' meal, among the less well-off, there was more concern with providing a meal that was sustaining and 'filling'.

Research in Britain has also shown that poverty has a direct effect on physical development. Long-term nutritional status influences physical development and thus nutritional disadvantage is established early in life. Height and physical stature can be regarded as a general indicator of this. Children of unemployed parents are shorter than children from households where the father is working (Rona et al

1978). A report published by the University of Ulster (Barker et al 1988) also showed evidence of a height gradient related to socioeconomic status. This report suggested that the children of manual workers were, on average, shorter. This was true for both sexes. The Glasgow Healthy City study (George 1993) highlighted the difficulties of achieving good nutritional status if you are poor. It found that poorer areas have fewer reasonably priced outlets for fresh food. To get good value and healthy food you need a car or good transport. Thus, healthy diets cost more.

REFLECTION POINT

We have seen that lifestyles and behaviours affect health. We have also seen that lifestyle choices are strongly influenced by levels of affluence or deprivation. Make a list of lifestyle choices which can have a negative impact on health. How might wealth or deprivation have an impact on these choices?

MATERIAL DEPRIVATION

The Black Report (Townsend et al 1992) identified material deprivation as the most important cause of heath inequalities as we noted earlier. Since then, a large number of studies have highlighted material and social deprivation as key determinants of ill-health (Wilkinson & Marmot 2003). Power (1994) illustrated the link between health and income distribution and suggested that the health gradient is not an anomaly but that in most European countries health has been shown to be linked to social circumstances. More recently, Gwatkin (2000) has demonstrated that this is a global problem.

The social context sets the parameters for behaviour, choice, access and use of resources. Health inequalities are linked to multiple factors, many of which locate the source of the problem in a lack of finance and an impoverished environment. Those from lower socioeconomic positions live in poverty with low wages, often enduring hazardous working conditions, poor housing and run-down neighbourhoods.

Living and working environments influence health. McCarthy et al (1985) discussed the health consequences of damp housing, mould and respiratory disease. This was supported by research which noted that mould growth produced by damp caused respiratory problems (Blackman et al 1989). The authors also observed significant health differences between inner and outer city children in Belfast and fixed the blame for this on bad heating and housing design. For example experience of the Divis Flats in Belfast is a case in point, which illustrates how reduced building costs (poor design and insulation, the use of toxic materials such as asbestos and calcium chloride in the cement to speed the drying process) are ultimately translated into subsequent medication and hospital costs (see Lowry 1990). Kogevinas (1990) in a longitudinal study also found a close link between housing tenure and the ability to cope with health threats. This study showed that housing tenure and cancer survival rates are related.

The type of local neighbourhood also influences health. Blaxter (1990) noted the importance of neighbourhoods suggesting that poor areas are health damaging. Macintyre et al (1993) argue for a more pragmatic approach to research suggesting that even if public servants cannot influence the economic status of the population, it might be possible for local authorities to upgrade the environment of poorer areas in ways which could promote health. They argue that there is a need to inspect poorer localities and evaluate the influence of environmental factors on health. For example, childhood accident rates are strongly influenced by environment.

The Macintyre et al (1993) study concluded that improving the local environment promoted better health. The authors discuss the findings from two areas of Glasgow. They look at the physical characteristics of each area such as safe and healthy environments, public and private services, sociocultural features and the reputation of the area. They showed that living in the better area meant better access to healthier and more affordable foodstuffs. Public services were better and there were more recreational facilities.

Despite suffering worse health, the working class receive inferior medical care. Tudor Hart (1971, 2006) argued that an *inverse care law* is operated in Britain, whereby the provision of services is inversely related to the need for those services, i.e. those areas in most need are worst served. Tudor Hart related this to the influence of a market economy on healthcare. The more disadvantaged have poorer access to the full range of medical services and they also tend to under-utilize healthcare resources. Survival rates may be poorer. For example, The Thames Cancer Registry (1994) showed social class to be a major factor in cancer survival rates. For most cancers, patients from lower socioeconomic groups have lower survival rates than patients from higher socioeconomic groups. Furthermore, consultation rates and GP attendance appeared also to be linked to social class and a difference in treatment and response from medical professionals has also been noted (Blaxter 1984, Cartwright & O'Brien 1976).

REFLECTION POINT

We have seen that most researchers believe that material deprivation is the most important factor causing inequalities of health between social classes. Make a list of the ways in which you think that a low income can negatively affect health.

SOCIAL CAPITAL AND THE SOCIAL GRADIENT

The social capital theory suggests that an individual's well-being is linked to social equality, social support and social cohesion (Kawachi & Kennedy 1997, Wilkinson 1994). We discussed social capital in Chapter 5 and are concerned here specifically with its impact on health. For example, Wilkinson (2005) suggests that socioeconomic differences do not simply cause damage to health through material deprivation. He says that inequality has damaging psychological effects by lowering self-esteem and increasing stress levels. Stress may have direct effects or may translate into unhealthy coping behaviours such as excess drinking or smoking. Using data comparing income differentials between different countries, Wilkinson (1992) suggests that, in developed countries, mortality is more closely related to relative income within countries than the absolute wealth of a country. In other words, how wealth is shared out can be more important than the overall wealth of a country. For example, the USA is four times as wealthy as Costa Rica but life expectancy for Black men in the USA is 9 years lower than in Costa Rica. More egalitarian societies therefore tend to be healthier and to have lower mortality rates (Wilkinson & Pickett 2006).

Support for this thesis also came from the studies of Whitehall civil servants conducted by Michael Marmot. These studies found that even among people who were not poor, there was a social gradient in mortality that ran from the top to the bottom of the civil service. Marmot thus concluded that health differences were not limited to poor health for the poor and good health for everyone else (Marmot 2003). He posited the existence of *pyscho-social pathways* to ill health which were linked to factors such as respect, autonomy and social support (Marmot 2004). For example, the Whitehall II study showed that low control in the workplace predicted coronary heart disease (Marmot et al 1997). Marmot & Wilkinson (2001) suggest that the pyscho-social effects of relative deprivation also involve 'insecurity, anxiety, social isolation, socially hazardous environments, bullying and depression'. Marmot argues that reducing the slope of the social gradient will achieve substantial health gains (Marmot 2003).

Robert Putnam (2000) highlights the negative effects of a breakdown of social cohesion and trust (see Chapter 5). Putnam argues that this is part of a wider social disengagement that is at the heart of many social problems. He argues that being a member of small organized groups that meet, face-to-face, on a regular basis, is one of the basic building blocks of social (and civic) cohesion. Further, he argues that social capital has a direct impact on a person's health. Reduced social capital, social cohesion and social solidarity are translated into increased crime and political conflict as well as higher mortality rates and poorer health. Kawachi and Kennedy (2002) argue that trust has a direct effect on the relation between income inequality and life expectancy. Thus, high levels of income inequality in a society produced low trust, and low trust creates a poor social environment that in turn impacts on health. Putnam's general thesis is that fostering social capital is good for society and individuals.

Some evidence from the USA supports the social capital thesis. Klinenberg (2002) argues that levels of social capital among vulnerable groups, particularly the elderly and infirm, was a predictor of their likelihood of surviving temperatures that reached over 120° Fahrenheit during the Chicago heat wave of July 1995. Distribution of deaths showed that fatalities came from mostly low income, elderly, African-American and from violent regions of the city. There was also a gender difference. When age was controlled for, it was found that men were more than twice as likely to die as women. It showed how social vulnerability as measured by social isolation accounted for the frequency and distribution of deaths during the heat wave. Men constituted 80% of the unclaimed bodies in the morgues during the heat wave. Thus, it was the low social capital of the poor elderly men that created their acute vulnerability when faced with an intense heat wave.

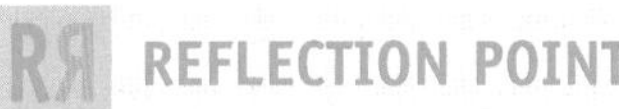

REFLECTION POINT

We have seen that the term *social capital* has been used to describe the ways in which social support and a sense of community can have a positive impact on health. Conversely, low *social capital* can have a negative impact on health. List some of the ways in which you think that low levels of social capital could adversely affect health.

Gender, poverty and health

Gender also appears to be an important determinant of health. The evidence suggests that females are born with a biological advantage; their chance of surviving the first year of life is higher than for males (Annandale 2003). While women have a higher life expectancy than men, overall, women appear to experience high rates of long-standing illness. It is important that nurses, if they are to understand the needs of women patients, look at some of the underlying reasons for women's illnesses which are often closely related to social circumstances. It is also important to be aware of the possibility of institutional discrimination in the provision of services to women. Numerous studies have indicated that gender may confer disadvantage in the utilization of health services.

Women are more likely to experience psychological illnesses than men and to be admitted to hospital for these illnesses. In terms of specific psychiatric disorders, morbidity is consistently higher for women with respect to psychological problems particularly depression and anxiety (Macintyre et al 1996). A ground breaking study of depression by Brown and Harris (1978) highlighted the role of social and economic circumstances in women's depression. They demonstrated the importance of stressful life events and a lack of social support in the aetiology of depression. Hunt and Annandale (1993) raise the issue of the social categorization of illness and argue that depression is often seen as a female problem. There may be gender differences in the diagnosis of mental illness by health professionals. For example, in a sample that met standardized criteria for depression, doctors were more likely to diagnose depression in women than in men (Potts et al 1991). Women with depressive symptoms (particularly in deprived areas) were also reluctant to seek help from mental health professionals (Jimenez et al 1997). Heart disease, on the other hand (which is a major mortality risk, particularly after the menopause) is not typically seen as a woman's problem and may be overlooked. Women also receive differential treatment after diagnosis. While women appear to present more to their GP both with physical and psychological complaints, GPs tend to refer a higher proportion of men to secondary care services (Johnson & Buszewicz 1996).

There is expanding literature on poverty and women's health. Payne (1991) illustrates the feminist critique, which underlines the failure to expose women's experiences of poverty and health. The relationship between socioeconomic status and health status among women is of central importance. Health authorities in Britain have now begun to take account of this link. Cohen (1994) looks in particular at the impact of poverty on women's health and the social disadvantages that they suffer, arguing that women bear the brunt of poverty problems. Cohen also argues that uptake of health screening and preventative measures are correlated with socioeconomic factors. For example, women from disadvantaged backgrounds were less likely to have a cervical smear, mammography or undertake breast self-examination. This points to the need to specifically target women from disadvantaged backgrounds. Blackburn (1992) argued that it is important to inform nurses and other healthcare practitioners about the link between family poverty and health. She underscores the need to create a data base on poverty and on health, arguing that unless information is gathered and analysed to show the impact of poor living conditions, health and social needs will not be adequately recognized or addressed.

RR REFLECTION POINT

We have seen that women have a higher life expectancy than men but more long-standing illness. We have also seen that a range of social factors affect women's health, particularly poverty. Make a list of the ways in which you think that social factors may affect women's health.

Ethnicity and racism

Modernization and globalization in recent decades has brought about major social and institutional challenges for British society. Inward migration, ethnic diversity and the implications for health have only relatively recently been addressed. However, the literature is growing and focuses on interpersonal interaction, communication, language, ethnic religious beliefs, cultural practices, treatment, compliance and issues of privacy (Karlson & Nazroo 2002, Kelleher & Hillier 1996, Nazroo 2003, 2004).

The literature suggests a link between ethnicity and health chances and between ethnicity and inferior healthcare treatment. There is evidence that different ethnic groups experience the health service differently, and that treatment and care is not equitable. Some ethnic groups have physical health problems and health needs specific to their ethnic background such as sickle cell disease. This lends support to the suggestion that there exist innate 'racial' differences which account for differences in the health chances of different ethnic groups. The danger with such an approach is that biological and cultural explanations may take primacy over other explanations of health inequalities which may result in the needs of these groups being disregarded or ignored (Karlson & Nazroo 2002). There is overwhelming evidence that the socioeconomic differences discussed at the start of this chapter play a major role in ethnic differences in health status. Nazroo (1997, 1998) has argued that members of ethnic minorities are often economically disadvantaged and this is a major contributing factor to their poorer health.

In London, minority ethnic groups make up 44% of the capital's population and a recent report pointed to worrying health inequalities between different ethnic groups (London Health Observatory 2005). The study looked at the health status of the capital's population, the impact of priority public health interventions, the effectiveness of health service partnerships, patients' experience of the NHS and how representative the NHS workforce was. The report showed that many ethnic minority groups fared badly. It showed higher levels of coronary heart disease, HIV/AIDS and tuberculosis in some of these groups. It also indicated that Chinese and Asians have a poorer experience of the NHS as patients compared with other Londoners. The causes are varied and include socioeconomic, genetic, cultural and organizational factors.

Various research accounts have pointed out shortcomings and deficiencies in health service provision for individuals from various ethnic groups whose culture, values and way of life may be different to mainstream British culture. Some research evidence has suggested that social and institutional discrimination limits access to healthcare (see Gerrish et al 1996, Smaje 1995). Ethnocentrism and racism have been highlighted as contributing factors for health inequalities (see Ahmad 2000, Ahmad & Jones 1998, Benzeval et al 1992). Bhui (2002) illustrates how various studies in a range of healthcare settings in Britain suggested negative attitudes among healthcare professionals and cultural stereotyping of patients from ethnic minority backgrounds.

Identity, including ethnic and religious identity has an important bearing on health even for those who might be regarded as being the closest migrant group. The Irish born in the UK continue to have (with the exception of schizophrenia) the highest rates of severe mental illness, suicide and self harm for all ethnic and migrant groups (Kelleher & Leavey 2004). Their physical health fares little better (see Kelleher & Hillier 1996). Observations through the 1970s through to the 1990s suggest that there are higher mortality rates for Irish people living in England. Also health disadvantage among the Irish born in England appears to be inexplicably reproduced through successive generations (Harding & Balajaran 2001).

It is tempting to assign culture as a key predictor of health status. Socioeconomic status, as we have seen is a major predictor of health chances and ethnic minority communities are economically disadvantaged (Karlson & Nazroo 2002). Socioeconomic position and institutionalized racism importantly contribute to lower health chances among ethnic minority groups. Ahmad (2000) suggested that professional ideologies have over-emphasized the differences in culture as a way of explaining health differences. A danger with assigning culture as an explanation is that it has the potential to excuse health inequalities. Nursing care and health services care for patients from different ethnic, religious and cultural backgrounds. The challenge for nurses is to endeavour to provide care on an equitable basis for all, irrespective of creed, colour, or 'race'.

REFLECTION POINT

We have seen that people from ethnic minorities frequently suffer worst health. We have also seen that cultural differences are a weak explanation of differences between ethnic groups. Material deprivation and racism are more important explanations of the poor health experiences of people from ethnic

Continued

RЯ REFLECTION POINT—cont'd

minorities. Make a list of the ways in which deprivation and the experience of racism might have a negative impact on the health of people from minority groups.

Older people and health: experiencing ageism and poverty

Older people are physically and socially vulnerable. They have been described in official literature as 'a demographic time bomb'. There is an inference that they constitute a major worrying drain on health resources. Much healthcare literature conveys the message that old people are unwanted as patients and they are frequently assigned pejorative labels such as 'bed blocker'. Such stereotyping has the effect of marginalizing this group (Ham 1992). It could be said that healthcare services display institutionalized *ageism*. The term *ageism* refers to systematic discrimination and stereotyping on grounds of age and refers mainly to discrimination against older people. According to Ragan and Bowen (2001: 511)

> *'Ageism often results in the attitude that older people are unproductive, sickly, depressing and that cognitive impairment is normative. A few of the most prevalent outcomes of ageism for older people are isolation from the community, inadequate housing and income, unnecessary institutionalization, untreated mental and physical illnesses and suicide'.*

But as Neave (1994) points out the majority of older people not only care for themselves but also contribute to the care of other family members such as grandchildren and as such provide an important role. This challenges the stereotype. Yet such stereotypes hold significant currency. In terms of medical care the medical model of care (with a focus on high technology and science) is seen as prestigious and important whereas the provision of services for the elderly including residential and community care for the old and chronically ill is regarded as of low status (Ham 1992).

Such stereotyping has also translated into ageist attitudes and these have been documented at both the individual and structural levels in the NHS (Neave 1994). Ryan underscores this adding that nurses and other healthcare professionals need to examine their own conscience in respect to this (Ryan 1998). Koch and Webb (1996) argue that older people using health services have negative experiences and feel powerless. Patients believed they were deprived of information, dominated by the demands of the work timetable and unable to have any influence on their care. They had low expectations of care and were stoic and apologetic.

> *'The congested routine appeared to stretch nurses to their maximum capabilities and patients felt that they could not complain'. (Koch & Webb 1996: 955)*

They argue that routine geriatric style and segregation arise from the history and culture of the wards and resulted in care deprivation and depersonalization as the needs of patients were ignored. Older patients became objects of inflexible routines within healthcare practice. They suggest that there is a need for a review of routine geriatric care of older people and a social gerontology programme for nurse education.

Many health problems in the elderly are either caused or exacerbated by poverty. A good example of this is fuel poverty. Allamby (1987) looked at the consequences of fuel poverty for old people. He argues that other countries which have a similar climate to Britain (Canada, Norway and Sweden for example) do not have the same rates of death because the house building, energy and healthcare policies are taken seriously by these countries. Allamby suggests that the true extent of hypothermia is not known and is under-estimated as hypothermia is often not listed as cause of death. Thus, it is difficult to get accurate figures on this. In assembling a number of studies, he illustrates the links between temperature, rainfall and social circumstances and illness and death from ischaemic heart disease. Those with coronary diseases were especially at risk. There is a linear increase in certain heart conditions (cerebral and coronary thrombosis) as temperatures fall. In other countries, high seasonal mortality rates are not as pronounced because of socially oriented domestic energy policies. Allamby argues that the problem is not seriously addressed by government and that severe weather payments are inadequate to reduce deaths due to hypothermia. Rather carefully planned housing and consultation would offset nursing and medical expenses. In this country fuel poverty is just one example of the ways in which poverty disproportionately affects the elderly and shows how the needs of older people are overlooked.

REFLECTION POINT

We have seen that older people are often negatively stereotyped and experience discrimination. List the ways in which older people may experience ageism. In what ways may health services be ageist? In your experience, do health professionals hold negative stereotypes of older people? What actions do you think would help to overcome ageism in healthcare?

Discussion points

1. What changes in society do you think would help to address inequalities of health? How do you think these could be achieved?
2. What do you think that you as a nurse could do to help to address health disadvantage?

CHAPTER SUMMARY

There has been considerable debate and argument associated with research and policy on health inequalities. Much of the debate has centred on competing claims as to the most important explanation of health inequalities. A major consensus of opinion accepts that material deprivation is a more important cause of inequality. In spite of this, culture and lifestyle change remain a central focus of government policy. This is not merely an academic issue as policy to tackle inequalities is shaped by these debates. This is not a neutral matter either as political ideologies and political expediency have a powerful influence on the explanations favoured by policy-makers.

Recently, the social capital thesis has enjoyed a certain amount of favour and there has been considerable interest in psychosocial pathways to ill health. However, policy initiatives inspired by this research have largely been limited to the promotion of civic engagement and the message about reducing inequality is frequently unheeded. But the evidence suggests that it is impossible to address social cohesion and social capital without also addressing inequality. Reducing health inequalities therefore inevitably means reducing poverty (Lynch et al 2001). There has been action to reduce gender discrimination, racism and ageism but poverty remains the most pervasive problem for many women, ethnic minorities and the elderly. Further, there has been considerable interest in promoting lifestyle change in the poorer classes but little effective action to reduce material deprivation. According to Gwatkin (2000), tackling health inequalities will require:

> *'An impressive degree of political will, including a firm determination on the part of national and international leaders to stand up to the interests of the 'haves' in order to advance the cause of the 'have nots'. Such considerations argue for health professionals being prepared to enter the political forum on behalf of social and economic equity, rather than limiting themselves simply to work within the health sector'. (Gwatkin 2000: 5–6)*

In the meantime, health inequalities are evident, continue to persist and have increased.

FURTHER READING

Tudor Hart J 1971 The inverse care law. Lancet i: 405–412e

Wilkinson R, Marmot M 2003 Social determinants of health: The solid facts. World Health Organization, Copenhagen

Wilkinson R 2005 The impact of inequality: How to make sick societies healthier. New Press, New York

REFERENCES

Acheson D (Chair) 1998 Independent Inquiry into Inequalities in Health. The Stationery Office, London

Ahmad W, ed. 2000 Ethnicity, disability and chronic illness. Open University Press, Buckingham

Ahmad W, Jones L 1998 Ethnicity, health and healthcare in the UK. In: Peterson A, Waddell C (eds) Health matters. Allen and Unwin, London, p 114–127

Allamby L 1987 Dying of cold: fuel poverty and ill health in Northern Ireland. Northern Ireland Council for voluntary action, Belfast

Annandale E 2003 Gender differences in health. In: Taylor S, Field D (eds) Sociology of health and healthcare, 3rd edn. Blackwell, Oxford, p 81–97

Barker M, McLean S, McKenna P et al 1988 Diet, lifestyle and health in Northern Ireland: a report to the Health Promotion Trust. University of Ulster, Coleraine

Benzeval M, Judge K, Soloman A 1992 The health status of Londoners. Kings Fund Institute, London

Bhui K, ed. 2002 Racism and mental health: prejudice and suffering. Jessica Kingsley, London

Black Report 1980 Department of Health and Social Security (DHSS) 1980 Inequalities in health: report of the Research Working Group, chaired by Sir Douglas Black. DHSS, London.

Blackburn C 1992 Improving health and welfare work with families in poverty: A Handbook. Oxford University Press, Buckingham

Blackman T, Evason E, Melaugh M et al 1989 Housing and health: a case study of two housing areas in West Belfast. Journal of Social Policy 18:1–26

Blaxter M 1984 Equity and consultation rates in general practice. British Medical Journal 288:1963–1967

Blaxter M 1990 Health and lifestyles. Routledge, London

Brown G, Harris T 1978 The social origins of depression. Tavistock, London

Carstairs V, Morris R 1989 Deprivation: Explaining differences in mortality between Scotland and England and Wales. British Medical Journal 299:886–889

Cartwright A, O'Brien M 1976 Social class variations in healthcare and in the nature of general practitioner consultations. In: Stacey M (ed.) The sociology of the NHS. Sociological Review Monograph 22. University of Keele, Keele

Chadwick E [1842] 1965 Report on the sanitary conditions of the labouring population of Great Britain. (1st edn. 1842) Edinburgh University Press, Edinburgh

Cohen M 1994 Impact of poverty on women's health. Canadian Family Physician 40:949–958

Department of Health 1991 The health of the nation. HMSO, London

George M 1993 Glasgow Healthy City Project 1992 – Food, poverty and health. Conference proceedings. Nursing Standard 7(49):21–23

Gerrish K, Husband C, McKenzie J 1996 Nursing for a multi-ethnic society. Open University Press, Buckingham

Graham H 1993 Hardship and health in women's lives. Harvester Wheatsheaf, London

Gwatkin DR 2000 Health inequalities and the health of the poor: What do we know? What can we do? Bulletin of the World Health Organization 78(1)3–18

Ham C 1992 Health policy in Britain: The politics and organization of the National Health Service. Macmillan, Basingstoke

Harding S, Balajaran R 2001 Mortality of third generation Irish living in England and Wales: Longitudinal study. British Medical Journal 322:466–467

Hunt K, Annandale E 1993 Just the job? Is the relationship between health and domestic and paid work gender specific? Sociology of Health and Illness 15(5):632–664

Jimenez A, Alegria L, Pena M et al 1997 Mental health utilization in women with symptoms of depression. Women and Health 25:1–21

Johnson S, Buszewicz M 1996 Women's mental illness. In: Abel K, Buszewicz M, Davison S et al (eds) Planning community mental health services for women. A multiprofessional Handbook. Routledge, London, p 6–19

Karlson S, Nazroo J 2002 Agency and structure. The impact of ethnic identity and racism on the health of ethnic minority people. Sociology of Health and Illness 24(1):1–20

Kawachi I, Kennedy B 1997 Socioeconomic determinants of health: Health and social cohesion:

why care about income inequality? British Medical Journal 314:1037–1040
Kawachi I, Kennedy B 2002 The health of nations: why inequality is harmful to your health. New Press, New York
Kelleher D, Hillier S 1996 Researching cultural differences in health. Routledge, London
Kelleher D, Leavey G 2004 Identity and health. Routledge, London
Klinenberg E 2002 Heat wave: The social autopsy of disaster in Chicago. University of Chicago Press, Chicago
Koch T, Webb C 1996 The biomedical construction of ageing: implications for nursing care of older people. Journal of Advanced Nursing 23:954–959
Kogevinas E 1990 England and Wales: Longitudinal study – sociodemographic differences in cancer survival 1971–1983. HMSO, London
London Health Observatory 2005 Indications of public health in the English regions 4. Ethnicity and Health: Key findings from the London Region. London Health Observatory, London
Lowry S 1990 Getting things done. British Medical Journal 300:390–392
Lynch J, Davy-Smith G, Hillimeier M et al 2001 Income inequality, the psychosocial environment and health: comparisons of wealthy nations. Lancet 358:194–200
McCarthy P, Byrne D, Harrison S et al 1985 Respiratory conditions: effects of housing and other factors. Journal of Epidemiology and Community Health 39:15–19
Macintyre S, MacIver S, Sooman A 1993 Area, class and health: should we be focusing on places or people? Journal of Social Policy 22(2):213–234
Macintyre S, Hunt K, Smeeding H 1996 Gender differences in health: are things as simple as they seem? Social Science and Medicine 42 (4):617–624.
McKeown T 1979 The role of medicine. Blackwell, Oxford
Marmot M, Shipley M, Rose G 1984 Inequalities in death: Specific explanations of a general pattern. The Lancet 1:1003–1006
Marmot M, McDowall M 1986 Mortality decline and widening social inequalities. Lancet ii:274–276
Marmot M, Bosma H, Hemingway H 1997 Contribution of job control and other risk factors to social variations in coronary heart disease. Lancet 350:235–240
Marmot M, Wilkinson R 2001 Psychosocial and material pathways in the relation between income and health. British Medical Journal 322:1233–1236
Marmot M 2003 Understanding social inequalities in health. Perspectives in Biology and Medicine 46(3): S9–S23
Marmot M 2004 Status syndrome. Bloomsbury, London
Marmot M 2005 Social determinants of health inequalities. The Lancet 365:1099–1104
Navarro V 2004 Inequalities are unhealthy. Monthly Review 56:2
Nazroo J 1997 The health of Britain's ethnic minorities. Policy Studies Institute, London
Nazroo J 1998 Genetic, cultural or socioeconomic vulnerability? Explaining ethnic inequalities in health. Sociology of Health and Illness 20(5):710–730
Nazroo J 2003 The structuring of ethnic inequalities in health: economic position. Racial discrimination and racism. American Journal of Public Health 93 (2):277–284
Nazroo J 2004 Ethnic disparities in ageing health: what can we learn from the United Kingdom? In: Anderson N, Bulatao R, Cohen B (eds) Critical perspectives on racial and ethnic differentials in health and later life. National Academies Press, Washington, DC, p 677–702
Neave J 1994 Older people. In: Gough P, Maslin-Prothero S, Masterson A (eds) Nursing and social policy: Care in context. Butterworth-Heinemann, London, p 193–212
Pappas G, Queen S, Hadden W et al 1993 The increasing disparity in mortality between socio-economic groups in the United States – 1960–1986. New England Medical Journal 329:103–108
Payne S 1991 Women's health and poverty: and introduction. Harvester Wheatsheaf, Hemel Hempstead
Phillimore P 1989 Shortened lives: premature deaths in North Tyneside. Bristol papers in Applied Social Studies 12, University of Bristol, Bristol
Phillimore P, Beattie A, Townsend P 1994 Widening inequality of health in Northern England 1981–1991. British Medical Journal 308:1125–1128
Potts, M K, Burnam M, Wells K 1991 Gender differences in depression detection: a comparison of clinician diagnosis and standardised assessment. Psychological Assessment 3:609–615 Cited in Ramsay et al 2001 Needs of women patients with mental illness. Advances in Psychiatric Treatment 2001 7:85–92
Power C 1994 Health and social inequality in Europe. British Medical Journal 308:1153–1156
Putnam R 2000 Bowling Alone: The Collapse and Revival of American Community. Simon and Schuster, New York
Ragan A, Bowen A 2001 Improving attitudes regarding the elderly population: The effects of information and reinforcement for change. The Gerontologist 41:511–515

Rona R, Swan J, Altman D 1978 Social factors and height of primary school children in England and Scotland. Journal of Epidemiology and Community Health 32:147–154

Ryan S 1998 Disadvantaged groups in healthcare. In: Birchenall M, Birchenhall P (eds) Sociology as applied to nursing and healthcare. Baillière Tindall, London, p 110–129

Shaw M, Dorling D, Gordon D et al 2000 The widening gap: health inequalities and policy in Britain. Policy, Bristol

Shaw M 2005 Labour's 'Black Report' moment? British Medical Journal 331:575

Smaje C 1995 Health 'Race' and Ethnicity: making sense of the evidence. King's Fund, London

Smith D 1989 Britain's growing divide: North and South. Penguin, London

Thames Cancer Registry 1994 Cancer in South England 1991: cancer incidence, prevalence and survival in residents of the district health Authorities in South East England. Thames Cancer Registrar

Townsend P 1979 Poverty in the United Kingdom. Penguin, London

Townsend P, Davidson N, Whitehead M 1992 Inequalities of health: the Black Report and the Health Divide. Penguin, Harmondsworth

Tudor Hart J 1971 The inverse care law. Lancet i: 405–412

Tudor Hart J 2006 The political economy of healthcare: A clinical perspective. Policy, Bristol

Whitehead M 1987 The health divide: inequalities in health in the 1980s. Health Education Council, London

Whitehead M 2000 William Farr's legacy to the study of inequalities in health. WHO Bulletin 78(1): 86–96

Wilkinson R 1992 Income distribution and life expectancy. British Medical Journal 304(6820): 65–68

Wilkinson R 1994 Unfair shares: the effects of widening income differentials on the welfare of the young: A report for Barnardo's. University of Sussex, Brighton

Wilkinson R, Marmot M 2003 Social determinants of health: The solid facts. World Health Organization, Copenhagen

Wilkinson R 2005 The impact of inequality: How to make sick societies healthier. New Press, New York

Wilkinson R, Pickett K 2006 Income inequality and population health: A review and explanation of the evidence. Social Science and Medicine 62(7): 1768–1784

Yuen P, Machin D, Balarajan R 1990 Inequalities in health: socioeconomic differences in self reported morbidity. Public Health 104:65–71

PART

2

Healthcare systems and nursing

CHAPTER

7

Healthcare policy and organizational change

Gillian Olumide and Hannah Cooke

KEY CONCEPTS

- Political beliefs and welfare
- The development of the welfare state
- The development of the NHS
- Contemporary issues in UK healthcare

Introduction

This chapter will put present-day healthcare into context by looking at the changing nature of UK approaches to healthcare. Social policy has reflected changing political and economic circumstances and the prevailing political debates of the time. We have discussed the theme of inequality in previous chapters and have noted that some groups in society are disadvantaged and lacking in power and influence. These inequalities of power and resources have also shaped the policy process with more powerful groups often more able to get their voices heard and to shape the direction of policy.

Nurses care for some of the most vulnerable members of society so nurses' work is profoundly affected by social policies over which nurses often have very little influence. Nurses also need to understand the policy context in which they work in order to understand how nursing is being shaped and directed. Only through greater understanding of the policy process can nurses begin to have a voice in the future direction of nursing.

In this chapter, we will first consider key concepts in welfare then we look at different political belief systems and what they say about welfare. We then consider the development of the welfare state before considering the origins and development of the National Health Service.

Key concepts in the provision of welfare

EQUALITY

Equality can take many forms. A concern with legal and political equality has involved issues such as voting rights. We are concerned here with social equality which relates to the distribution of social goods such as education and health services.

Political beliefs about equality vary. *Egalitarianism* involves a commitment to equality in its purest form and underlies some religious and political ideologies such as socialism. Egalitarianism involves some attempt to achieve equality of *outcome* – for example in life expectancy or health status. Egalitarianism appeals to ideas of brotherhood, sisterhood and social solidarity (Blakemore 2003). Social policy theorists who have advocated egalitarianism include R H Tawney (1931) and T H Marshall (1963). These theorists believed that a commitment to egalitarianism would create a society in which everyone felt valued and that this would reduce social problems such as crime and mental illness. Authors such as Marshall saw the unfettered free market as socially destructive (Barry 1990). According to Marshall:

> *'What matters is that there is a general enrichment of the concrete substance of a civilized life, a general reduction of risk and insecurity, an equalization between the more and less fortunate at all levels'.*
> *T H Marshall (1963: 107)*

Criticisms of egalitarianism tend to focus on *differences* between people arguing that egalitarianism is either unachievable or undesirable. Critics believe that egalitarianism creates unwanted uniformity. Critics of egalitarianism thus offer market ideas such as choice as an alternative value (Barry 1990). Whilst there may be general consensus that complete equality of outcome is unachievable, ideological differences centre on the question of whether it remains a desirable goal; should we try to reduce inequalities in society or accept that in a competitive society there are winners and losers?

A second version of equality is the idea of equity. This idea modifies the idea of equality in ways that are intended to take account of the differences between people. Thus, instead of equality of outcome we have ideas of *fairness* and *justice* (Blakemore 2003). Equitable policies tend to favour improving access and delivering targeted rather than universal services based on individual needs and circumstances. This does however, depend heavily on having a fair and accurate assessment of needs and this is where policies based on equity often have difficulties since concepts of need are often disputed.

Proponents of market approaches to welfare tend to favour *equality of opportunity* rather than equality of outcome. This involves removing barriers to access so that everyone has the same chance at the outset; the idea of fair competition. This has frequently involved a legislative framework establishing formal equality such as the Disability Discrimination Acts of 1995 and 2005 discussed in Chapter 14. Political differences tend to centre on whether establishing formal equality of opportunity is enough on its own. Arguments depend on whether a 'level playing field' really exists and thus on the extent to which structured inequalities limit individual's life chances as we saw in Chapters 5 and 6. Critics argue that positive action is also needed, for example, tackling prejudice and unfair practices and helping disadvantaged groups to access services (Lister 2001).

HUMAN NEEDS

We said in our discussion of equity that some notion of need often underpins ideas about the equitable distribution of resources. We also noted that conflicts can arise about the assessment of human need. Of particular interest to healthcare professionals is the distinction between *needs, wants* and *desires.* Take for example the provision of fertility treatment – is having a child something that we should consider as a *need* or as a *desire*?

There are a number of different theories of human need. The one most familiar to nurses is the psychologist Maslow's (1943) hierarchy of need. His hierarchy is a theory of human motivation. He believed that needs were arranged in a hierarchy with physiological and safety needs at the base and 'self actualization' at the pinnacle. He argued that lower needs had to be satisfied for higher ones to become motivators. Maslow's theory has many critics. Arguments have centred on the limited evidence base for his theory. It has also been criticized for basing ideas about human nature on US society and culture.

A more recent theory of particular relevance to welfare policy has been Doyal and Gough's (1991) *theory of universal human needs.* Doyal and Gough criticize the idea of a hierarchy of needs and say that there are two basic and universal needs – *health* and *autonomy*. Following on from this premise, they say that it is relatively easy to establish a list of universal human needs on the basis that any society will need to provide these in order to provide for these two basic needs. Their list is as follows:

- Nutritious food and clean water
- Protective housing
- A non-hazardous work environment
- A non-hazardous physical environment
- Appropriate healthcare
- Security in childhood
- Significant primary relationships
- Physical security
- Economic security
- Appropriate education
- Safe birth control and child bearing.

Doyal and Gough say that their list is based on research evidence and that governments should be judged on how well they provide for the needs of their people. They suggest that being deprived of any of the needs that they describe will lead to measurable harm. Their theory has led to comparative research to judge how well different countries provide for the needs of their citizens and their work has been influential in the study of health inequalities.

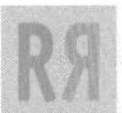

REFLECTION POINT

We have discussed different authors' beliefs about human needs. Make your own list of those things that you believe are fundamental human needs.

HUMAN RIGHTS

Another important set of values which have influenced health policy are values concerned with human *freedom* and human *rights*. T H Marshall made a classic distinction between *civil, political* and *social* rights. Marshall believed (based on the history of the UK) that as society developed these rights should develop (Marshall 1950).

- *Civil rights* – rights under the law such as freedom from arbitrary arrest, right to a fair trial, freedom of speech, freedom to join groups such as trade unions
- *Political rights* – right to vote and to join political parties, right to political representation
- *Social rights* – rights to welfare and health such as a right to receive healthcare, a right to have access to clean water.

Debates about rights have involved arguments about specific groups whose access to rights has been unequal, for example women, ethnic minorities and people with disabilities. More recently, the 'animal rights' movement has tried to extend the notion of rights to include the animal kingdom. Political differences have centred on the relative importance of civil, political and social rights with the existence of social rights being the most contentious issue. Since social rights have been eroded by neo-liberalism Marshall's theories have been challenged by some theorists while others believe that they are still worth defending (Bulmer & Rees 1996).

A related concept is that of *citizenship*. Citizenship involves membership of a society which confers both *rights* and *responsibilities*. The definition of citizenship can both *include* and *exclude* people. Debates about *citizenship* have often concerned groups that have been *excluded* or denied some of their rights such as women, people with disabilities and migrant labourers (Lister 1997).

There has also been concern over the nature of the *rights* that citizens should enjoy. The strong version (associated with social democracy) says that citizens should have social rights such as healthcare and relief from poverty. The weak version confines *citizenship* rights to *civil* and *political* rights.

The first clear statement of human rights by an international body was the United Nations' Universal Declaration of Human Rights in 1948. This was closely followed in the European Convention on Human Rights, which was enshrined in British legislation in 1998.

REFLECTION POINT

We have discussed different ideas about human rights. Make your own list of what you consider should be fundamental human rights.

Political ideologies influencing welfare

Policies that attempt to meet the health and welfare needs of the population depend on underlying political beliefs. It is important to be able to distinguish between some of these beliefs as the policy that flows from them sets out to achieve different social outcomes. The following sections present key political approaches to welfare which have been influential during the history of the welfare state. Differences in political positions tend to reflect alternative views about how society should be managed and the needs of the people catered for. Beliefs about values such as equality and human rights and about how and why these will be achieved vary considerably between political positions. There are other important differences such as philosophies concerning the role and size of the state and the extent of its responsibilities. Even state provision of free nursing services is a point of political debate.

SOCIAL DEMOCRACY

The thinking behind the welfare legislation of the 1940s was broadly social democratic. Social democracy in the UK was influenced by Fabian socialism which argued that social justice could be achieved by an enlarged (welfare) state for the benefit of all citizens rather than through the revolutionary changes advocated by many Marxists. Another philosophical contribution to the origins of the welfare state was ethical socialism, which had Christian roots and provided a critique of the social inequality produced by industrial capitalism. Thinkers, such as Tawney (1931) saw the exploitation of labour as an indignity that needed to be addressed to achieve a more equal and just society.

The idea that the state should be involved in protecting and providing for the welfare of its citizens is sometimes called a *collectivist* approach, indicating that the welfare of all is the responsibility of all. Collectivists tended to argue for the reduction of inequalities through the redistribution of resources (see Chapters 5 and 6). The welfare state, funded from taxes, was one important means of achieving this aim. Higher earners are expected to pay more in taxes and make a greater contribution to welfare services than those with lower incomes.

CONSERVATISM

Conservatism stems from Edmund Burke's 'two principles of conservation and correction'. ([1790] 1968). In this thinking, society should preserve the traditions of the past whilst improving the life of the nation. According to Fitzpatrick (2005), Conservatism focuses on the fragility of social order seeing human society as a 'rudderless ship on a harbourless ocean'. The most important question for government then becomes how to avoid 'rocking the boat'. Conservatism therefore values the lessons of experience and advocates incremental rather than radical change. Thus it has tended to support the status quo and as a result has often been seen as associated with the defence of privilege and the perpetuation of social inequality.

However, Conservatism has adapted to social changes such as the Industrial Revolution and the creation of the welfare state and is not without a reforming element. Disraeli (Conservative prime minister during the 1860s and

1870s) was a notable social reformer who formulated 'one-nation conservatism' which was committed to national unity and the building of social consensus.

Collectivist views had gained support during the early twentieth century but the Conservative Party opposed many of the Beveridge proposals for welfare reform, leading to its defeat in the 1945 election. Subsequently, the Conservative Prime Minister, Harold Macmillan, showed during the 1950s, that a Conservative government could adapt to the existence of the welfare state. Health and housing services in particular were improved and extended under conservatism. This was a revival of 'one nation conservatism' which held to a vision of a society which, while not aspiring to equality, acknowledged the inter-connectedness of all citizens. The Conservative leader, David Cameron, has recently tried to re-invent some of the ideas of 'one nation conservatism'.

NEO-LIBERALISM

In 1976, when Margaret Thatcher became Conservative party leader, anti-collectivist opinions within conservatism came to the fore and the party turned its back on 'one nation conservatism'. Traditional conservatism was challenged by neo-liberal (or 'new Right') ideas. Briefly, these ideas concerned a determination to 'roll back the state', reduce the burden of taxation and promote 'freedom' and 'efficiency' through the introduction of market forces into public services. Economic liberalism was, however, accompanied by a commitment to social conservatism with a stated aim to restore 'Victorian values' of individualism and self help and to strengthen 'family values' (Clarke & Newman 1997).

We discussed the idea of the market in Chapter 4. The 'new Right' believe in the ability of free markets to organize choices about welfare far more effectively than the state. The political instincts of the 'new Right' have been to decrease state intervention in private matters in order to avoid a 'nanny state', which they suggest limits freedom and creates dependency. Thus in Hayek's (1944) famous words the welfare state is regarded as the 'road to serfdom'. Neo-liberal governments have tended to reduce taxes, limit public spending and introduce charges for welfare services. They have emphasized the use of market mechanisms in the provision of public services arguing that these promote freedom of choice. They have promoted a 'mixed economy' of welfare services in which state services compete with charitable and private providers. They argue that 'managed competition' encourages providers of services to become more efficient in order to compete for business.

THE 'THIRD WAY'

Social democracy envisaged a welfare state as achieving greater equality through state sponsored collectivist policies. By contrast the 'Third Way' initiated by Clinton's New Democrats in 1992 and promoted by the 'New Labour' administration has dwelt more on removing barriers to individual achievement (equal opportunities) than on achieving equality of outcomes or a more even distribution of resources. Giddens (1998) suggested a new approach to welfare, which enabled people to make their own estimations of need rather than having these defined by the state. The 'Third Way' marked a drift away from a concern with social inequalities. Instead, the 'Third Way' has been preoccupied with 'social exclusion', a term much used by *New* Labour which tends to refer to a lack of ability or willingness to participate in the labour market (Lister 1998). The emphasis has thus moved away from equality of rights towards an equality of obligations (Fitzpatrick 2005) with an attempt to extend the obligation to participate in the labour market to, for example, single parents and people with disabilities.

Powell (2000) points to the fact that terms, such as 'welfare' are being given new meanings under *New* Labour's administration. The older understanding of welfare as a safety net for all citizens is transformed into a situation where citizens may expect 'a hand up not a hand out'. Echoing many of the ideas of the neo-liberals, education, good health, the acquisition of skills and hard work are seen as the main routes away from poverty and exclusion.

'Third Way' politicians have embraced the use of market mechanisms in the provision of welfare services. There is, however, more emphasis on state regulation of managed markets than under neo-liberal Conservative governments (Cutler & Waine 2000). For example, new Labour's 'modernization' of the NHS has emphasized on the one hand competition and choice but on the other hand, has introduced a highly centralized framework of regulation and performance targets. Although there has been disagreement as to where the balance lies, many critics have argued that the 'Third Way' lies closer to neo-liberal approaches than to social democracy (Baggott 2004).

The creation of the welfare state

Before considering the creation of the welfare state after the Second World War, we outline the provision of welfare prior to this period. According to Blakemore (2003) there are some enduring themes in welfare provision. Furthermore, historical approaches to welfare, such as the 'poor laws' and the workhouse have had a lasting impact on cultural attitudes to welfare. Laws to help the poor in Britain dated back to the Tudor period, as we noted in Chapter 6. However, the 1834 Poor Law Reform Act marked a radical break with the past. The Act associated 'pauperism' with shame and stigma and introduced the principle of 'less eligibility', which decreed that welfare conditions should be worse than the worst paid job available in the labour market. This led to the creation of the 'workhouse test' in which 'paupers' were expected to forego their liberty and civil rights and enter an institution if they wished to receive relief. This system of 'indoor relief' set up the conditions for widespread institutionalization of problem populations during the nineteenth century as we discussed in Chapter 4.

The legacy of the Poor Law remained until the start of the Second World War, although poor law institutions had been handed over to local authority control during the 1920s. Arguably, the cultural legacy of the poor law remains today with poverty and welfare dependency still attracting shame and stigma even when associated with unavoidable causes such as disability and chronic illness.

In the UK, Lord Beveridge and a small committee provided, in 1942, the blueprint for a comprehensive system of welfare organized by the state and paid for through taxation. Beveridge's original brief was to regularize the patchy social insurance system that had grown up to provide limited welfare benefits to some sections of the population. The Committee however delivered a much bolder plan which alarmed the serving Conservative administration because of its cost implication. The proposal included welfare services for all citizens and a national health service which served the entire population and which was free at the point of delivery. This plan for state sponsored welfare was taken up by the post war Labour Government and implemented in 1948.

Areas envisaged in this post-war settlement as being in need of attention, referred to by Beveridge as the five giant social evils (Timmins 2001), were ignorance, want, idleness, disease, squalor. In response, education, employment, income maintenance, housing and health became the concern of the state at local and national levels. These are also now routinely acknowledged to be amongst the key social determinants of health.

> *'The plan for social security is put forward as part of a general programme of social policy. It is only part of an attack upon the 5 giant evils: upon physical want, with which it is directly concerned; upon disease which often causes that want and brings many other troubles in its train; upon ignorance which no democracy can afford amongst its citizens; upon squalor which arises mainly through the haphazard*

distribution of industry and population; and upon idleness which destroys wealth and corrupts men, whether they are well fed or not, when they are idle'. (From the Beveridge Report 1942)

The development of the national health service

HEALTHCARE BEFORE THE NHS

Prior to the development of the NHS, healthcare was provided by a mixture of institutions. Self-governing 'voluntary hospitals' often founded by charitable subscription existed alongside municipal hospitals run by local authorities. Many of the latter were remnants of the old workhouse system although some enlightened local authorities had developed new hospital services. A social insurance system founded in 1911 gave workers access to GP services but their families were not covered by this system. Free care was not universally available and cost was a barrier to treatment for many people. In the inter-war years, there was increasing concern about the chaotic nature of UK health services as UK health indicators began to lag behind other countries (Webster 2002). There was a recruitment crisis in nursing due to poor conditions, low pay and long hours. An influential survey in 1939 found that there was a 'chaotic jumble' of services with no overall standards, too many services in some places and huge gaps in others (Herbert 1939).

THE CREATION OF THE NHS

At the outbreak of the Second World War, there was enormous concern about the ability of Britain's disorganized healthcare system to cope with wartime casualties. The Emergency Medical Service was set up by the government to coordinate and plan wartime healthcare. The experience of war led not only to the promise of new social welfare services offering a better future after the war as outlined in the Beveridge report. It also led to an appreciation of the benefits of better coordination and planning of healthcare services at both a regional and national level.

The 1946 general election brought a Labour government to power with a mandate to implement the Beveridge report. The new health minister Aneurin Bevan had a clear vision for the National Health Service. He believed that all citizens should have a right to free healthcare. He rejected the idea of local councils running the health service. He believed that only central government control and regional coordination would overcome the unacceptable variations in care that existed in the pre-war period (Willcocks 1967). Bevan held extensive negotiations with the medical profession over the new service but it seems to have been assumed that nurses would simply have to accommodate themselves to whatever arrangements were agreed (Dingwall et al 1988).

1946 NHS ACT

The passing of the National Insurance Act in 1946 created the structure of the welfare state and state benefits. The government also announced plans for a National Health Service that would be, 'free to all who want to use it'. The NHS Act 1946 made this a reality. The principles had been stated in 1944 (Box 7.1).

In July 1948, the NHS was founded. The Act provided free diagnosis and treatment of illness, at home or in hospital, as well as dental and ophthalmic services (Box 7.2).

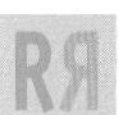

REFLECTION POINT

We have discussed the ideas and principles that underpinned the creation of the NHS. The aims of the NHS are listed under the heading 'Objects in view', Box 7.1 above. Do you think that these are appropriate aims for the NHS today? If not how would you change them? To what extent do you think that the NHS has achieved the aims set out in 1944?

Box 7–1 Objects in view (Ministry of Health 1944)

1. To ensure that everyone in the country – irrespective of means, age, sex or occupation – shall have equal opportunity to benefit from the best and most up-to-date medical and allied services available.
2. To provide, therefore, for all who want it, a comprehensive service covering every branch of medical and allied activity from the care of minor ailments to major medicine and surgery; to include the care of mental as well as physical health and all specialist services, e.g. for tuberculosis, cancer and infectious diseases, maternity, fracture and orthopaedic treatment, and others; to include all normal general services, e.g. the family doctor, the midwife and nurse, the care of the teeth and of the eyes, the day-to-day care of the child; and to include all necessary drugs and medicines and a wide range of appliances.
3. To divorce the care of health from questions of personal means or other factors irrelevant to it; to provide the service free of charge (apart from certain possible charges in respect of appliances) and to encourage a new attitude to health – the easier obtaining of advice early; the promotion of good health rather than the treatment of bad.

Box 7–2 Key principles of the 1948 NHS

- The service was comprehensive (everyone was eligible for care) and funded out of central taxation
- The service was free to all at the point of use
- It was a genuinely national service so anybody could be referred to any hospital regardless of where they lived
- Coordination was through 14 regional hospital boards who oversaw local hospital management committees. Wartime experiences had convinced the government of the need for a regional tier of the service
- The service had a 'tripartite' structure with GP services, hospital services and community services all organized separately – this would prove to be the main drawback of the new service as it made coordination between the three 'arms' of the service difficult.

In the next section, we review the development of the NHS from the 1940s to the 1990s, highlighting some key milestones in its history.

The development of the NHS 1948–1997

THE GUILLEBAUD REPORT

Concerns about the cost of the NHS surfaced early in its history, even Aneurin Bevan worried that there would be 'cascades of medicine' pouring down British throats (Foot 1997). In the 1950s, the new Conservative government cast doubt on the rising cost of the NHS. It instituted the Guillebaud report (Ministry of Health 1956) to look at NHS finance. It found that NHS spending as a proportion of GDP had declined and that the service was, if anything under funded. During the 1950s the first NHS charges were introduced – a prescription charge of 1 shilling was introduced in 1952 and a flat rate dental charge of £1. The cost of the service as a proportion of GDP remained stable until 1973. Attempts to develop the service were made throughout the 1950s and 1960s.

THE 1962 HOSPITAL PLAN

In 1962, the health minister Enoch Powell instituted a hospital building programme under the Hospital Plan. This envisaged the creation of a district general hospital in every district that would provide a comprehensive range of services to a population of approximately 125 000. At the same time, Powell began the closure of long-stay mental hospitals, instituting the policy of care in the community. A number of attempts to improve the administration of the service took place in the 1960s. For example, the Salmon report (Ministry of Health 1966) modernized the nursing management structure replacing matrons with 'nursing officers'. It was heavily criticized at the time for distancing nurse managers from clinical care (Bellaby & Oribabor 1980).

THE 1974 REORGANIZATION

Administrative reform of the NHS had been on the agenda of the 1964–70 Labour government and Green Papers were issued in 1968 and 1970 suggesting unification of the three 'arms' of the service, improved coordination between health services and local government social services and a clearer management structure. However, after Labour lost the election of 1970 the new Conservative Secretary of State, Sir Keith Joseph, employed an American firm of management consultants, McKinsey & Co, to reorganize the NHS leading to a much higher profile for managerialism within the 1974 reorganization (DHSS 1972). An extra 'area' tier of management was added with 'consensus teams' of managers working at every level. As a concession to democratic accountability, Community Health Councils were introduced as a watchdog body to represent patient and public interests in each health district.

There was a detailed blueprint for the reorganized NHS laid down in the 'Grey book'. Disillusionment with the 1974 reorganization was rapid (Strong & Robinson 1990). Ironically, for a reform designed to introduce a sound financial structure to the NHS it was followed by a sharp rise in NHS expenditure as a proportion of Gross Domestic Product (GDP). The DHSS acknowledged to the Public Accounts Committee that the cost of reorganization had been unexpectedly high creating 16 400 new administrative posts. Nurse managers consolidated their position under the 1974 reorganization gaining a place in the newly created consensus management teams at each level in the new structure.

However, the unwieldy new structure led to persistent calls for reform. In 1979, the 'Patients First' reform simplified the organizational structure The 1970s was characterized by economic crises over oil prices and the development of the service started by the 1960s hospital plan ground to an abrupt halt. Cuts and hospital closures began in the late 1970s and accelerated through the 1980s with approximately half the inpatient capacity of the service being closed over a 20-year period (Pollock 2004) leading among other things to a steady increase in nurses' workloads. Cost pressures led to increased desire to strengthen the NHS management function with increased emphasis on financial management (Webster 2002).

GRIFFITHS REPORT 1983

Under the administration of Margaret Thatcher, an inquiry under the leadership of Sir Roy Griffiths (then managing director and deputy chairperson of Sainsbury's) reported in 1983, on management within the NHS. The Griffiths NHS Management Inquiry took little formal evidence, involved only four people and resulted in a report only 25 pages long. Its lack of consultation became the hallmark of NHS decision-making in the Thatcher era. Griffiths had a simple central message which was that 'if Florence Nightingale were carrying her lamp through the corridors of the NHS' she would be 'searching for the people in charge' (Griffiths Report 1983: 12).

Perhaps the most striking aspect of the recommended changes was the introduction of business methods into the NHS. The new system of 'general management' was intended to establish clear lines of responsibility and accountability for the running of the health service. Planning, budgeting and evaluation of services were all supposed to improve under the leadership of general management.

Florence Nightingale was the only nurse mentioned by Griffiths in his report. Doctors were to be involved in management in order to hold them responsible for their expenditure but overnight nurses had lost their managerial authority (Dingwall et al 1988). After Griffiths, the bulk of nurses would be managed by general managers. The number of senior managers in the NHS would increase from 1000 to 26 000 and management costs would more than double (Pollock 2004). According to Harrison and Wood (1999) the Griffiths Report marked a break with the detailed planning of NHS reform. The 1974 reorganization was the last time there would be a fully worked out blueprint for reorganization. From Griffiths onwards, reforms would be set in motion by simple policy ideas easily conveyed in sound-bites but short on detail. It would be left to managers on the ground to work out the detail in a process that Harrison and Wood describe as 'manipulated emergence'. This would considerably increase the role of managers and multiply their numbers.

1989 WORKING FOR PATIENTS

Cultural change had been taking place in the NHS with a growth of managerialism from the 1960s onwards. The Griffiths reforms accelerated this process but the biggest change followed the introduction of the 'internal market' in 1989. The 1989 White Paper, Working for Patients, proposed the introduction of a 'managed market'. Described as the 'Americanization' of the NHS (Walker 1999), this would embed the principles of private enterprise in the NHS and further strengthen the powers of managers. The introduction of a form of 'managed care' in the NHS was based on the ideas of former US nuclear war strategist, Alain Enthoven (1985), who was asked by Margaret Thatcher to advise on the reorganization of the NHS (Box 7.3).

Box 7–3 Managed care

Managed care was introduced in the USA in the 1970s to reduce the costs of healthcare. Most healthcare in the USA is provided privately and paid for by private insurance companies. Under traditional 'fee for service' models, hospitals were reimbursed the costs of the actual care given. Managed care replaces this with a flat rate of payment per patient which gives healthcare providers an incentive to reduce the costs of care. The most common model under managed care is for patients to enrol in a 'Health Maintenance Organization' (HMO). HMOs are given a prepaid fee to cover the cost of care for enrolled members. Any specialist care has to be agreed in advance by a primary care physician working for the HMO. There is therefore an incentive for the HMO to reduce the use of hospital care and HMOs were believed to have the advantage of increasing efficiency, reducing costs and encouraging primary and preventive care (Baggott 2004). 'Care pathways' were introduced to manage patient's journeys through the healthcare hospital efficiently especially in order to keep down length of hospital stay.

Hospitals are reimbursed at a standard rate for a particular type of diagnosis; patient care is organized by 'diagnosis related groups' (DRGs) and standardized protocols of practice are increasingly applied to DRGs. It was felt that managed care would put more pressure on health professionals to provide cost-effective care and managed care has been associated with a growth in performance management systems such as benchmarking and clinical audit (Fairfield et al 1997). However, a drawback of this system is that it may discourage hospitals from dealing with more complex cases.

Managed care has been advocated as offering higher quality care for patients at reduced cost. Managed care does result in shorter hospital stays, lower hospital admission rates and fewer hospital tests and procedures but there is no conclusive evidence of improved outcomes. There is some evidence of lower patient satisfaction (Miller & Luft 1994). Healthcare costs in the USA have continued to increase in the managed care era and managed care appears to be associated with high administrative costs (estimated as at least 25% of US health spending).

Concerns about managed care have centred on the provision of care to vulnerable groups such as the elderly, chronically sick, disabled and mentally ill. There has been some evidence of HMOs refusing to enrol patients from vulnerable groups due to the high costs of their care and access to care seems to be poorer for disadvantaged groups. There is also evidence that disadvantaged groups receive worse care from secondary services and thus managed care appears to increase inequities in healthcare provision (Sullivan 2000).

Managed care has been said to reduce clinical freedom since doctors must increasingly practice according to protocols and be subject to managerial scrutiny. It has thus been described as 'fish-bowl medicine' (Le Grand 1998). It is also said to have the potential to undermine trust between patients and physician (Mechanic 1996) since doctors have financial incentives to practice cost effectively and this may include limiting or refusing care to patients. Thus, many health professionals have perceived managed care very negatively as the poem below describes ...

I used to be a doctor
Now I am a Healthcare Provider
I used to practice medicine
Now I function under a managed care system
I used to have patients
Now I have a consumer list
I used to diagnose
Now I am approved for one consultation
I used to treat
Now I wait for an authorization to
  provide care
I used to have a successful people practice
Now I have a paper failure
I used to spend time listening to my patients
Now I spend time justifying myself to the
  authorities
I used to have feelings
Now I have an attitude
Now I don't know what I am

(Quoted in Fairfield et al 1997: 1895)

Working for Patients introduced a form of managed care by introducing an 'internal market'. Hospitals and community services were to be run by self-governing Trusts organized along corporate lines with a board comprised of executive and non-executive directors. Nurses would have a place on the Trust board but would not necessarily manage the nurses in the Trust. Health authorities would purchase services from Trusts under contracts and would be free to purchase services from other providers such as the private and voluntary sector, thus the intention was to stimulate a 'mixed economy' in healthcare (Levitt et al 1995). GPs would be able to apply for their own budget and as 'fundholders' would be able to purchase a range of services for their patients based partly on the HMO model.

The NHS 'internal' market was supposed to produce cost savings for the NHS by encouraging purchasers to seek out the cheapest forms of healthcare provision (Webster 2002). Breaking up the service into separate Trusts was also intended to produce greater financial flexibility by allowing for local decision-making and in particular local pay bargaining. Ostensibly, these decisions were now left to the responsibility of local Trust boards and purchasing authorities whilst discipline was maintained through the workings of the market. However, from the outset the government retained a firm grip on the internal market. Concerns about negative publicity led to a strong emphasis on the need for stability and a 'smooth take off' of the reforms (Timmins 2001).

Following the example of managed care in the USA, quality assessment became an issue of rising importance within the new NHS contract culture. This spawned a variety of initiatives to measure standards of care. According to Rivett (1998) throughout the 1990s, hospitals had never been so efficient nor under such strain. Nurses began to complain both about increased workloads and also about the negative impact of market principles on nursing culture (Traynor 1999). Sweeping managerial changes were accompanied by continued downward pressure on resources.

REFLECTION POINT

We have seen that from the 1980s onwards, the NHS was increasingly organized along the principles of a 'managed market'. What are the advantages and disadvantages of a market approach to healthcare?

'NEW LABOUR' HEALTH POLICY

The first phase 1997–2000

The 1997 Labour Party manifesto stated that New Labour would 'save and modernize' the NHS. The government white paper 'The New NHS: Modern, Dependable' (DoH 1997) laid out the New Labour plans for reform of the NHS. In line with the rhetoric of the 'Third Way' they were not going to return to the 'Old Labour' NHS but were going to 'modernize' the NHS for the twenty-first century. In practice, this meant continuing the internal market introduced by the previous government but renaming the process 'commissioning'. New Labour introduced primary care-led commissioning, abolishing GP fundholders and phasing out health authorities. They were replaced with Primary Care Groups who would later be upgraded to the status of Primary Care Trusts. The incoming Labour government had committed themselves to the previous government's spending plans, so that pressures on resources continued. This led to negative media coverage of problems such as staff shortages and long waits in accident and emergency departments.

The second phase 2000–2002

The government responded in 2000 with The NHS Plan (DoH 2000). The Plan was subtitled 'A Plan for Investment. A Plan for Reform', and envisaged some expansion of NHS capacity including 20 000 extra nurses. In return, the government expected NHS staff to commit to its reforms. An extensive performance assessment system was introduced with Trusts expected to meet an elaborate range of centrally set targets. Most important were targets for waiting lists and waiting times. An initial 'traffic light' system was later replaced by a 'star rating' system. Poor performing Trusts were threatened with sanctions. In spite of these reforms, negative publicity about the cash-strapped NHS continued to threaten the government.

The third phase 2002–present

A series of three reports was commissioned by the UK Treasury and headed by former banker Derek Wanless. The first of these reports, 'Securing Our Future Health' (Wanless 2002), suggested that the UK was behind comparable health services on a range of indicators such as health outcomes and time spent waiting for treatments. Further, because the NHS had received too little investment, both short- and long-term investment would be required to catch up with the best of European health provision. As well as a need for increased funding, Wanless suggested that more reforms were needed in the way health services were used and made available with increased emphasis on primary care and prevention.

Following Wanless, there was a period of increased investment in the NHS to bring NHS spending nearer to the European average which it had lagged behind for many years. The government continued its commitment to reform and the pace of change has become 'increasingly frantic' (Greener 2004) since Wanless. In particular, there has been increased emphasis on consumerism and a more explicit use of market approaches to healthcare. Components of recent reforms include those listed in Box 7.4.

Box 7-4 Key components of NHS reform in England

Primary Care Trusts

Primary Care Trusts (PCTs) are responsible for planning and commissioning NHS care, and control 80% of the NHS budget. After two rounds of reorganization there are now 152 PCTs, each covering a population of around 300 000. PCTs are managed by executive directors and a board which includes representatives of primary care professionals and non-executive directors appointed by the NHS Appointments Commission.

Strategic health authorities

Founded in 2002, strategic health authorities have replaced the regional tier in previous NHS structures. They are responsible for the oversight of primary care and hospital trusts. They have an important role in strategic planning, particularly workforce and capacity planning. Originally there were 28 but reorganization has reduced their number to 10.

Foundation Trusts

Hospitals given Foundation Trust status have greater financial independence (including over staff pay). They can vary the range of clinical services they provide and are regulated by a body called 'Monitor'. They are managed by executive directors advised by a board elected by Trust members. Foundation Trust members can be drawn from service users and carers, local residents and staff but uptake has been extremely poor. In 2006, there were 40 Foundation Trusts but numbers were planned to increase.

Payment by results

Payment by results is a new funding system which requires PCTs to pay for itemized services according to a 'national tariff' set by the government which lays down a fixed cost for every treatment episode. Healthcare providers will be able to make a profit if they can provide actual care more cheaply than the tariff. They will lose money if their actual costs are higher than the tariff.

Patient choice

The new 'choose and book' service now allows patients a choice of hospital from a fixed menu when they are referred to hospital by their GP. This is intended to stimulate competition between providers and will include private providers.

Practice-based commissioning

Similar to the HMO system, General Practices can now manage their own 'indicative budget' from which they commission care for patients. They will be encouraged to reorganize services to make 'efficiency' savings. However, practices will not have complete freedom, as PCTs retain overall control of budgets. Practices who make savings from practice-based commissioning will get 70% of their savings but will have to spend them on priorities agreed with their PCT.

Continued

Box 7–4 Key components of NHS reform in England—cont'd

Patient and public involvement

The government abolished Community Health Councils in 2000. They have been replaced by a variety of bodies including Patient Advice and Liaison Services (PALs), Local Involvement Networks (LINKS) and local authority scrutiny committees. The Commission for Patient and Public Involvement in Health coordinates the system and advises the government on public involvement. Although the government has emphasized their commitment to patient involvement, the new bodies have fewer powers and the new system has been criticized as weak and fragmented (Baggott 2004).

Devolution

Since 1999, the NHS in Scotland, Wales and Northern Ireland has been organized separately from the NHS in England. The Scottish Parliament and the Welsh and Northern Ireland Assemblies have varying legislative powers, so have moved away from the English model to differing degrees (Talbot Smith & Pollock 2006). Scotland has moved furthest away from the English model by abolishing the internal market and returning to an integrated, directly managed service. Wales has retained the internal market but has not introduced Foundation Trusts and has made a much more limited use of the private sector than in England. Northern Ireland has diverged least since devolution and largely follows the English model.

The mixed economy of care

The creation of a managed market in the NHS has opened up opportunities for non-NHS organizations, such as the private and voluntary sectors to compete for business with NHS Trusts particularly in England. The government has encouraged a mixed economy of care and has become increasingly committed to the use of market mechanisms to improve efficiency in healthcare. England's convergence with the US system has been suggested by many commentators (Ham 2004). Key developments include the private provision of Walk in Centres and independent sector diagnostic and treatment centres. Independent sector treatment centres provide fast track access to routine surgery and concerns have been expressed about the negative financial consequences for NHS providers who are then left to provide for higher risk patients and the more complex and costly procedures.

The Private Finance Initiative (PFI) has involved the private sector in new NHS capital projects. Essentially, the private sector finance and carry out NHS building projects on the basis of a long lease, which the NHS will have to repay. Advocates have argued that this has allowed the government to build new hospitals while controlling public spending. Critics have pointed to the high overall cost of PFI projects arguing that PFI has mortgaged the future of the NHS (Pollock 2004). The commercial secrecy surrounding PFI has made it difficult to evaluate the value for money of PFI projects (Baggott 2004). Recent plans to involve the private sector in commissioning in England (such as franchising PCTs to private organizations) could, if carried out, make substantial inroads into the public nature of the NHS.

Performance management and regulation

Concerns about variations in care across an increasingly fragmented system of providers have led the government to commit heavily to a centralized system of regulation and performance measurement. The 1999 Health Act laid a duty on NHS organizations to monitor the quality of service provision. Clear lines of accountability for service quality were supposed to be established through 'clinical governance' arrangements. Initially the government focused heavily on performance targets set by the Department of Health. Over time, the government has added a number of new organizations who set standards and monitor NHS performance (Talbot Smith & Pollock 2006).

Performance targets are set by the Department of Health, and Strategic Health Authorities play a major role in performance managing local organizations. In addition, the Department of Health produce National Service Frameworks which lay down national protocols for a range of conditions (such as heart disease, cancer and diabetes) and population groups (children, older people).

The Healthcare Commission is the health watchdog in England. The Healthcare Commission sets national standards and checks that healthcare services are meeting its standards. These include safety, cleanliness and waiting times. The Commission has statutory duty to assess the performance of healthcare organizations and award annual performance ratings for the NHS. The creation of foundation Trusts led to the creation of an additional watchdog body, Monitor, specifically to regulate Foundation Trusts.

The National Institute for Health and Clinical Excellence (NICE) provides national guidance on the effectiveness of services and treatments. While all NICE guidance applies in England, in Wales and Scotland uptake of NICE guidance is more selective. NICE produces guidelines through three centres. The Centre for Public Health Excellence provides guidance on effective health promotion and public health in England. The Centre for Technology Evaluation issues guidance on the use of new and existing medicines and treatments. In making assessments NICE is required to take into account both clinical effectiveness and value for money. Thus, NICE operates as a rationing body for new treatments. It had been hoped that by basing rationing decisions on 'expert' judgement political controversy would lessen. This has not been the case as NICE decisions have frequently been disputed by patient groups such as the recent decision to limit use of drugs for Alzheimer's disease. The Centre for Clinical Practice issues clinical guidelines on the treatment of people with specific conditions.

In addition, the reform of professional regulation has led to the creation of The Council for Healthcare Regulatory Excellence to oversee professional regulation and the National Patient Safety Agency monitors patient safety. The NHS Institute for Learning Skills and Innovation now takes forward the 'modernization' of the NHS.

The huge increase in regulatory activity over the last few years has led to complaints about a confusing, burdensome and constantly changing performance management system. There are now a total of 38 'arms length bodies' in the NHS, many of which are concerned with regulation. Klein (2003) has described it as a 'cacophony of accountabilities'.

RR REFLECTION POINT

We have seen that the health service has been organized as a 'managed market'. This means that in addition to being subject to market pressures, it is also subject to increased regulation and performance management. Think of examples of performance management and regulation that you have come across in your own experience. Some health professionals believe that increased audit, target setting and measurement improves standards while others believe that it distracts attention from care giving. What do you think?

Discussion points

1. What do you think should be the fundamental values and principles of the NHS today?
2. What do you think should be the key priorities of contemporary healthcare?

CHAPTER SUMMARY

In this chapter, we have discussed some key concepts underpinning health policy and have reviewed the political ideologies that have shaped health policy in the post-war period. We have reviewed the origin and development of the NHS and described the key themes of recent reform.

Over the last 20 years, the NHS has experienced a period of unprecedented change which Webster (2002) has summed up as 'continuous revolution'. Such change has largely been motivated by political ideologies and its evidence base is frequently questionable. The overall direction of change has been towards a mixed economy of care although there have been increasing variations between the four countries that make up the UK. In England, the NHS seems to be moving inexorably towards a US-style managed market in healthcare. In such a system, professional practice is intensively regulated and prescribed with a declining role for individualized care and clinical judgement.

The administrative costs of managed markets are high. The USA has the most expensive healthcare system in the world but it fails to address the human needs of a significant portion of its population due to its serious inequities. It has some of the worst health indicators in the developed world. It remains to be seen whether efforts to address health inequalities in the UK are confounded by emerging structural inequities in the 'New NHS'. Nurses, who have traditionally cared for some of the most vulnerable members of society, must be concerned about the impact of policy changes on their future roles and we will return to this issue in Chapter 9.

FURTHER READING

Baggott R 2004 Health and healthcare in Britain. Palgrave Macmillan, Basingstoke.
Talbot Smith A, Pollock A 2006 The New NHS: A Guide. London, Routledge.
Webster C 2002 The National Health Service: A political history. Oxford University Press, Oxford.

All of the above provide clear accounts of recent NHS policy.

REFERENCES

Baggott R 2004 Health and healthcare in Britain. Palgrave Macmillan, Basingstoke

Barry N 1990 Welfare. Open University Press, Buckingham

Bellaby P, Oribabor P 1980 Determinants of occupational strategies adopted by British hospital nurses. International Journal of Health Services 10 (2):291–309

Beveridge Report 1942 Social insurance and allied services. HMSO, London

Blakemore K 2003 Social policy: An introduction. Open University Press, Buckingham

Bulmer M, Rees A 1996 Citizenship today: The contemporary relevance of T H Marshall. Routledge, London

Burke E 1968 Reflections on the revolution in France. Penguin, Middlesex

Clarke J, Newman J 1997 The managerial state. London, Sage

Cutler T, Waine B 2000 Managerialism reformed? New Labour and Public Sector Management. Social Policy and Administration 34 (3):318–332

DHSS 1972 National Health Service Reorganization, England. HMSO, London

Department of Health 1997 The New NHS: Modern dependable. HMSO, London

Department of Health 2000 The NHS plan. HMSO, London

Dingwall R, Rafferty A, Webster C 1988 An introduction to the social history of nursing. Routledge, London

Doyal L, Gough I 1991 A theory of human needs. Macmillan, London

Enthoven A 1985 Reflections on the management of the NHS London. Nuffield Provincial Hospital Trust, London

Fairfield G, Hunter D, Mechanic D 1997 Managed care: Implications of managed care for health systems, clinicians and patients. British Medical Journal 314:1895

Fitzpatrick T 2005 New theories of welfare. Palgrave Macmillan, Hampshire

Foot M 1997 Aneurin Bevan 1897–1960. Victor Gollancz, London

Giddens A 1998 The Third Way. Polity, Cambridge
Greener I 2004 The three moments of New Labour's health policy discourse. Policy and Politics 32 (3):303–316
Griffiths Report 1983 NHS management inquiry. DHSS, London
Ham C 2004 Health policy in Britain. Palgrave Macmillan, Hampshire
Harrison S, Wood B 1999 Designing health service organization in the NHS 1968–1998: From blueprint to bright idea and manipulated emergence. Public Administration 77(4):751–767
Hayek F 1944 The road to serfdom. Routledge, London
Herbert S 1939 Britain's health. Penguin, Middlesex
Klein R 2003 Governance for NHS Foundation Trusts. British Medical Journal 326:174–175
Le Grand J 1998 US managed care: has the UK anything to learn? British Medical Journal 317:831–832
Levitt R, Wall A, Appleby J 1995 The reorganised National Health Service, 5th edn. Chapman and Hall, London
Lister R 1997 Citizenship: Feminist perspectives. Macmillan, Hampshire
Lister R 1998 From equality to social inclusion: New Labour and the welfare state. Critical Social Policy 18(2):215–225
Lister R 2001 New Labour: a study in ambiguity from a position of ambivalence. Critical Social Policy 21 (4):425–447
Marshall T H 1950 Citizenship and social class. Cambridge University Press, Cambridge
Marshall T H 1963 Sociology at the crossroads. Heinemann, London
Maslow A H 1943 A theory of human motivation. Psychological Review 50:370–396
Mechanic D 1996 Changing medical organization and the erosion of trust. Milbank Quarterly 74:171–189
Miller R, Luft H 1994 Managed care plan performance since 1980: a literature analysis. Journal of the American Medical Association 271:19
Ministry of Health 1944 A National Health Service, Cmnd 6502. HMSO London
Ministry of Health 1956 Report of the Committee of Inquiry into the Cost of the NHS (Guillebaud Inquiry Report). HMSO, London
Ministry of Health 1966 Report of the Committee on Senior Nursing Structure (Salmon Report). HMSO, London
Pollock A 2004 NHS plc: the privatization of our healthcare. Verso, London
Powell M 2000 New Labour, New Welfare State? Policy Press, Bristol
Rivett G 1998 From cradle to grave: fifty years of the NHS. Kings Fund, London
Strong P, Robinson J 1990 The NHS – under new management. Open University Press, Buckingham
Sullivan K 2000 Pull the plug. Washington Monthly 1 April
Talbot Smith A, Pollock A 2006 The New NHS. A Guide. Routledge, London
Tawney R H 1931 Equality. Allen and Unwin, London
Timmins N 2001 The five giants: A biography of the welfare state. Harper Collins, London
Traynor M 1999 Managerialism and nursing. Routledge, London
Walker R 1999 The Americanization of British Welfare: A case study of policy transfer. International Journal of Health Services 29(4): 679–697
Wanless D 2002 Securing our future health: Taking a long term view. HM Treasury, London
Webster C 2002 The National Health Service: A political history. Oxford University Press, Oxford
Willcocks A 1967 The creation of the NHS. Routledge and Kegan Paul, London

CHAPTER

8 Power and communication in healthcare

Martin Johnson

KEY CONCEPTS

- Nurses are weak in relation to medicine
- Patients often fail to exploit their power
- Goals of care are based on a balance of power
- Power is complex
- The effects of power cannot always be seen

Introduction

This chapter is about the relationship between nurses and their patients and the power that holds it together. It also considers some of the wider issues of power as an aspect of professionalism. We considered professionalism in Chapter 4 and examine nursing professionalism in Chapter 9. In particular, we will examine how it is that nursing care, as currently conceived, can effectively 'disempower' patients, despite the official desire to increase their independence. The place of nurses in relation to other professionals is examined briefly; this is developed further in Chapter 9. We then look at the ways in which nurses and patients negotiate, and sometimes collude, in seeking to influence events. In particular, we examine the strategies that patients and their nurses may use to access power and achieve objectives. Sometimes these goals are less in tune with patient preferences than we would like to think. The chapter concludes with a discussion of particular views of power which, though not new, have perhaps been neglected in nursing literature.

The concept of power

Although we all probably imagine that we have an idea of what power means, a concrete definition is usually found wanting.

The great British philosopher, Bertrand Russell (Russell 1938) argued that it is 'the production of intended effects', which seems reasonable. If we want to achieve something and we can make it happen, then we must have had the 'power' to do so. Unfortunately, this view now seems rather oversimplified. Our actions and those of others may also have unintended effects that illustrate our 'power'. For example, when nurses put on a uniform it may not be directly to create obedience in their patients, but it often has this type of effect, and of course the nurse's power to influence the patient's behaviour increases accordingly.

Both philosophers and sociologists have wrestled with clarifying the concept of power. One of the most widely respected of these, who is seen as both sociologist and philosopher, is Steven Lukes (1974, 2005). His and other theories of power are examined at the end of this Chapter, but to give a flavour of the complexity, he describes power as 'ineradicably value-dependent' and 'essentially contested'. By this, he means that Russell and others had failed to take into account the history and culture that people bring to the use and the understanding of power.

Nurses and power

Many books address the question of the power of the nurse but it may be fair to say that this is often in the context of leadership and the simplistic Russell-type view prevails. Bryan Turner (1987) however, makes the important point that, in the context of work, nurses are for the most part instruments of the power of at least one other occupational group: the doctors. This builds upon the earlier, but still very relevant analysis by Eliot Freidson (1970), in which he argues that all occupations whose work is essentially 'medical' in character cannot fail to be subordinate in authority and responsibility to the medical profession. Turner goes on to illustrate how it is that what dentists are allowed to do is very tightly controlled by the medical profession. In this 'control by limitation', dentists, despite a 6-year training, are confined to work on the teeth, and may practise wider 'surgery' only under strict control. Turner shows how other occupations with claims to manage illness, such as the clergy and practitioners of alternative therapy are controlled largely by 'exclusion'. The excluding profession maintains a register of legally licensed practitioners to which only the properly qualified are admitted. Turner argues that the strategy through which the medical profession controls nurses is by 'subordination'. Taking an historical perspective he seems to mean that, partly by means of their status as educated men, doctors successfully convinced not only a willing public and government, but nurses themselves (less well-educated women), that medicine rightfully controls all medical work and that much of this that is mundane should be delegated to 'inferior' occupations while physicians and surgeons retain overall 'responsibility'. If this analysis is correct, we must conclude that much of what nurses do will be, whether they realize it or not, in pursuit of medically desired objectives. This view casts doubt on the validity of much of the rhetoric on the nursing process which speaks of nurses and patients agreeing mutually acceptable goals for which the nurse will be accountable (Roper et al 1996).

Another dimension to the question of nurses' power base is that they are also subordinated to another group: the professional health service managers, who increasingly have business-related objectives (Traynor 1999). Nurses have begun to sense an important constraint to the development of autonomy in the face of targets set by managers who, for the most part, are not nurses (see Chapters 4 and 9). Overall, the resultant picture is one where Conrad (1979) feels that nurses can best be described as 'captive professionals'.

Service users, patients and power

A good deal of the language of the last decade has been in terms of service user, client, or patient empowerment. Even the increasing use of the term 'service users' for health service consumers reflects this trend, despite little evidence that patients or clients actually prefer it. The term 'service user' generally refers to a person who makes use of the services of health and social care services delivered by professional and related support staff. The term 'client' became fashionable in the 1990s. In the case of legal or accounting services, it implied a more equal relationship between the professional and the purchaser of a service. In principle, if unsatisfied, the client can take their money elsewhere. In the private health sector, this could increasingly describe the situation accurately, even though the majority of patients are still paying via a once-removed bureaucracy, such as an insurance plan (rather than with cash). More recently, the words 'service user' have become popular (DoH 2005) to imply even greater autonomy of those who might use and benefit from health and social care services. A term more appropriate than 'patient' or even 'client' seemed to be a good idea, particularly in mental health and learning disability services, as it might remove some of the stigma from holding this status. How equal the professional–service user relationship actually is remains in some doubt, as I hope to show. This section examines the ways in which service users could, and sometimes do, exploit what power is available and how, perhaps more commonly, they comply with nursing and medical goals. I will make no effort, however, to modernize terms such as 'client', 'patient' or 'inmate' when they are used by researchers and theorists. I take the view that in general, the social definition of a word, such as service user, is determined by the use of the word by real people rather than by Government Policy.

WORK

At first glance, work has little to do with the patient's experiences of healthcare, especially if we accept Parsons' (1951) view of the sick role in which ill people are exempted from their normal work and responsibilities, provided that they want to get well and comply with medical instructions (see Chapter 13). However, in Chapter 4 we discussed the fact that work can mean more than paid employment and noted that the boundaries of care work were ambiguous. On closer analysis, work is a key source of power and influence for patients. Strauss et al (1982) suggest that using a 'sociology of work' perspective can illuminate much in the social relations between patients and their care in hospital. They identify the place of 'work' carried out by patients in hospital in providing a basis for negotiation on other dimensions of social relations. Indeed, they note that the staff's opinion of patients may depend on the nature of the work that they (patients) are prepared to do. Strauss et al (1982) identify as work, many activities which take place in hospitals and in which patients are involved. They suggest that some work is officially recognized in the hospital division of labour, such as diabetics injecting their own insulin. Other work is not so recognized and may include patients reporting mistakes or deterioration in their patient colleagues. Of particular interest, is the interpersonal dimension in which Strauss et al identify patients' endurance of painful or uncomfortable procedures as work through which the patient can then negotiate in other domains. Another area of work that if not done properly gets patients 'into trouble with staff', is the case of the very ill person who knows she or he is dying. Strauss et al suggest that the patient is expected to do (unrecognized) work to maintain reasonable control over reactions, which might be excessively disturbing of the staff's work, or disruptive of other patients' poise.

This unrecognized work has been called sentimental work (Strauss et al 1982) or emotional labour (Hochschild 1983, James 1989). James' paper analyses the notion of largely unpaid and 'invisible' emotional work from the viewpoint of the female health worker. She argues from an explicitly feminist perspective that women are socialized into providing unpaid labour without which the elite aspects of care, such as medical work, could not take place. Strauss et al (1982), however, focus on the role of the patient in the ward division of labour illustrating that they too contribute an untold amount of emotional labour (which they term sentimental work). They argue further that this work contributes to the development of the professional–patient relationship or its deterioration. It seems particularly relevant today to examine the nature of patient work in all or any of its forms, since independence and 'self care' are increasingly aspects of both nursing and government ideology. The part this work (or its absence) plays in the management of human relations and the use and abuse of power are examined again later.

Case study

Consider the case of Nick, who was terminally ill. Nick had lung cancer which had spread seriously. He had agreed to radiation therapy, which both he and nursing staff knew was probably futile. Nick was able to get away with disturbing a ward report to get medication, usually an unacceptable behaviour, perhaps because he was careful in his control of the more emotive consequences of his diagnosis. Publicly, he did not challenge the decision of the doctors that he should have more treatment.

This insight is useful because it also identifies patient work as a source of power, or a legitimate negotiating resource. It is a source of patients' control over their social situation; in this case, getting his medication early. It also shows that on the 'big issues' he was relatively powerless (Johnson 1997).

REFLECTION POINT

In the case study above, Nick felt powerless to negotiate his treatment. To what extent do you think that patients find it difficult to influence their treatment and care?

COMPLAINING

Another opportunity to exploit the limited power available to patients is the complaint. Much complaining in hospital is 'off stage' and out of earshot of the nurses. It happens in the day rooms and toilet areas and health professionals often have little knowledge of it.

What is known comes largely from the work of sociologists, like Benyon (1987), who have been patients and, when well enough, have realized that they could learn much from observing and recording the insights available as opportunistic participant observers. Benyon noted the 'grumbling' of patients in a surgical ward, which was not meant to be heard by the staff. Such behaviour helps to relieve frustration and gives a degree of social support to otherwise vulnerable persons in an anxiety-laden atmosphere, especially of the surgical ward.

Some formal complaints are made, however, and can present a threat to nurses who may perceive their image of competence to be under attack. The problem for the patient is often the judgement of the moment when a complaint really is the best course, in a context in which complaining can be labelled as 'difficult behaviour'. According to English and Morse (1988: 28), in their ethnography of 'difficult' elderly patients, nurses said that 'complaining patients made them feel they could never do anything right'. Clearly, patients do complain both about day-to-day concerns like the tea being too hot, or too cold. On the other hand, patients can be motivated to 'risk' their social reputation by complaining, especially where they feel that they have nothing to lose because they feel that their social reputation is already damaged. They are, as Goffman (1968) would put it, 'stigmatized' or 'with spoiled identity'. Sometimes, the criticism is more personal as in the following case study.

Case study

Charles, who had very serious chronic airways obstruction, and was constantly weak from lack of oxygen and carbon dioxide excess, had apparently lost confidence in Paula, one of the junior nurses on the ward. Charles asked the staff nurse to arrange for his care to be carried out by someone else as he felt that Paula was slow and clumsy. At one level, he was expressing a legitimate preference if, indeed, Paula had caused him previous discomfort. At another level, he must have assumed that 'reporting her' to a staff nurse might be a sanction both for her and an example to others.

Consider the view that he had power over both the staff nurse and Paula, at that and subsequent moments. Charles had long since given up trying to be popular; his condition of chronic airflow limitation was too discomforting and frightening to allow him to keep up appearances of 'niceness'. So, in complaining he had less to lose, and something to gain. At least he did not 'suffer' Paula's care, which in his eyes was inadequate to his needs at that time. Such a tactic illustrates how patients can resort to conflict if necessary.

The case study illustrates a patient exploiting a localized complaint mechanism to influence events as they affect him. Objectively speaking this is legitimate, but is nevertheless seen as a course of last resort by many patients. It also points out the accountability that student nurses are subject to. Despite being only a relatively inexperienced student, Paula was directly accountable both to the staff nurses and to the patient for the care that she gave. This illustrates the way in which much discussion of accountability, as a thing that goes hand in hand with autonomy, may be misguided. The rhetoric of professionalism is that with accountability comes autonomy; however, this sort of example shows that being answerable for actions (accountable) in this potentially painful way is rather a feature of the least powerful of healthcare professionals than of the elite, such as the consultant physician, the clinical nurse specialist, or the university lecturer. To return to Freidson's (1970) brilliant analysis (which nurses have largely ignored in their own claims to professional status), true professionalism means 'legitimate organized autonomy' and this is not the same thing as accountability as the ward nurse experiences it. In other words, autonomy can imply not being accountable in any meaningful way to the patient (see Chapter 4 for a more detailed discussion).

EXCHANGE

Another attempt to restore the balance of power between nurse and patient is the exchange of services and, to a limited extent, of gifts. Officially discouraged from accepting 'substantial' gifts, nurses are often offered small tokens of appreciation by patients. Sweets, chocolates and tights seem to be popular. Janice Morse (1989), identifying the importance of gift-giving in the anthropological literature, suggests that the giving of care by nurses creates a further imbalance in an already unequal relationship between nurse and patient. Patients commonly wish to reciprocate by giving 'gifts' to attempt to equalize things. Although this notion may seem at first sight relatively inconsequential, the point is that the 'gift relationship' is a concept of some importance in the understanding of service relationships such as exist between patients and nurses. The anthropologist Marcel Mauss (1990), who was an associate of Durkheim, analysed the gift relationship. Like Durkheim (see Chapter 3) he was interested in the rituals and symbolic acts that help to forge social bonds. He described the ways in which gifts create a sense of reciprocity and hence community. Goffman has similar concerns about reciprocity in human relationships and suggested that: 'It is this spark not the more obvious kinds of love that lights up the world' (Goffman 1957). In his work on total institutions, Goffman (1968) was concerned with the way in which institutional rules and routines undermined reciprocity in human relationships as we saw in Chapter 4.

Malcolm Johnson (1975), drawing on Marcel Mauss, argues that the giving and receiving of gifts is symbolic rather than economic. It is a confirmation of reciprocity that exists between individuals and can symbolize a sense of community within a ward environment. Johnson's thesis is that the elderly are frequently disempowered in these terms by being systematically excluded from the possibility of reciprocity, for example by being rendered poor and socially isolated, as we noted in Chapter 6.

Such a notion is one possible explanation of the weak power-base of patients. Generally, the range of 'gifts' available is small. Indeed, it may be that the offering of such relatively insubstantial items as sweets is a modest attempt to fill the gap left by the minimal opportunity for a truly balanced exchange of services or other 'gifts'. Where 'patient work' in the terms of Strauss et al (1982) can be seen as an aspect of this 'gift exchange' idea, it becomes clear how those who cannot offer even this will be seriously disempowered in their presentation of themselves as 'socially worthwhile'. 'Exchange theory' has been influential in most of the social and behavioural sciences. One key idea, apart from the giving of services and actual gift artefacts, is that individuals also bring aspects of their background, culture and class into any relationship, all of which helps to bring either balance or disorder to social interaction (see also Bourdieu's concepts of social and cultural capital discussed in Chapter 5). Simplistically therefore, young university-educated nurses might have little in common with the elderly retired bus conductor, and so will spend little enough time interacting with this person except at a very instrumental level of 'routine care'. Although studies show that this can determine some aspects of care (Stockwell 1972), Kelly and May (1982) argued that such a view fails to recognize the true complexity of human interaction in specific circumstances. In a study of my own, for example, one elderly man was failing to comply with medication, smoked despite being an oxygen user, was quite elderly and seemed to meet the criteria for being a 'social problem' (Johnson 1997). As it happened this person, who exchange theory would have predicted to have been unpopular and with little influence over his care, was quite the reverse. He was able, through his manifest bubbly personality and stoic acceptance of discomforts, to win respect and concessions from the nursing staff.

CONFLICT

The 'gift' relationship can be seen as an attempt to create a moral bond between staff and patient and hence create a sense of moral obligation. However, often such an agreeable approach fails to maintain consensus between staff and patient. It is probably true to say that texts on nursing care emphasize consensus and mutual goal setting in planning care. Conflict is not seriously considered as an aspect of 'nursing models' which purport to explain and predict patient behaviour and nursing care. An example is that of the popular Roper Model (Holland 2003) which, although produced by British academics, has a good deal in common with its American counterparts. In contrast to 'nursing theory', much important sociological theory has identified conflict as a fundamental concept. According to Lukes (1974, 2005) the presence of conflict is a key test of power in any relationship but it should not be seen as the only test. Conflict has been seen as a struggle between competing classes or groups in society. Here we will discuss conflict in a fairly small-scale way as representing the struggle between individual patients and health professionals for the achievement of day-to-day goals rather than political objectives.

In an analysis of the strategies of clients in an alcohol treatment facility, Fineman (1991) presents categories at variance with the prevailing consensus view of professional–client relations. He argues that clients frequently resort to the subversive to achieve their own, rather than the health professionals', goals. Under a category of 'manipulation', he lists 'sabotage', where clients deliberately frustrate the professionals' intentions. One strategy might be failing to turn up for group meetings, being late for therapy sessions or failing to supply specimens for investigation. Think about the following case study, which is taken from practice.

Case study

Bob was a very ill patient with alcoholic cirrhosis of the liver and tuberculosis from living rough. He was acutely ill but was able to get the less experienced nurses to give his sedative medications earlier than the prescription sheet allowed. This was because they seemed afraid that if he did not get his own way some of the time, he would fail to stay on his side when he was turned and so the staff would be blamed for failing to keep him off his pressure areas. He knew that they were nervous of being 'accountable' for the worsening of his pressure areas.

Bob is a good example of a patient who has 'nothing to lose' by being openly in conflict with the nursing staff. He would make promises that if left in bed all morning, he would get up for an hour in the afternoon but later nurses would find that he had told the afternoon shift that he had already been exhausted by the morning staff getting him out.

Under a second category of 'working the system' Fineman lists 'doctor-shopping', seeking undeserved services, and provoking fights among the staff. Doctor-shopping amounts to recruiting multiple staff members to work toward contradictory ends.

COMPLIANCE

It would be wrong to overestimate the ability of service users to utilize these strategies in achieving their own goals in defiance of those of the nursing and medical staff. Very frequently, patients will hold out for the unimportant, such as an extra cup of tea or the right not to be bathed first thing in the morning, only to comply with the health professionals' wishes on the 'big' issues, such as whether to undergo uncomfortable and even dangerous treatments. Freidson (1970) drew attention to the theoretical point of great relevance here. There are objective differences in perspective between the patient and the professional (in this case the nurse). Therefore, whatever the patient may do to impose their view, any success erodes claims to professionalism.

Frequently, nursing and other health occupations will recruit extra-professional support for their intentions, such as appeals to relatives. Many people would take no issue with Parsons' (1951) view that compliance with medical instructions is in everyone's interests. The study by Waterworth and Luker (1990) showed that, at least in one Liverpool hospital, many patients were keen to 'toe the line' because they saw no reason to be involved in decisions about their care. They assumed that the professions knew best and that, in any case, they felt vulnerable, like being in a dentist's chair. That is to say, they perceive a physical or emotional threat of discomfort which renders them compliant. Nurses, like dentists, have a wide range of very uncomfortable or embarrassing procedures at their disposal, a point we shall expand on later.

Interestingly, most medical research literature on compliance sees it uncritically as something to be achieved in societal interests. Sociologists on the other hand have taken the opposite view with perhaps a most ardent (if polemical) advocate Ivan Illich (1976) arguing that compliance with medical care is dangerous to health on a number of levels. His polemic *Limits to Medicine (Medical Nemesis)* (outlined in Chapter 4) is essential reading in order to develop a really critical appreciation of the role of medicine in healthcare.

We will now give some attention to the ways in which nurses exercise power over patients.

Nurses' power and the patient's response

A wide range of strategies are available to health professionals in general, and nurses in particular, which enable the effective control of patients in the direction of professional goals. Here we will discuss a selection of those which may perhaps seem controversial or that you may not have thought of as aspects of social control. Think critically about the suggestions made in relation to your own practice experiences.

CONTROL OF INFORMATION

Nurses control most of the information flow in relation to the care of patients. They maintain the main record systems, control telephone and other information media in most if not all clinical areas, and even decide who may and may not enter clinical areas and the times when this will be allowed. They frequently act as gatekeeper to other professionals, notably the doctors. The Sister's or Ward Manager's Office, or its equivalent, is a place where personal and clinical information is centralized under the control of specific nursing staff. Given their structural control over communications, nurses are also well versed in the arts of secrecy. Building on the work done in the USA in the 1960s by Glaser and Strauss, David Field (1989) argued that despite some changes from the systematic lying to virtually all patients about serious diagnoses, a good deal of information of concern to the very ill patient is still kept hidden in a 'silent conspiracy'. Despite some progress in disclosure of malignant diagnoses, many patients are still deprived of information about their prognosis, whatever progress has been made on the front of openness about diagnosis (Costello 2001). Of course, it can be argued that this is done for the best of reasons, that the paternalism here is justified on the grounds of saving patients unnecessary anxiety and allowing hope where none may be possible. Whether or not it is finally in the patient's interests, this strategy emphasizes the power of the doctors compared with the patient. It can only be concluded that nurses collude substantially in this. Given that nurses operate in a mode of only guarded release of information, they are in a position which inevitably disempowers their patients. They manage the uncertainty patients have about their future.

DEPERSONALIZATION

More controversially, it can be argued that nurses maintain a strategy of disempowerment of their patients which, although not deliberate as such, has evolved to play a major place in the achievement of medical and increasingly managerial objectives in health service provision. One of the tactics in this strategy is depersonalization. Goffman (1968) and others have noted that excessive routine, wearing of night clothes at most times of the day, deprivation of usual privacy and the systematic changing of daily routine from the personal to the institutional are key factors in the causation of patterns of behaviour which engage the compliance of 'inmates' for the nurses (see Chapter 4 for a more detailed discussion). Whatever the rhetoric of individualized care, many of these features remain in mainstream hospital practice. Furthermore, the procedures for the delivery of 'individualized care' have contributed systematically to the collection and centralization of sensitive patient data in nursing process cardexes, care plans and computerized patient administration systems.

Case study

Drawing on a number of sometimes distressing examples, Lawton (2000) brilliantly illustrates depersonalization in the hospice setting. Despite the aims of the hospice to confront death as part of life, and to maintain personal individuality, the particular problems accompanying a protracted death from cancer can lead to a loss of personhood. Lawton gives one detailed example of Annie, a woman with cancer of the cervix which has spread to involve the bladder, rectum and vagina. Annie is concerned that caring for her has

> exhausted her husband, and together with leakage of faecal and other body fluids, this leads to her admission to the hospice and admission to a shared ward.
>
> At first, she was 'self-caring' but after a few days, her fistula enlarged so that whenever she got up out of bed, diarrhoea and urine would 'pour out of her body'. It is very hard to imagine how this must have felt, but Annie felt she was losing her personal dignity, and over coming weeks she lost all control over her bowel and bladder functions as she 'rotted away below'. At first she resisted staff attempts to move her to a single room for the benefit of the other patients sharing her room. Eventually, however, she is moved into one. Sadly at this point, visits from her family reduced as they felt she was barely aware of their presence.

Although permission for the study was gained from all concerned, to use this woman's suffering to make a theoretical point can seem uncaring. However, I believe that Lawton considered this a good deal before discussing these people and their situation. She discusses Annie's case in great detail and with much sensitivity. She does not treat her plight lightly, and yet is able to make a number of important points. Most germane of these is the degree to which Annie loses her autonomy and is gradually sequestered (hidden away) from the world, first in the hospice itself, and then in a single room. Lawton argues that fundamental to this is the persistent 'unboundedness' of the body, that is the uncontrolled loss of bodily contents without suitable privacy. Also giving other examples, she shows how people begin to disengage from normal interaction. Despite even the best efforts of hospice staff they become effectively depersonalized, they experience a 'loss of self'.

SOCIAL JUDGEMENT

Much of what I have said bears upon the social reputation of the patient and the nurse. Labelling, or the process of social judgement, is another dimension of the disempowerment of patients by nurses in the healthcare context. First described substantially by Roth (1972) and Stockwell (1972), the process of labelling people as 'good', 'bad', 'popular' or 'unpopular' has been examined more closely from an interpretive perspective in Kelly and May (1982) and Johnson and Webb (1995). Generally, it can be argued that most patients and their nurses are aware of the differing social judgements that each makes of the other, and that this viewpoint can become part of the bargain for cooperation in achieving goals of care. Often, staff views of a patient vary; indeed, they may be re-negotiated by the patient in relation to new 'evidence' or behaviour. The 'official' or dominant view of a patient can be an important backdrop to the type of decision made about their care and can even play a part in important moral decisions. Some nurses report having to 'like people secretly' because they do not feel ready to challenge the prevailing view of a patient. Nurses even adopt strategies of secret caring to 'compensate' or advocate for the patient they feel is unfairly seen in a bad light (Johnson 1997). It is important however, to avoid the assumption that certain characteristics necessarily lead to 'unpopularity'. Like access to 'power', many factors are involved and there is much that depends on the social context of the time, place and people involved.

These are illustrations of the source of nursing power in relation to service users, both for their benefit and occasionally for abuse. It is important to remember that in reality more factors come into play. You may be able to identify others, or you may feel that the view portrayed here is rather pessimistic and sees health professionals in too sinister a light. The provision of excellent care probably does depend on professionals having a certain amount of authority to act and to make decisions based on their extensive professional knowledge. This view is now examined in more detail, by discussing this 'functional' view of health professional power and two of its competitors.

Theoretical issues

You will recall that we can see power as a very complex notion. This section reviews some key views of power to examine their ability to illuminate some of the issues and examples discussed earlier. Russell's (1938) view of the production of intended effects is clearly too simple. Because many patients are socialized to accept the authority of the professional, nurses may be more powerful than they intend to be. A small study by Waterworth and Luker (1990) illustrates how many patients do not wish or expect to be involved in decisions about their care, but the explanation probably lies in the powerful socialization to accept professional authority to which, throughout their lives, they have been subject.

POWER AS FUNCTIONAL

Nursing authors have realized the importance of power. Benner (1984) is widely influential and is arguably more credible than some other nursing theory because her work is drawn from direct observation of practice. In her book, she argues consistently that experience and reflection combine to produce expertise and the ability to wield clinical power in an 'excellent' way. The following direct quote from Benner's research illustrates her viewpoint fairly well:

> *'The nurses who took part in this study have offered us glimpses of the nature of the power that resides in caring, They have used their power to empower their patients – not to dominate, coerce or control them. But this relationship is highly contextual. To empower, nurses, sometimes border on coercion as they coach and prompt the patient to engage in painful tasks that patients would not readily undertake on their own. The difference between empowerment and domination can be understood only if the nurse–patient relationship and the situation are understood. Caring out of context will always be controversial, because caring is local, specific and individual'. (Benner 1984: 209)*

RЯ REFLECTION POINT

Analyse this quote and try to decide which kind of view of power Benner has. Keep it in mind when we look at theories of power from the wider philosophical and sociological literature. Does it have anything in common with Parsons? Compare it with the views of Foucault and Lukes later in this Chapter.

PARSONS' VIEW OF POWER

Parsons (1951) viewed socialization as necessary to a functioning social system (see Chapter 2 for an introduction to Parsons and a discussion of the role of the family in socialization). Through the media of education, religion, the law and medicine, Parsons saw the exercise of power merely as a proper tool of social control to avoid anarchy and inefficiency. Power, in a later work by Parsons (1963 cited by Lukes 2005), is simply a system resource (not unlike money) to be used, preferably by those properly so authorized (professionals) to return the sick to 'normal functioning' (see Chapter 13). Parsons saw professional power as derived by legitimate consensus and therefore necessarily good. This view of power could be described as 'power to'. Parsons does not see any possibility of the use of power for illegitimate purposes, and so from a modern perspective, we must see this view as perhaps too conservative. As we have seen, self-regulation – a key attribute of a profession as Parsons saw it – can sometimes be seen manifestly to fail to protect the public.

To recapitulate, Parsons' (and arguably Benner's) view, in assuming experience and expertise are necessary and sufficient conditions for practice, which is entirely in patients' interests, may be insufficiently cognisant of dangers of malpractice. Parsons' view may seem dated, but something like it underlies much paternalistic thinking among health professionals and it could be said to be an influence behind concepts of 'general management', efficiency and effectiveness, and the current fashion for educating for purpose. The view is flawed because it assumes that each professional is altruistic and generally acts primarily in patients' interests alone.

MICHEL FOUCAULT'S VIEW OF POWER

A more complex view of power, which has received remarkably little attention in nursing literature given its impact elsewhere, is that of Michel Foucault (1991).

As with Parsons, a brief introduction to Foucault's ideas risks injustice to them, but his perspective is so challenging (especially to health professionals) that it is worthy of some discussion. He takes a historical approach to the evolution of ideas and social relations, examining in his various books, psychiatry, medicine, legal systems and the theory of knowledge. He notes that in order to wield power over people those in authority used to have to use torture, restraint, imprisonment and incarceration to control those in society who presented some kind of threat to the dominant order. Some of his text makes very emotive reading, such as his graphic account of hanging, drawing and quartering.

Although we imagine that such methods are no longer used to subdue society to the will of those in authority, it might be argued that the recent television and internet broadcasts of horrific executions by terrorists serve a similar long-term purpose, to instil a perception of power beyond mere military might, which many terrorists lack.

In relation to the health professions, Foucault shows how, at first, lepers were seen as a threat to society so that they were excluded from 'society' by incarceration in 'colonies'. Later, as leprosy became less important, other previously well-tolerated groups were marginalized and

BIOGRAPHY Michel Foucault (1926–1984)

Michel Foucault was born in France in 1926 to a middle class French family. He became an established academic in the 1960s and was elected to the prestigious College de France in 1969. Foucault resisted biography as irrelevant to his work saying 'do not ask me who I am'. Foucault was active in radical politics and was also a homosexual. He was an early victim of AIDS dying of an AIDS-related illness in 1984. In spite of his injunction to ignore his biography, the link between his work and his life has been the subject of much speculation and debate. It has been suggested for example that an impetus for his work was the sexism and homophobia that he encountered in French radical politics in the 1950s and 1960s. As a result, his work has been animated by a concern for human rights and has been particularly central in the study of sexuality and gender (see especially his last unfinished work, *The History of Sexuality*).

Foucault's main objective in his work was to provide a critical history of the present. Foucault is often described as a post-modernist or post-structuralist. Foucault analysed the history of thought and practice (which he called discourse) and the ways in which discourses shaped reality. He famously stated in *The Order of Things* that 'man' was a discourse that would soon be 'erased, like a face drawn in the sand at the edge of the sea'. Foucault's ideas are explored further below. His major works include:

Madness and Civilization 1961
The Birth of the Clinic 1963
The Order of Things 1966
The Archaeology of Knowledge 1969
Discipline and Punish 1977

incarcerated, such as the mentally ill and, in the nineteenth century, the poor. It is no coincidence, and nonetheless shameful, that people with frequent and disabling epilepsy were kept in 'colonies' until the 1970s. Lawton (2000) implies, I think with some cause, that despite its aims of openness about death, the hospice has become a place to hide and manage the increasingly 'unbounded' and difficult death which takes place there (we will discuss this debate further in Chapter 15).

Foucault is not arguing that modern health professionals, nor even prison officers, now undertake these approaches to the exercise of power. Rather he argues that over time we have subtly absorbed such events (as torture and execution) into our collective consciousness. They have become the legitimation for our preparedness to be subject to the authority of others. We remain conscious that these brutal physical methods are available were it ever necessary. Now, those in authority can usually control the behaviour of others by much more subtle means. These gentler but just as effective means he describes collectively as 'The Gaze'.

HIERARCHICAL OBSERVATION

Through what Foucault (1991) calls surveillance, information is collected about those to be subjugated and controlled. Systems are developed (e.g. the nursing process) more effectively to collect and distribute this information among those who may need it. Foucault observed that the ideal prison (called the panopticon) is one where all the inmates can be seen by just one officer, not unlike the 'Nightingale' ward in a hospital. As subjects become accustomed to their position in this social order, they can even be relied upon to undertake self-surveillance, which emphasizes Foucault's point that power is as much given up by the subjects as taken by the powerful. Burden (1998), studying a maternity unit, reports the stress experienced by midwives when women and their partners take control of the bed screens and exclude the professionals from visual observation of their activities.

NORMALIZING JUDGEMENT

Powerful people, in this case nurses, monitor the behaviour of their patients, executing penalties for infringements of acceptable behaviour and, most importantly, controlling the social reputation of their patients. It is in this way that the opinions of the 'powerful' nurse carry weight in decisions about the patient's future. Detailed knowledge of activity, speech and particularly the body is maintained.

THE EXAMINATION

This is the ritual collection of appropriate data, but it also acts as the symbolic act of disempowerment. Just as executions in the Middle Ages were undertaken with the subject naked, specifically to enhance the humiliation (if this were possible), the ritual of nakedness and detailed examination of the body and (increasingly) of the personality is maintained. It is particularly important to the idea that it is only the patient that submits to 'the examination'. Health professionals go to considerable lengths to avoid their private circumstances becoming known to patients as this would provide access to 'power' for patients and would erode claims to professionalism.

Foucault's view of power is nothing if not interesting. He defied requests to define power absolutely, preferring it to be seen as in a diffuse conjoint relationship with knowledge, which as can be seen is integral to the maintenance of, or rather access to, power. He argues that power is as much given up by the weak as taken by the strong, and that all have access in certain contexts. There is no doubt that Michel Foucault is commonly regarded as taking an extreme view, polemical if you will, and is comparable with the influential (but equally extreme) Ivan Illich. On the other hand, nurses are vulnerable to criticism that their education in sociology, philosophy and other 'liberal' disciplines tends to be sanitized and rendered 'safe' for their consumption. Much that is of value in feminist discourse is marginalized for the same reason.

STEVEN LUKES' STUDY OF POWER

The last 'theorist' we will examine is Steven Lukes (1974, 2005). He argues that many conceptions of power are simplistic. He typifies the Russell view, for example, as one-dimensional. He suggests that such views as the production of intended effects are dependent on both the relevant actions and the effects being observable and able to be determined in advance. Any view in which power needs to be exercised presupposes a conflict of interests between the parties concerned. Such a view is not common in the health professions, as most practitioners argue that they only act in the interests of the patient. A second approach to the analysis of power would be a two-dimensional view. Here, one face of power would be based in the observable actions and effects of decisions based on power. The second face of this more complex view of power is what Lukes loosely calls 'bias'. It is the extent to which a person or group consciously or unconsciously creates obstructions to openness. Here, he seems to suggest that together with open use of control measures goes a more sinister, less open form of power analogous to coercion. He notes that this view of power still has conflict at its roots, and that the 'bias' or coercive element can best be revealed by discovering 'grievances' (complaints) that the disempowered may hold; however, he remains unsatisfied by this 'extended behavioural' view of power.

Because he is dissatisfied with the 'individualistic' nature of the previous views of power, Lukes proposes a three-dimensional view of power that incorporates a systemic or organizational dimension. The key aspect that he adds to his view of power can be illustrated as follows. He draws upon a Marxist concept analogous to hegemony to argue that people make their own history but they are not fully in control of it. They do not choose the circumstances of their birth or, to a large extent, their socialization. Rather, the extra dimension is the sense in which power can be used to shape the very needs, wants and preferences of those we would subjugate. This is particularly apposite in the analysis of healthcare where patients' needs and wants are primarily determined by health professionals. To put it another way, health and healthcare are defined by health professionals who then wholly control access (or not) to it.

Lukes' (1974, 2005) radical model of power goes beyond that of Parsons to examine what the exercise of power prevents people from doing and even thinking. The model is 'radical' because it makes the assumption that individuals or groups have responsibility for the exercise (or not) of their power. This view of power has a certain appeal in healthcare because it brings into focus what in ethics is called the acts and omissions doctrine. This states that just as much responsibility attaches to a decision not to act as is attached to a decision to act in a given circumstance. This may be as simple as failing to make a contrary opinion known about the plan of care for a patient, or failing to strike someone from the register to protect the public. In the 2005 edition of his book, Lukes is at pains to review evidence for and against his theory of a third dimension of power, and examines in particular, why it is that individuals and groups subject themselves to the domination of others, whether politicians, industrial capitalists, or professionals. Building on, but also sceptical of the work of Pierre Bourdieu, another important French thinker who we review in Chapter 5, he discusses the degree to which domination, through what Bourdieu called 'symbolic violence' (see Chapter 5), remains a key feature of disempowerment.

Case study

On a medical ward-round, Bill, an elderly man with a severe arthritic condition of the feet, was authorized to go home at the earliest convenience because his medication was now stabilized and no further treatment was possible. He did not live far away, but could walk only with considerable discomfort. It was late afternoon and the newly qualified staff nurse knew that it was too late to order an ambulance for that day. She had the option of authorizing a hospital taxi, but she decided that, since Bill would probably manage without one once he got home, she would ask him to find his own way home by bus or pay for a taxi himself. This decision is routine enough, but became problematic when she asked a male staff nurse (who did not really agree) to tell Bill the decision because 'he'll take it better from a man'. This second staff nurse did tell him, and with a little persuasion and the offer of a wheelchair to the door, he agreed to go. The male staff nurse felt guilty at failing to act as an advocate for Bill and particularly for failing to discuss the issue more forcibly with the staff nurse. In this case, 'loyalty' to the new staff nurse and a wish to maintain her confidence was, perhaps, misplaced when Bill's interests were considered.

According to Lukes (1974, 2005) view, the male staff nurse in the Case study is responsible (negatively if you like) for the situation of the patient in having to find his own way home, perhaps in discomfort. By doing nothing, he is just as powerful in the interests of the hospital rather than the patient. This can be even more important on issues arguably of greater consequence, such as whether to continue painful treatments for the very ill.

REFLECTION POINT

Can you think of incidents in your own experience where the interests of the institution were in conflict with those of the patient? To what extent did you as a nurse try to promote the interests of the patient? To what extent do you think that nurses should act as patient advocates?

Discussion points

1. What are the main sources of influence that nurses have in relation to their patients?
2. What do you feel may be some of the reasons that service users in healthcare fail to be assertive in asking for information or making clear their views about treatment and care?
3. How much does the rather pessimistic view of Michel Foucault fit with your experiences as a health professional?

CHAPTER SUMMARY

Power can be understood at many levels. The concept is complex, and yet examples can help to identify aspects such as social judgement, coercion, authority, humiliation, force, restraint, surveillance and incarceration which are among many devices we all use to access power and the ways in which both patients and nurses may gain access to it in order to influence events. It is certainly important to think more critically about such matters than may have been evident in nursing textbooks in the past. Power has consistently been seen as a legitimate professional resource based on knowledge and altruism of the nurse or doctor. Very frequently, individual nurses and other health professionals clearly have patients' interests at heart. This may not, however, prevent them frustrating patients' preferences and goals because they are different from those the professionals have in mind. In order to discuss power at all, it is necessary to leave some of the conceptual complexities to one side, since the notion is so contested. What may be important, however, is to be aware of competing notions of power so that contemporary healthcare practice may be analysed in relation to each. Observing the context of a patient receiving an enema through the perspective of Michel Foucault produces a very different analysis than, say Parsons or even Benner. Their views seem essentially flawed in the direction of experienced nurses always being 'nice people'. A critical appreciation of the sources of influence in healthcare is important. It has the implication for practice that nurses could effectively act as advocates for their patients when necessary and more importantly, will refrain from doing so when this is, in itself, a disempowering act.

FURTHER READING

Johnson M 1997 Nursing power and social judgement. Ashgate, Aldershot

Developing substantially some of the ideas in this Chapter, this book draws upon ethnographic research into the social context of decision making by nurses and others in healthcare. The book concentrates on how labelling forms a basis for the construction of nurses' and patients' relative use of and access to power.

Lawler J 1991 Behind the screens: nursing, osmology, and the problems of the body. Churchill Livingstone, Melbourne

Joclyn Lawler's book is a very stimulating and readable account of her research as a participant observer in Australian hospitals. She recounts detailed examples of how it is that nurses 'manage' the bodies of those in their care, giving in my view a realistic picture of many 'taboo' areas for discussion. She takes a pragmatic approach to the method she uses, even 'deceiving' her respondents for some of the time. Overall, one gains a sense of reality from the book which many academics fail to portray.

Lawton J (2000) The dying process: patients' experiences of palliative care. Routledge, London.

Julia Lawton's account of her doctoral study working in a UK hospice as a full time research student is exemplary. She deals with the difficult material of the experiences of people dying sensitively, yet draws out important theoretical and practical insights. She combines very moving and detailed ethnographic description with a high level of theoretical analysis.

Street AF 1992 Inside nursing: a critical ethnography of clinical nursing practice. State University of New York Press, New York

Annette Street's account of nursing practice (which, along with Lawler's is also Australian) has an explicitly feminist and critical-theory orientation. Like Lawler's book it helps to throw into stark relief the ways in which nurses and patients manage their different power bases.

REFERENCES

Benner P 1984 Novice to expert: excellence and power in nursing. Addison-Wesley, Menlo Park, CA

Benyon J 1987 Zombies in dressing gowns. In: McKeganey NP, Cunningham-Burley S (eds) Enter the sociologist, reflections on the practice of sociology. Avebury, Aldershot, p 144–173

Burden B 1998 Privacy or help? The use of curtain positioning strategies within the maternity ward environment as a means of achieving and maintaining privacy, or as a form of signalling to peers and professionals in an attempt to seek information of support. Journal of Advanced Nursing 27:15–23

Conrad P 1979 Types of medical social control. Sociology of Health and Illness 1(1):1–11

Costello, J 2001 Nursing older dying patients: findings from an ethnographic study of death and dying in elderly care wards. Journal of Advanced Nursing 35 (1):59–68

Department of Health 2005 The National Service Framework for long term conditions. Department of Health, Leeds

English J, Morse JM 1988 The 'difficult' elderly patient: adjustment or maladjustment? International Journal of Nursing Studies 25(1):23–29

Field D 1989 Nursing the dying. Routledge, London

Fineman N 1991 The social construction of non-compliance: a study of healthcare and social service providers in everyday practice. Sociology of Health and Illness 13(3):354–374

Foucault M 1991 Discipline and punish. Penguin, Harmondsworth

Freidson E 1970 Profession of medicine: a study of the sociology of applied knowledge. Dodd Mead, New York

Goffman E 1957 Alienation from Interaction. Human Relations 10:47–59

Goffman E 1968 Asylums. Penguin, Harmondsworth

Hochschild A 1983 The managed heart: Commercialization of human feeling. University of California Press: Berkeley

Holland K, ed. 2003 Applying the Roper, Logan and Tierney Model to Practice. Elsevier, London

Illich I 1976 Limits to medicine. Marion Boyars, London

James N 1989 Emotional labour: skill and work in the social regulation of feelings. Sociological Review 37(1):15–42

Johnson ML 1975 Old age and the gift relationship. New Society 31(649):639–641

Johnson M, Webb C 1995 Rediscovering unpopular patients: the concept of social judgment. Journal of Advanced Nursing 21:466–475

Johnson M 1997 Nursing power and social judgment. Ashgate, Aldershot

Kelly MP, May D 1982 Good and bad patients: a review of the literature and a theoretical critique. Journal of Advanced Nursing 7:147–156

Lawton J 2000 The dying process: patients' experiences of palliative care. Routledge, London.

Lukes S 1974 Power: A radical view. Macmillan, London

Lukes S 2005 Power: A radical view, 2nd edn. Palgrave Macmillan, Basingstoke

Mauss M (1990) The gift: Forms and functions of exchange in archaic societies. Routledge, London

Morse JM 1989 Gift-giving, reciprocity for care: gift giving in the patient – nurse relationship. Canadian Journal of Nursing Research 21 (1):33–45

Parsons T 1951 The social system. Free Press, Glencoe, IL

Roper N, Logan W, Tierney AJ 1996 The elements of nursing. Churchill Livingstone, Edinburgh

Roth JA 1972 Some contingencies of the moral evaluation and control of clientele. American Journal of Sociology 77:839–856

Russell B 1938 in Lukes S 1986 Power: The forms of power. Blackwell, Oxford

Stockwell F 1972 The unpopular patient. Royal College of Nursing, London

Strauss AL, Fagerhaugh S, Suczek B et al 1982 The work of hospitalised patients. Social Science and Medicine 16:977–986

Traynor M 1999 Managerialism and nursing. Routledge, London

Turner BS 1987 Medical power and social knowledge. Sage, London

Waterworth S, Luker K 1990 Reluctant collaborators: do patients want to be involved in decisions concerning care? Journal of Advanced Nursing 15:971–996

CHAPTER

9

Nursing and nursing professionalism

Hannah Cooke

KEY CONCEPTS

- The origins and development of modern nursing
- Nursing as women's work
- Nursing and professionalism
- The changing boundaries of nursing work

Origins and development of modern nursing

Nursing as an occupation has been carried out throughout history. We have records of nursing from ancient Greece and Rome, as well as in early Islamic society. Nursing as a separate occupation often formed part of domestic service but soon also became part of a religious vocation. Within Christianity, nursing formed part of the work of religious orders and these were to have a decisive influence on the creation of the modern occupation of nursing. It is clear that in earlier times, there were no rigid divisions between nursing and other forms of healing in the same way that there was no rigid distinction between care and cure (Stacey 1988). Stacey classifies healers as domestic, folk or professional but the boundaries between these three categories were often blurred. Much healing occurred in the domestic sphere and women learnt home remedies as an integral part of learning to manage the home. In addition, a variety of paid healers might also be consulted. For example, a wide range of different types of healer existed in Tudor England including physicians, apothecaries, barber surgeons, bone-setters and folk healers (described as 'cunning men' and 'wise women'). Approximately one-third of healers were women (Stacey 1988). Although professional physicians were the elite, even the wealthy sometimes made use of folk healers whose traditional techniques had often been tried and tested over centuries, and thus were sometimes more effective than the physicians' remedies.

Nursing as we know it today began with the nineteenth-century reforms of nursing which established what at that time was described as the 'new model nurse'. Nursing reform was closely linked to the rise of the medical profession and the creation of modern scientific medicine. The rise of modern medicine began in the eighteenth century and was closely associated with the French revolution and the period that we now describe as the 'Enlightenment' (Porter 2003). Gradually, other forms of healer (especially women) were driven out of the marketplace culminating in the Medical Registration Act in 1858, which established medicine as a state regulated profession.

The growth of modern medicine was associated with the growth of the hospital system which began in France and continued throughout the nineteenth century. Doctors were now often working in an institutional rather than a domestic sphere. Furthermore, Jewson (1976) argued that modern scientific medicine marked the death of 'bedside medicine'; a process which Foucault has described as a change in the medical 'gaze' (Foucault 1973, see Chapter 8). The new public hospitals in France allowed mass observation of the sick and for the first time a patient's symptoms could be correlated with pathological findings after death. This was the beginning of the new anatamo-clinical medicine (Porter 2002) and as doctors moved the focus of their attention from the bedside to the laboratory, the need for a reliable worker at the bedside, to observe the patient and carry out doctors' instructions, became apparent. Doctors thus wanted a better educated helper who could, for example, read medical prescriptions and drug labels.

Opinions have been divided as to the quality of nursing prior to the reforms of Florence Nightingale and her contemporaries. According to Abel Smith (1960), prior to nursing reform, hospitals employed women of the 'charwoman class' and their limited abilities reflected their poor pay and conditions. He records that provincial hospitals at this time offered nurses a weekly wage of 2s 6d at a time when a wage of 9s 6d could be obtained for work in a cotton mill. It was small wonder therefore that many hospital nurses during this period were old, infirm and illiterate. Florence Nightingale and her fellow reformers portrayed the nurses of their times in the worst possible light in order to engage support for their political project. Nevertheless, Dingwall et al (1988) suggest that their claims may have been exaggerated. They record that doctors had begun to reform the education and working conditions of nursing staff prior to the reforms of Florence Nightingale and her contemporaries and that by no means all nurses

BIO GRA PHY

Mary Seacole (1805–1881)

Mary Seacole was born Mary Grant, in Jamaica. She was the daughter of a free-born Black Jamaican woman and a Scottish soldier. She learnt nursing skills by working with her mother, who ran a boarding house for invalid British soldiers. She travelled widely in the Caribbean and Central America and became well versed in both traditional and modern medicine. She married Edwin Seacole in 1836 but was widowed in 1844. In 1854, she travelled to England to offer her services as a nurse in the Crimea, hoping her many years' experience nursing British soldiers could be put to good use. Her services were refused by the War Office and it seems likely that this refusal was motivated by racism. Undaunted, she travelled to the Crimea and set up her own hotel for wounded soldiers. She was notable for her presence on the battlefield and the war correspondent W H Russell described her as 'a warm and successful physician, who doctors and cures all manner of men with extraordinary success. She is always in attendance near the battle field to aid the wounded, and has earned many a poor fellow's blessings'.

She returned to England destitute in 1857 and a charitable subscription was set up for her by her supporters who were angered that Florence Nightingale had been feted, while she had been forgotten. She published her memoirs in 1857. She spent the rest of her life in Britain, dying in obscurity in 1881. Mary Seacole was forgotten for many years but there was a recent revival of interest in her life and her memoirs have been republished.

were the illiterate drunkards portrayed by nurse reformers, such as Nightingale and immortalized by Charles Dickens in the characters of Mrs Gamp and Betsy Prig (Dickens 1844). For example, Mary Seacole whose story has recently been rediscovered (Seacole 2004) has been described as the 'black Florence Nightingale'. She worked on the front line in the Crimea and was plainly a skilled and dedicated nurse. By contrast, Nightingale's ladies worked in the safety of a hospital and there were strict limitations to their role in 'hands on' care.

A variety of motives inspired the nursing reform movement. We can see that there was a distinct demand for a new type of hospital nurse to act as an adjunct to medicine. Some nursing reformers, although worried that nurses were incompetent, were even more preoccupied by their moral failings. This reflected wider concerns about the growth of the urban working class and the threat that they represented to the new economic and social order as Kay's contemporary report illustrates.

> *'The evils affecting the working class so far from being the necessary results of the commercial system, furnish evidence of a disease which impairs its energies if it does not threaten its vitality ... Want of cleanliness, of forethought and economy, are found in almost invariable alliance with dissipation, reckless habits and disease. The population gradually becomes physically less efficient as producers of wealth – morally so from idleness – politically worthless as having few desires to satisfy, and noxious as dissipaters of capital accumulated' (Kay 1832).*

Nursing reformers wanted the sick poor to be nursed by obedient and respectable women who would remind them of their Christian duties. The reform of nursing was seen as an important factor in the attempts to cleanse and moralize the poorer classes and thus can be seen as part of the new institutions of social control that grew up in the industrial era (Dingwall et al 1988). The growth of the industrial working class during the nineteenth century was seen as a pressing social problem. This was partly based on compassion for the conditions of the working class and concern at their appalling conditions, but perhaps even more due to a desire to contain the poor for fear that they might riot or spread immorality and disease. As we noted in Chapter 4, the discipline of the new industrial system was often resisted and draconian social measures, such as the workhouse, were employed to ensure its success. This was what Scull (1977) has called the 'era of incarceration' when the poor, the sick and the deviant were locked away in a wide variety of specialist institutions such as prisons, workhouses, asylums and sanitaria. The 'discovery of the asylum' (Rothman 1971) during this era created institutions where the poor were expected to learn new habits of cleanliness, order and obedience. Nurses played an important part in the growth of these new institutions but they also played an important role in the regulation of the poor in their homes, communities and workplaces. A number of schemes were organized to arrange 'lady visitors' to the poor to impart lessons in Christian morals and domestic economy. We can trace modern health visiting back to these early schemes.

So far, we have seen that modern nursing owes its origins to the need for a new more skilled helper for the medical profession and also to a Victorian preoccupation with the moral reform and containment of the urban poor. According to Dean and Bolton (1980: 80):

> *'The nurse was to be one element in the rich ensemble of techniques which were elaborated in the later nineteenth century so that the health, sexuality, sanitation and moral behaviour of the population could become an essential part of the art of government'.*

A further factor in the rise of modern nursing was the need of many middle and upper class spinsters to find careers which freed them from their dependence on male relatives. Women who were unwilling or unable to find husbands had few opportunities to earn a respectable living. In the mid-nineteenth century, there was a very real concern about the 'problem' of 'surplus women'. Many of the early nurse reformers were 'surplus' middle class spinsters and these lady reformers aspired to a new career directing the lower orders of nursing just as their married sisters directed their household servants. The links to domestic service were strong. Summers (1989) has suggested that the rise of the middle classes brought changes to domestic service which fed the demand for a new class of nurse in the private sphere as well as in the hospital:

> *'In the 1840s and 1850s new conventions were being established for the hierarchy, dress and behaviour of female domestic servants. They were to wear the uniform of the household, to speak only when spoken to, to know their place and to answer, very often, to a name of their employer's choosing. Gamp, Prig and Woodward represented a survival of earlier conventions: their clothes did not blend with the décor, they occupied no fixed rung in the service hierarchy, they were addressed by their own names, and they expected to be able to voice, and even enforce, their own opinions'. (Summers 1989: 373)*

Thus, the faults of nineteenth century private nurses included their 'vulgarity' which caused offence to their middle class employers and their alleged ignorance and insubordination which offended both the doctor and employer. Summers suggests that the movement for nursing reform was 'many stranded', bringing together:

> *'male physicians and surgeons, religious reformers of both sexes, and all those anxious to expand professional opportunities for women' (Summers 1989: 365).*

Thus, the demands of doctors and middle class employers for a more reliable and biddable employee became linked to social and religious reformers' attempts to cleanse and moralize the poor and also, ironically perhaps, to the movement for female emancipation. Since so many contending interests became involved in the reformation of the nurse it is not surprising that the 'new model nurse' was to be all things to all people as is manifest in the lengthy list of virtues that reformers of this era expected her to display. For example, Eva Luckës, Matron to the London Hospital, required the following:

> *'Nurses are required to be truthful, obedient, punctual, calm, cheerful, pleasant, clean and neat. It is important that they should bring the valuable qualities of memory, forethought, and method to bear upon their work, in addition to the essential characteristics of unselfishness and a genuine sympathy with suffering ... Well-managed hospitals afford abundant opportunities for the necessary exercise of the very qualities that need strengthening and developing in the characters of most women. By faithfully carrying out the rules laid down for her guidance, an intelligent nurse will soon appreciate the fact that many of them are calculated to help her far more than she would have imagined possible. But it is only those who are prepared to accept this temporary rule of life in the right spirit who will derive full benefit from it'. (Luckës 1899: 11)*

We can sum up the contradictory expectations imposed on the 'new model nurse' in the phrase 'intelligent obedience'. Nurses were expected to exercise independent judgement but also to know when to be submissive. They were expected to be intelligent but not too intelligent. They were expected to have a degree of medical knowledge but never to question a doctor's judgement. These contradictory expectations have continued to influence the development of nursing as an occupation to this day. The rationale behind these contradictory ideas was the 'separate spheres' theory of a gendered division of labour (Rafferty 1996). Men and women in the workplace should have different roles and areas of jurisdiction just as they did in the household.

REFLECTION POINT

The nineteenth century nursing leader, Eva Luckes, listed a formidable list of virtues that she expected of nurses. What do you think are the qualities expected of nurses today? Traditionally nurses were expected to display 'intelligent obedience'. To what extent do you think that this quality is expected of contemporary nurses?

The woman credited with the creation of the nursing profession was Florence Nightingale. She subscribed firmly to the doctrine of 'separate spheres' stating that 'nursing and medicine must never be mixed up' (cited in Rafferty 1996). We can see many contradictory ideas expressed in her writings and more starkly in the myths that have come to characterize the many and varied stories of her life.

According to Whittaker and Oleson (1964), the story of Florence Nightingale's life has become a 'heroine legend' and Dingwall et al (1988) note the difficulty of separating myth from reality. Different aspects of the Nightingale myth appeal to different groups and her story has been used to lend support to a multitude of conflicting causes. Early popular biographies claimed that she had an innate desire to care and nursed and bandaged her dolls from the earliest age, thus emphasizing her support for traditional female roles. By contrast, other authors have presented her as an early feminist and seen her nursing reforms as 'an instalment of the emancipation of women' (Abel Smith 1960). Nursing traditionalists presented her as 'the lady of the lamp', selflessly devoting herself to the care of her patients and used her story to justify long hours and poor working conditions (Godden 1997). In contrast, her administrative rather than

BIOGRAPHY Florence Nightingale (1820–1910)

Florence Nightingale was by no means the only important nurse reformer of the nineteenth century, but her name has become synonymous with the creation of the profession, due to the enormous influence which she wielded following her work in the Crimea (Baly 1997).

Nightingale was born in Florence in 1820 to an affluent and influential family. She expressed an interest in nursing during her 20s and developed a connection with religious Sisterhoods, which led to her studying with a Protestant nursing order at Kaiserwerth during 1850 and 1851. In 1853, she became superintendent of a charitable institution for sick 'gentlewomen'. According to Dingwall et al (1988), she modelled her superintendence on the management of a large household and had strict ideas about economy, discipline and moral order. The results of her superintendence were sometimes unfortunate. During her 12 months stay, she imposed rigid rules and economies on the inmates whom she regarded with deep suspicion. She is also said to have got through two complete sets of servants. Her ideas nevertheless impressed social reformers of the time, leading to her being asked to lead a party of nurses to go out to the Crimean war. Her impact remains controversial. She and her supporters claimed that her intervention was an astounding success leading to a dramatic fall in the death rate. Detractors expressed reservations about these claims (Summers 1988). Whatever the facts of the case, following her return from the Crimea,

Nightingale was treated as a national heroine who came to have an enormous influence over the reform of nursing, even though she spent most of the rest of her life confined to bed by a mystery illness. She was asked to oversee the reform of nurse training at St Thomas' Hospital, and the 'Nightingale School' became the pattern for the training of the 'new model nurse'. Nightingale was a prolific writer and her ideas remain influential. She believed in 'sanitary' reform, saying that hospitals should 'do the sick no harm'. Light, quiet, cleanliness, fresh air and good diet were central to the fight against disease. She was a keen statistician and saw statistical analysis as essential to hospital administration. She pioneered the comparison of hospital death rates and is credited with the invention of the pie chart (Maindonald and Richardson 2004).

nursing skills have been emphasized by those advocating increased managerialism. The Griffiths report (1983) which introduced 'general management' into the NHS stated:

> *'If Florence Nightingale were carrying her lamp through the corridors of the NHS today she would almost certainly be searching for the people in charge'. (Griffiths report 1983: 12)*

Ironically, Griffiths used the Nightingale myth to justify axing nursing managers and putting nurses under the control of 'general' managers. More recently, Nightingale's 'passion' for statistics has been highlighted to claim her as a founder of the 'evidence-based practice' movement (McDonald 2001). Her religious writings still attract the attentions of evangelical Christians and some contemporary supporters of evidence-based practice might be surprised to learn that she regarded statistics as a 'religious service', which enabled statisticians to know the 'character of God'.

If the story of Nightingale is riven with contradictions then so also is the development of nursing from its earliest origins to the present day. We will consider these contradictions throughout this chapter beginning by looking at the gendered nature of the occupation. To what extent is nursing 'women's work' operating in a 'separate sphere' from medicine as Nightingale suggested?

REFLECTION POINT

In the next section, we are going to think about nursing as 'women's work'. Early nursing leaders thought that feminine qualities were essential to nursing. Before you go on to the next section, think about your own experience of nursing. To what extent is it still regarded as 'women's work'? What impact has this had on the professional status of nurses?

Nursing as women's work?

According to Eva Gamarnikow (1978), early nursing theorists based their ideas on biological determinism. They believed it was 'natural' for women to care and for men to take charge. The division of labour between doctors and nurses was based therefore on the 'natural' order of things. Writing from a feminist perspective Gamarnikow challenged these ideas. She saw the division of labour between doctors and nurses as social and not biological. She said that doctors had 'defined femininity in terms of the patriarchal feminine subordination to safeguard their own dominance'. She pointed out that the roles assigned to doctor, nurse and patient replicated the roles of father, mother and child within the Victorian household (for a further discussion of roles within the family, see Chapter 2). The doctor gave the orders, the nurse carried them out, the patient did as he was told and like the Victorian child, was expected to be 'seen and not heard'. We can see therefore that this division of labour had many drawbacks for patients as well as nurses.

According to Hart (2004), this association with the 'oppressed mother' has long oppressed nursing. Just as the father was defined by his work, so the doctor has clear parameters to his role. The nurse however just like the mother must always 'be there' and is thus expected to get on and cope with anything and everything else. This 'unlimited liability' (Aldridge 1994) has had a profound and often negative impact on the status and working conditions of nurses. In particular, it has made it extraordinarily difficult for nurses themselves to define the boundaries of nursing. We will return to this issue later.

Extending this domestic metaphor, Stein (1967) described a ritual of nurse–doctor interaction which he called the 'doctor–nurse game'. Nurses and doctors played out traditional gender roles in the workplace. The nurse had to learn to make suggestions to the doctor without undermining his authority or appearing to be openly assertive. She learnt to make treatment recommendations covertly in such a way that they appeared to be initiated by the physician. Nurses were therefore expected to adopt a role which conformed to the stereotype of the wife who used 'feminine wiles' to get round her husband rather than being allowed to adopt the role of an assertive and respected professional. To put it in the language of Hochschild (1983), the nurse was expected to engage in emotional labour (see Chapter 4) in order that the physician could save face. In 1990, Stein 'revisited' the 'doctor–nurse game' and noted that nurses had 'decided to stop playing the game' and had become more openly assertive (Stein 1990). What had changed to bring this about?

The nineteenth century nurse reformers were trying to build a professional career for nurses at a time when few other occupational opportunities for women existed. Given the attitudes to women at that time, this was no mean achievement. A century later, economic and social conditions had changed dramatically. New rights for women in the workplace were coupled with a growth in service sector employment where 'soft' skills such as caring and communication traditionally associated with women workers were in high demand. Nursing was only one career out of many that women could choose to pursue.

The gender structure of healthcare changed markedly in the late twentieth century. Male nurses were not admitted to the Royal College of Nursing until 1960 and prior to this period, male nurses were concentrated in mental health nursing and were members of trade unions. Gradually, general nursing began to open up to male nurses who quickly came to assume a disproportionately higher number of senior positions than their numbers would merit (Hart 2004). Men make up around 10% of the nursing workforce but occupy approximately 40% of senior posts. Male nurses are over-represented in nursing management, research and education (Miers 2000). During the late twentieth century, the numbers of women in medicine began to climb, and by the 1990s, 50% of medical students were women. The traditional 'doctor–nurse game' had become outmoded and in many situations, nurses had become more assertive (Allen 1997). This did not necessarily imply an end to gender inequalities in healthcare but that they were no longer ordered simply around the doctor–nurse relationship.

In these circumstances, the nurse's role as a doctor's 'handmaiden' had come to be openly questioned and nurses had developed a range of strategies to assert their professional independence. Education was seen by many as the key to professional advancement and by the end of the century, nurse education had transferred to the university sector and nurses had developed their own body of theory and research. However, the impact of these changes on the realities of nursing at the bedside was a matter of some debate (Dingwall & Allen 2001). What exactly was the nature and purpose of nursing professionalism?

REFLECTION POINT

In the next section, we are going to look at nursing professionalism. You were asked to think about what professionalism meant, in Chapter 3. You may wish to go back to Chapter 3 to remind yourself of this. Think about what professionalism means to you before reading on.

Nursing professionalism

We noted in Chapter 4 that occupational groups often pursue the traits of professionals in order to try to claim the advantages that go with professional status and that professional 'traits' included the following:

- Skill based on theoretical knowledge
- The provision of education and training
- The testing of member competence
- The existence of a professional body
- Adherence to a code of conduct
- Emphasis on altruistic service.

Early nurse reformers were preoccupied with establishing nursing as a respected occupation. Nursing was described as altruistic service; a 'vocation' and the high moral character of the nurse was emphasized. Indeed 'character' was central to the development of the 'new model nurse' (Rafferty 1996). Thus, early in its development nurses made moral claims about their occupation. It was an occupation which claimed the ethical standards of the professions; an occupation which demanded respect.

For some nurses, this led to the demand for professional registration similar to that achieved by doctors in the 1858 Medical Registration Act. This was an issue which divided nursing for 30 years. The leading advocate of state registration was Ethel Bedford Fenwick who founded the British Nursing Association. She saw state registration of nurses as facilitating independent careers for nurses. Many of the bigger training institutions opposed state registration. The voluntary hospitals maintained their own register of the nurses that they had trained and this list gave these institutions considerable control over the nursing labour market. Without state registration, nurses were dependent on the hospitals in which they trained to recommend them for work. Florence Nightingale opposed nurse registration on the grounds that the moral character of the nurse could not be taught, examined or regulated by the state. Thus, from its earliest origins, some nursing leaders expressed ambivalence about nursing's professional status.

State registration was first proposed in the 1880s and six Bills were unsuccessfully brought before parliament between 1904 and 1918. The Nurses Act which established state registration was finally passed in 1919. It was successful at this time largely because of wider social changes in the position of women due in part to the First World War and also partly due to the Suffragettes' successful campaign for votes for women. According to Hart (2004), state registration was also seen as a way to prevent nurses from joining the trade union movement. Nursing has had three successive professional bodies. The 1919 Act established the General Nursing Council. This body was replaced in 1983 by the United Kingdom Central Council for Nursing Midwifery and Health Visiting (UKCC). This body introduced the Code of Conduct in 1992. The UKCC was replaced by the Nursing and Midwifery Council in 2002 and a revised code of conduct was produced in the same year only to be revised again during 2007. During this period, professional self-regulation had come under hostile public scrutiny. Nursing has found itself defending its recently acquired professional traits at a time of growing managerialism. As we discussed in Chapter 4, as a result of the growth of managerialism, professionalism has come under attack and professions have become increasingly fragmented. These recent developments have also tended to fragment the nursing profession.

Witz (1994) has described nursing's pursuit of professional registration as the 'legalistic' approach to professionalization. At the same time, nursing pursued a 'credentialist' approach to professionalization through the reform of nurse education. A key demand of Ethel Bedford Fenwick had been for 3-year training for nurses. This was opposed at the time by many training institutions who considered 1 year to be an adequate training period. Thus, from its earliest origins, there were demands to strengthen and improve nurse training; demands which were often resisted by those in authority, usually for reasons of cost. In 1972, the 'Briggs report' advocated reform of nurse education but this was not taken forward until the 1990s although a small number of nursing degrees were set up from the 1960s onwards. The 'Project 2000' reforms removed student nurse training from hospitals into higher education. Basic training would be through a new 3-year undergraduate diploma in nursing which also removed nurses from service provision.

Members of the profession such as the UKCC had intended that this would lead to more patient care being carried out by qualified nurses but they were to be disappointed (Davies 1995). The government acceptance of Project 2000 was conditional on nurses accepting the training of a new grade of 'support worker' by the National Council for Vocational Qualifications that would be outside the profession's control. Soon after the implementation of Project 2000, there was evidence of skill-mix dilution as students and qualified nurses were replaced with NVQ-trained support workers or unqualified care assistants. According to Thornley (1996), the reforms have led to greater 'segmentation and inequality' in the nursing workforce. The introduction of support workers lowered the pay floor in nursing (Grimshaw 1999) and offered alternative qualifications in competition with professional qualifications (Allen 2001).

A key demand of Project 2000 was that programmes were educationally driven and students' experiences based on their educational needs rather than service needs. However the government's 'Working for Patients' market reforms were extended to nurse education and local service managers were given a decisive role in the commissioning of nurse education. This has had a devastating effect on the stability of nurse education leading to dramatic year on year fluctuations in the numbers of places funded (Allen 2001, Hart 2004).

The success of the 'Project 2000' reforms in raising the status of the profession has therefore been mixed. However, even though the reforms were diluted by government interventions the introduction of university nurse education led to much hostile criticism of nurses. Healthcare was undergoing many changes during this period with the introduction of the internal market, increased managerialism and massive cutbacks in inpatient services. Placing the blame for a perceived decline on standards on university nurse education offered an easy target and a convenient one for those in power. Meerabeau (2004) has described a 'counter reformation' in English nurse education. Press commentators suggested that nursing was a practical occupation that required 'motherly souls' not 'college girls'. Nurses were accused of being over educated and these criticisms led to the 'Making a Difference' reforms which further strengthened the Department of Health's control over the nursing curriculum (Meerabeau 2004).

Latterly, nurses have been accused of being 'too posh to wash' and 'too clever to care' (Scott 2004). At the same time, growth in the employment of NVQ-trained support workers and untrained care assistants has eroded nurses' jurisdiction over hands on care and fragmented care delivery. This has been compounded by the invention of the concept of 'social care' which places much of what would once have been considered nursing care entirely outside the domain of nursing. The debate about whether it was possible for nurses to be 'too clever to care' went to the heart of the debate about nursing professionalism. It is impossible to think about this issue without referring back to the gendered nature of nursing (Witz 1994). These recent debates have their roots in the earliest debates about how nursing should develop. Is 'caring' something that can be taught or a natural attribute of individual (normally female) 'character' as critics of Project 2000 have implied? Should nursing education restore the 'domestic academy' advocated by Florence Nightingale and give up its pretensions to professional status? If 'caring' is a matter of 'character', then on what basis do nurses lay claim to professionalism?

REFLECTION POINT

In this section we have looked at the changing nature of nursing professionalism. We have considered in particular the role of contemporary nurses in delivering bedside care. To what extent do you think that modern nurses have become 'too posh to wash' and 'too clever to care'?

Defining nursing

Critics of Project 2000 saw a binary division between cleverness and caring. Nurses did not need to be clever to care. Many went further; cleverness was an impediment to caring (Meerabeau 2004). By contrast, nurses themselves were beginning to articulate professional aspirations which put caring at the centre of nursing's professional identity and which identified caring as a highly skilled activity.

Skeggs' (1997) study of care assistants found that care assistants 'celebrated the practical not academic self'. Care assistants described caring as a 'natural' attribute of personality and claimed caring as an unlearned activity. Care work offered working class girls a sense of self worth inasmuch as they could identify themselves as a 'caring person'. However, studies of care assistant work frequently show care assistants conforming to industrial models of work with a focus on routines and on 'getting through the work' (Clarke 1978). This depersonalizes patients by treating them as work objects to be processed. For example Lee Treweek's (1994, 1997) study of nursing homes shows care assistants engaged in the production of the 'lounge standard patient' (clean, tidy and ready to be wheeled out and parked in the lounge area of the home). This led to 'bedroom abuse' as care assistants delivered care as if working on a production line. Lee Treweek says that we need to look to studies of factory work to understand working conditions in nursing homes. Thus, the domestic ideologies which construe care as 'natural' also help to construct care as routinized, low paid and low status work.

By contrast, nursing theorists have tried to articulate the importance of skilled and knowledgeable caring which recognizes the 'unique needs' of each individual patient. According to nursing theorists effective caring, particularly of the very ill, required more than a kind heart and a willing pair of hands. In the 1970s, Mcfarlane (1970) identified caring as the 'proper study' of the nurse and stressed the value of giving attention to the minutiae of basic nursing care. The feminist writer, Ann Oakley (1984) (see Chapter 2) also defended the importance of what nurses do and suggested that feminists needed to assert the value of caring. In the 1980s, theorists such as Patricia Benner emphasized the ways in which nurses combined moral commitment, skill, academic knowledge and experience to produce 'expert' nursing care (Benner 1984, Benner & Wrubel 1989). For the care assistants studied by Skeggs caring was simply a matter of 'character' but for nursing theorists character was insufficient; in depth knowledge and the refinement of clinical skills were also required. Furthermore, nurse researchers were able to establish empirically that skilled care by registered nurses improved outcomes in acutely ill patients (Needleman 2001).

Nurses themselves have been much exercised by the problem of defining nursing. There have been many definitions of nursing, the most widely accepted of which is that of Virginia Henderson. In 1964, Virginia Henderson defined the 'unique function' of the nurse:

> *'The unique function of the nurse is to assist the individual, sick or well, in performance of those activities contributing to health or its recovery (or peaceful death) that he/she would perform unaided if he/she had the necessary strength, will or knowledge. And to do this in such a way as to help him/her gain independence as rapidly as possible' (Henderson 1964: 63).*

In 1987, Reverby said that nurses had been 'ordered to care' by a society which did not value caring. Much of the recent professional energies of nursing have concentrated on 'recentring' caring and asserting its value. Increasingly nursing theorists presented 'caring' as the unique and autonomous domain of nurses.

BIO GRA PHY Virginia Henderson (1897–1996)

Virginia Henderson has been described as the 'foremost nurse of the twentieth century'. She was born in Kansas and enlisted in the army school of nursing during the First World War. After practicing in New York she taught nursing at Columbia University from 1930–1948. She began to research nursing at Yale University in 1953. Her *Principles and Practice of Nursing* has become a nursing classic and her definition of nursing has been widely adopted. She continues to be an important influence on nursing research, education and practice.

Since the 1960s the study of professionalism had moved on from the trait approach to highlight, above anything else, the 'autonomous and self directing' nature of professional work (Freidson 1970). Nursing leaders would begin to see that the trappings of professionalism were necessary but not sufficient for occupational advancement. According to Freidson:

> *'By the turn of the century nursing had become a full fledged occupation rather than a sideline of gentility or charity, and a fairly dignified occupation with a status independent of the clientele it served. As first established its 'code' stressed skilful and intelligent execution of the doctor's orders but in time the question came to be raised, 'Are we still subservient or do we make intelligent responses to instructions?' The leaders of nursing came to be concerned that nursing be neither a dilution of medicine or an accretion of the functions medicine had sloughed off. While nursing originally established itself as a full-fledged occupation of some dignity by tying itself to the coat-tails of medicine, it has come to be greatly concerned with finding a new independent position in the division of labour' (Freidson 1970: 63).*

Thus, nursing leaders came to be much pre-occupied with nurses' occupational subordination to medicine and this has been frequently linked to gender politics (Davies 1995). The attempt to develop nursing 'theories' and 'models' emphasized both the esoteric nature of nursing knowledge and its independence from medicine. Nursing models were linked to the development of new methods of organizing nursing, such as 'primary nursing' and the 'nursing process' which emphasized the professional autonomy of the nurse.

These developments were described by Salvage (1992) as the 'new' nursing. They offered a private practice model of nursing similar to that advocated by Mrs Bedford Fenwick. Nursing would be oriented around an individualized professional–client relationship between and nurses would give 'holistic' care. Psychological care was given a new prominence alongside physical care. 'New' nursing was contrasted with 'traditional' nursing which was described as dominated by tradition, routine and 'task allocation', all of which were seen as unworthy of an occupation aspiring to be an independent profession. Thus, nursing was trying to model itself on what Krause (1996) has described as the 'guild' model of the established professions (see Chapter 4). Unfortunately, nursing chose to pursue the 'guild' model at a time when according to Krause the 'last guilds' such as medicine were under severe attack from corporate interests.

What Krause describes as the corporate attack on the 'last guilds' is characterized elsewhere as the conflict between managerialism (see Chapter 4) and professionalism (Traynor 1999). Nurses have increasingly come under the control of lay managers first by the introduction of general management in the 1980s and more recently by the steady move towards US-style 'managed care' (see Chapter 7). The managerialist vision for nursing has largely entailed the extension of Taylorist controls over the nursing workforce in order to get 'more for less' from nurses. Following the 'Babbage principle' (see Chapter 4), managers have increased nurses' workloads and where possible replaced registered nurses by cheaper grades of staff. Managed care increasingly delivers 'McDonaldization' (Ritzer 1996), which extends assembly line techniques into the care sector. Work intensification has been a very real experience for many nurses (Adams et al 2000). In many instances, work intensification has involved simply increasing workloads and leaving nurses to 'cope' with the consequences (Ackroyd & Bolton 1999). However, there have also been active attempts to increase labour flexibility and productivity in nursing by for example, manipulating shift patterns, changing role boundaries and diluting skill mix (Cooke 2006). At the same time, registered nurses have been offered opportunities to act as doctor substitutes carrying out routine technical tasks such as intravenous cannulation and minor surgery. The recent attempts to 'modernize' nurses' careers have ratcheted up the pressure for labour flexibility in nursing promising 'a competency based work system to drive service and role redesign' (DoH 2006).The effects on care at the bedside have seldom been evaluated (Calpin-Davies & Akehurst 1999).

Managerialism has also led according to Lawler (1999) to a pressure to render nursing work 'transparent, observable, explicit and costable in economic terms'. Nursing has become increasingly subject to rigid protocols of practice, performance measurement, audit and target setting. We noted in Chapter 4 that the recognition of the indeterminacy of professional work was an important mark of professionalism. Nurses' work has always contained a high degree of indeterminacy and uncertainty as is apparent in Henderson's description of the 'unique function' of the nurse. However, the indeterminacy of nursing work has been neither recognized nor rewarded. As Reverby (1987) has said nurses have offered a caring service in a society that did not value caring. As nursing has acquired more of the traits of a profession so nurses have sought the public recognition of caring as a valuable activity. Nursing leaders such as Henderson have articulated a claim for professionalism based on the provision of 'holistic' or 'individualized' caring which recognizes the unique needs of each individual patient. The provision of individualized care is the cornerstone of nursing's contemporary professional identity. Sadly, it is debatable whether employers have been willing to recognize and value the unique contribution of the nurse. The hostile public reaction to some aspects of nursing advancement such as nursing degrees suggest a society that still wants to see caring as a gendered activity which requires little skill or reward. The contemporary ethos of economic rationalism and managerialism has created healthcare systems that place even less value on caring than they did formerly. Thus, according to Henderson (1986: 1):

> *'With more and more health agencies and institutions coming under the dominion of corporate industrialised management it is increasingly difficult to preserve the humane values in healthcare'.*

According to a number of nursing authors (Wigens 1997) managerialized systems leave less and less space for nurses to offer individualized care to patients. Henderson also notes:

> *'Ours is the 'worst of times' for nurses because it is a period of accelerated technological change in healthcare and nurses (who are with the sick, the handicapped and the dying more hours of the day than any other category of health worker) bear the brunt of trying to make these changes constructive rather than destructive. Nurses everywhere are frustrated because within existing systems they are so often unable to give the supportive care that they believe would enable people to recover from disease, cope with a handicap or die peacefully when death is inevitable'. (Henderson 1986: 1)*

Recent studies of bedside nursing have confirmed that nurses have been under considerable pressure to move away from supportive care. According to Latimer (2000), care at the bedside is becoming 'less and less visible' and nurses are being forced to take on more and more technical and managerial work. She suggests that nursing will thus become a less desirable occupation for those with a traditional vocation to care for others. The question that has to be asked is whether nurses should still pursue these vocational ideals.

According to Dingwall and Allen (2001), nurses need to re-think the future of nursing in response to recent reforms. Nurses need 'a little more realism' about the nature of nursing and should give up their dream of offering holistic care. They employ Everett Hughes' theories about professional work. According to Hughes a profession has first, a *licence*, which specifies what society allows it to do. The licence therefore describes the constraints of an occupation's work situation – what it is allowed to do. Second, a profession has a *mandate* which expresses the culture and ideals of the profession. In setting out its *mandate*, a profession states what it believes it ought to be able to do. A large gap between an occupation's *licence* and *mandate* is a recipe for dissatisfaction and low morale. Aspirations are thwarted by the realities of the work situation. Dingwall and Allen blame nurse educators for fostering 'self-indulgent' myths about the mandate of nursing. In focussing on holistic care, they say that nurse educators prepare nurses 'to do a job that did not exist in the past, does not exist in the present and may never exist in the future'. Nurses instead need to recognize that nursing's *licence* has always been as an adjunct to medicine and that nursing has the scope to extend its licence primarily as an auxiliary to medicine as technology advances. It needs therefore to give up its 'mandate claim' to offer holistic care and embrace the new technical roles that have been offered. What happens to care in this scenario is unclear. Presumably, it returns to the domain of untrained 'motherly souls'.

Discussion points

1. To what extent is caring still the 'unique contribution' of nurses?
2. What do you think that nurses could do to promote the value of caring?
3. To what extent do you think that nurses should move into new technical roles such as surgeon's assistant?
4. To what extent do you think that nurses require an academic education? Do you think that the move into higher education has helped or hindered the professional status of nurses?

CHAPTER SUMMARY

This Chapter has outlined the development of nursing and has described some of the historical events which have influenced the creation of the occupation we know today. It has considered the extent to which nursing can be considered as 'women's work' as well as the extent to which nursing can be considered to be a profession.

A fundamental problem for nurses has always been that care work has always been carried out by the untrained and unpaid. It has therefore been difficult for nurses to assert the value of their expertise and to define the boundaries of the profession. The gendered nature of care work has meant that caring is too easily construed as a 'natural' activity requiring little training or reward. Nevertheless by the twentieth century, nursing had succeeded as establishing itself as a 'profession of some dignity', as Freidson (1970) noted.

By the mid-twentieth century, nursing had established caring as its unique domain (Henderson 1964). However, recent reforms have tended to fragment care and to remove much care work from the jurisdiction of the nursing profession. The question for nurses to ask in future is whether nurses continue to defend their traditional vocational ideals or move with the times and develop more technical roles as an adjunct to medicine. Dingwall and Allen (2001) make a credible, pragmatic case for taking the latter option. However, these are matters not just of pragmatism but of values and beliefs. How we value and reward caring tells us how much value we as a society place on the most vulnerable members of our society. Traditionally, nurses were expected to make sacrifices on society's behalf and rightly came to object to being 'ordered to care' by a society which did not value care. The question now for nurses is do we continue to assert the value of care in a society which may turn a deaf ear on our arguments or do we abandon our defence of care and develop new roles? This is an ethical question that each and every nurse needs to contemplate.

FURTHER READING

Allen D 2001 The changing shape of nursing practice. Routledge, London.

Discusses recent changes in nursing.

Dingwall R, Rafferty M, Webster C 1988 An introduction to the social history of nursing. Routledge, London.

A good introduction to nursing history.

Hart C 2004 Nurses and politics: the impact of power and practice. Palgrave Macmillan, Basingstoke.

Discusses the relationship between nurses and politics.

Latimer J 2000 The conduct of care. Blackwell, Oxford.

Gives an interesting ethnographic account of contemporary nursing.

Miers M 2000 Gender issues and nursing practice. Macmillan, Basingstoke.

Discusses gender issues in nursing.

Seacole M 2004 [first published 1857] The wonderful adventures of Mrs Seacole in many lands. The X Press, London.

A wonderfully fascinating account of the life of an early nurse.

REFERENCES

Abel Smith B 1960 A history of the nursing profession. Heinemann, London

Ackroyd S, Bolton S 1999 It is not Taylorism: Mechanisms of work intensification in the provision of gynaecological services in a NHS hospital. Work, Employment and Society 13(2): 369–387

Adams A, Lugsden E, Chase J 2000 Skill mix changes and work intensification in nursing. Work, Employment and Society 14(3):541–555

Aldridge M 1994 Unlimited liability, emotional labour in nursing and social work. Journal of Advanced Nursing 20(4):722–728

Allen D 1997 The nursing-medical boundary: a negotiated order. Sociology of Health and Illness 19(4):498–520

Allen D 2001 The changing shape of nursing practice. Routledge, London

Baly M 1997 Florence Nightingale and the nursing legacy. Whurr, London

Benner P 1984 From novice to expert: Excellence and power in clinical nursing practice. Addison-Wesley, CA

Benner P, Wrubel J 1989 The primacy of caring: Stress and coping in health and illness. Addison-Wesley, CA
Calpin-Davies P, Akehurst R 1999 Doctor-Nurse substitution: The workforce equation. Journal of Nursing Management 7:71–79
Clarke M 1978 Getting through the work. In: Dingwall R, McIntosh J (eds) Sociology of Nursing. Churchill Livingstone, Edinburgh p 67–86
Cooke H 2006 Seagull management and the control of nursing work. Work, Employment and Society 20(2):223–243
Davies C 1995 Gender and the professional predicament of nursing. Open University Press, Buckingham
Dean M, Bolton G 1980 The administration of poverty and the development of nursing practice in nineteenth century England. In: Davies C (ed.) Rewriting nursing history. Croom Helm, London, p 76–102
Department of Health 2006 Modernising nursing careers. Department of Health, London
Dickens C 1844 (1982 World's Classics Edition), Martin Chuzzlewit. Oxford University Press, Oxford
Dingwall R, Allen D 2001 The implications of healthcare reform for the profession of nursing. Nursing Inquiry 8(2):64
Dingwall R, Rafferty M, Webster C 1988 An introduction to the social history of nursing. Routledge, London
Foucault M 1973 The birth of the clinic: An archaeology of medical perception. Tavistock, London
Freidson E 1970 Profession of medicine: A study in the sociology of applied knowledge. Dodd & Mead, London
Gamarnikow E 1978 Sexual division of labour: The case of nursing In: Kuhn A, Wolpe A (eds) Feminism and materialism. Routledge and Kegan Paul, London, p 96–123
Godden J 1997 'For the benefit of mankind'. Nightingale's legacy and hours of work in Australian nursing 1868–1939 In: Rafferty A, Robinson J, Elkan R (eds) Nursing history and the politics of welfare. Routledge, London, p 177–192
Griffiths Report 1983 NHS management inquiry. DHSS, London
Grimshaw D 1999 Changes in skill mix and pay determination among the nursing workforce in the UK. Work, Employment and Society 13(2):295–328
Hart C 2004 Nurses and politics: the impact of power and practice. Palgrave Macmillan, Basingstoke
Henderson V 1964 The nature of nursing. American Journal of Nursing 64(8):62–68
Henderson V 1986 Some observations on healthcare by health services or health industries. Journal of Advanced Nursing 11:1–2
Hochschild A 1983 The managed heart: The commercialization of human feeling. University of California Press, Berkeley
Jewson N 1976 The disappearance of the sick man from medical cosmology. Sociology 10:225–244
Kay J P 1832 The moral and physical condition of the working classes employed in the cotton manufacture of Manchester. Reprinted in Evans E (ed.) 1978 Social policy 1830–1914. Routledge and Kegan Paul, London, p 73
Krause E 1996 The death of the guilds: Professions, states and the advance of capitalism, 1930 to the present. Yale University Press, New Haven
Latimer J 2000 The conduct of care. Blackwell, Oxford
Lawler J 1999 De(con)struction of nursing work: economic rationalism and regulation. Nursing Inquiry 6(2):141
Lee Treweek G 1994 Bedroom abuse: the hidden work in a nursing home. Generations Review 4:2–4
Lee Treweek G 1997 Women, resistance and care: An ethnographic study of nursing auxiliary work. Work Employment and Society 11(1): 47–63
Luckës E 1899 General nursing. Kegan Paul, Trench, Trubner, London
Maindonald J, Richardson A 2004 This passionate study: A dialogue with Florence Nightingale. Journal of Statistics Education 12:1
McDonald L 2001 Florence Nightingale and the early origins of evidence based nursing. Evidence Based Nursing 4:68–69
McFarlane J 1970 The proper study of the nurse. RCN, London
Meerabeau E 2004 Be good, sweet maid, and let who can be clever: a counter reformation in English nursing education? International Journal of Nursing Studies 41(3):285–292
Miers M 2000 Gender issues and nursing practice. Macmillan Press, Basingstoke
Needleman J 2001 Nurse staffing and patient outcomes in hospital. US Department of Health and Human Services and Harvard School of Public Health, Boston
Oakley A 1984 The importance of being a nurse. Nursing Times 80(50):24–27
Porter R 2002 Blood and guts: A short history of medicine. Penguin, Harmondsworth
Porter R 2003 Flesh in the age of reason. Allen Lane, London
Rafferty A 1996 The politics of nursing knowledge. Routledge, London

Reverby S 1987 Ordered to care: the dilemma of American nursing 1850–1945. Cambridge University Press, Cambridge

Ritzer G 1996 The McDonaldization of society. Pine Forge Press, Thousand Oaks

Rothman D 1971 The discovery of the asylum. Little Brown, Boston

Salvage J 1992 New nursing: Empowering patients or empowering nurses? In Robinson J et al (eds) Policy issues in nursing. Open University Press, Buckingham, p 9–23

Scull A 1977 Decarceration. Prentice Hall, NJ

Scott H 2004 Are nurses 'too clever to care' and 'too posh to wash? 'British Journal of Nursing 13(10):581

Seacole M 2004 [first published in 1857] The wonderful adventures of Mrs Seacole in many lands. The X Press, London

Skeggs B 1997 Formations of class and gender. Sage, London

Stacey M 1988 The sociology of health and healing: A textbook. Routledge, London

Stein L 1967 The doctor–nurse game. Archives of General Psychiatry 16:699–703

Stein L 1990 The doctor–nurse game revisited. New England Journal of Medicine 322:546–549

Summers A 1989 The mysterious demise of Sarah Gamp: The domiciliary nurse and her detractors c. 1830–1860. Victorian Studies, Spring:365–386

Summers A 1988 Angels and citizens: British women as military nurses. Routledge and Kegan Paul, London

Thornley C 1996 Segmentation and inequality in the nursing workforce. In Crompton R, Gallie D, Purcell K (eds) Changing forms of employment: Organization, skills and gender. Routledge, London, p 160–182

Traynor M 1999 Managerialism and nursing: Beyond oppression and profession. Routledge, London

Whittaker E, Oleson V 1964 The faces of Florence Nightingale: Functions of the heroine legend in an occupational subculture. Human Organization 23:23–30

Wigens L 1997 The conflict between "new nursing" and "scientific management" as perceived by surgical nurses. Journal of Advanced Nursing 28(2):419–427

Witz A 1994 The challenge of nursing. In: Gabe J, Kelleher D, Williams G (eds) Challenging medicine. Routledge, London, p 23–46

CHAPTER

10 Partnerships and care in the community

Susan Lambert

KEY CONCEPTS

- The policy context of social care
- The mixed economy of care
- Partnership working
- The care divide and the 'social bath'
- Informal care

Introduction

This chapter will explore policies underpinning service developments in community settings for service users with complex care needs for example older people, people with learning or physical disabilities, mental health problems or chronic long-term illness. Landmark developments will be discussed including the 'cascade of change' introduced following the 1990 National Health Service and Community Care Act. Continuities and differences in Conservative and Labour governments' approaches to reforming community care will be discussed. Over many decades, policy-makers have urged health organizations and local authority social services departments to work more closely together in order to provide seamless care for patients. Models of partnership working will be discussed together with examples of policy initiatives to foster partnerships between professionals working in health and social care together with service users and carers.

Community care

The term community care is a contested, value laden and idealistic concept. As Titmuss (1968) remarked:

> *'Does it not conjure up a sense of warmth and human kindness, essentially personal and comforting?' (Titmuss 1968: 3)*

Community has been described by Raymond Williams (1976: 66) as a 'warmly persuasive' keyword to describe an existing or alternative set of relationships. He argues that each generation grieves for the passing of a golden age. Politicians draw on the myth of caring, integrated communities to propose replacements to current systems of care. 'Community' is used at one and the same time to describe a network of people with common interests; as a place where participation is to be found and where services are located and where change in social circumstances may be effected. We noted in Chapter 7 the increased development of a 'mixed economy' of care. Increasingly, community care has come to mean the provision of services by a variety of different agencies and individuals. Thus, effective links between agencies (inter-agency collaboration) and between professional groups (inter-professionalism) have become increasingly pressing issues. Community support is now provided by:

- Statutory or formal sector: such as staff employed in the NHS or local authority social services or housing departments
- Voluntary sector agencies: such as MIND, the mental health charity; Age Concern or Help the Aged; Care and Repair; Crossroads Caring for Carers
- Private or independent sector: such as care homes, private hospitals, private domiciliary care agencies and registered social landlords
- Informal carers including spouse, other family members, friends or neighbours.

The 1989 White Paper on community care, *Caring for People*, stated:

> *'Community care means providing the right level of intervention and support to enable people to achieve maximum independence and control over their own lives ... These services form part of a spectrum of care, ranging from domiciliary support provided to people in their own homes, strengthened by the availability of respite care and day care for those with more intensive care needs, through sheltered housing, group homes and hostels where increasing levels of care are available, to residential care and nursing homes and long-stay hospital care for those for whom other forms of care are no longer enough' (DoH 1989a: 9).*

This general definition continues to underpin policy developments although the emphasis on 'services' in the extract above has been replaced with a focus on the provision of 'person-centred' care.

REFLECTION POINT

Consider the ways in which the various social networks which make up a community may support people and protect their health and well-being.

The policy context and the 'cascade of change' 1990

The NHS and Community Care Act 1990 introduced a 'cascade of change' into health and social care services (Audit Commission 1992). It was preceded by the publication of two White Papers – one for health called *Working for Patients* (DoH 1989b) and a second for local authorities entitled *Caring for People* (DoH 1989a). A common feature of both sets of guidance was that they promoted the development of internal markets in the health and social care sectors. Local authority social services departments were given the lead role for the main groups of service users in the community. *Caring for People* was underpinned by the concepts of autonomy and choice for service users and 'seamless' delivery of care by professionals and providers. It set out six key objectives:

- To make the assessment of an individual's needs and good case management the cornerstones of high quality care and resource allocation
- To enable people to live in their own homes wherever possible through the development of day, domiciliary and respite services
- To raise the standards of public sector care alongside a dynamic independent sector
- To make clear the responsibilities of health and social care agencies and to hold them to account for performance
- To encourage service providers to priorities support services for carers
- To introduce a funding structure for social care and thus offer taxpayers better value for money.

The achievement of these objectives became – and continues to be – the focus of attention for policy-makers and care professionals, as this chapter will show.

BACKGROUND TO THE REFORMS

It is useful to outline the patterns of care provision that existed prior to the watershed community care reforms of 1990 in order to understand the reasons for the changes and to assess their impact upon patterns of care delivery. Up until the mid-1970s, the district nursing service was funded by local government and nurses were able to respond to a wide variety of patient needs in the community. They carried out tasks ranging from making breakfast to managing complex end of life care for their patients, and many of course still do (Griffiths 1998). The separation of health and social care began in 1974 when the NHS took over responsibility for district nursing services. The gap between the professions of local government based social workers and nurses employed by the NHS widened, leading eventually to demands for improved interagency and interprofessional working to close the divide between the professions and to provide holistic, coordinated services in order to enhance care for patients and service users in the community.

Community care occupies a central point in the continuum of care between informal care provided by family members in a person's own home and the provision of formal care by paid staff in a hospital or long stay institution. Until the 1960s and 1970s care of the most highly dependent people including older people, people with mental illness or physical and learning disabilities was provided in the main at the expense of the state in a care home or long stay hospital setting. A series of trenchant critiques of this type of institutionalized provision catalogued many examples of physical neglect and abuse (e.g. Goffman 1968, Morris 1969, Robb 1967, Townsend 1962). A growing understanding of the extent to which institutionalized communal living created psychological dependency and loss of individuality led to further demands for reform (see Chapter 4). A parallel development was the 'planning for priority groups' movement that developed during the 1970s.

Case study

De-institutionalization – discharging mentally ill patients into the community

Traditionally many people who were mentally ill, disabled or frail because of old age were segregated in institutions such as special hospitals or residential homes. Asylums were built in the nineteenth century for those people believed to be mentally ill in order to remove them from society. This approach was considered by some at the time to be in the person's own good as it kept them away from unregulated 'madhouses' and squalid workhouses for the destitute poor. The number of asylum inmates increased dramatically from 16 000 patients in 1859 to 132 000 'lunatics' and 32 500 'mental defectives' in 1939 (Dingwall et al 1988). However, in the post-war period, developments in drug regimes and talking therapies led to a belief that many conditions could be cured and that mental illness should be treated as an illness and therefore people did not require to be locked behind closed doors for the rest of their lives. During the 1960s, a growing body of professional opinion argued that asylums themselves compounded mental illness by compelling inmates to live abnormal lives. Goffman (1961) argued that the regime of hospitals was designed to meet the aims of the institution rather than the needs of the individuals who lived there as we discussed in Chapter 4.

The worst fears of critics of the long-stay institutions were confirmed during the 1960s and 1970s by a series of scandals over the treatment of people living in special hospitals (Martin 1984). A growing emphasis on respecting the rights of patients was reflected in the content of the Mental Health Act (1983). By the 1980s, the policy of discharging more and more mentally ill patients back into the community – known as de-institutionalizing them – was well under way. Custodial care remained to deal with chronic long-standing mental disorders but therapeutic services in the community were developed for acute, less serious mental disorders. De-institutionalization has not been without problems. Cutbacks in local government expenditure led to difficulties in developing adequate community-based support services in the community. Staff working in welfare agencies faced new demands for which they had been inadequately trained. Concerns grew about the fate of the many people who were discharged from institutions. We noted in Chapter 4 that the creation of asylums in the nineteenth century was intimately linked with the restructuring of the labour market during the industrial revolution and with the desire to discipline the poor and indigent. According to Scull (1977), this era of incarceration was superseded in the late twentieth century by an era of 'decarceration' when the labour costs of institutional care became prohibitive. Thus, it was always questionable whether community care would be adequately funded.

Slowly the shift began towards the provision of small group homes in the community. Initially Conservative and Labour governments continued to accept a major role for public services in supporting highly dependent people whether in hospital or the community however during the 1980s this was to change. The emphasis on publicly provided care *in* the community was replaced by an emphasis on care *by* the community (DHSS 1981).

The closure of long-stay hospitals and the transfer of patients into the community was expected to lead to a diffusion of responsibilities for funding and provision of care between private, public and voluntary sectors. However, the cost of private care provision continued to be borne by the public sector because older people on low incomes could have their costs met by their social security housing benefit payments instead of the NHS. The private care home sector expanded to accommodate older people and other individuals for whom hospital-based care was no longer considered appropriate with their fees funded mainly out of welfare benefits. For local authorities, there were 'perverse incentives' to discontinue providing residential care themselves and to place people instead in private care homes since private nursing home care came out of the central government social security budget not out of their budgets. For older people and their families there were financial incentives to sell the family home, pass capital and savings to relatives and thus be eligible for welfare benefits to cover their fees. During the 1980s, the Social Security budget increased from £500 million in 1986 to £2.5 billion in 1992 (Timmins 2001). This led to demands for reform. It was the desire to cut costs more than any other factor that caused the government to act (Lewis & Glennerster 1996).

The expansion of the private care home market funded at the expense of the public purse, also contradicted the government's ideological approach to family values and overall intention to reduce dependency on the welfare state (see Chapter 7). The government sought to encourage the development of private alternatives based on care funded out of personal income and savings or provided by relatives.

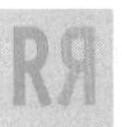

REFLECTION POINT

Consider the ways in which nursing work in the community is influenced by the key objectives outlined in *Caring for People* (DoH 1989a).

The mixed economy of care

The Conservative government's remedy to reverse these trends was set out in the 1989 plans for health and social care. Policy-makers wanted to see the development of needs-led services, based on assessment and care management and internal markets in health and social care. Local authority social services departments were to be responsible for coordinating the assessments of individuals to establish whether they were in need of services. Prior to the reforms older people entering residential care had not always had their needs for such care professionally assessed. After the reforms, health and social care staff would act as professional gatekeepers to these services. Packages of care based upon a personal plan of care, would then be purchased from private, statutory or voluntary agencies for people deemed to meet eligibility criteria. A range of services would be developed to sustain people in their own homes, to offer day or respite care, sheltered housing or residential and nursing home care. The encouragement of such independent or voluntary sector provision within the community, alongside statutory services, became known as the mixed economy of care (see Chapter 7). The relationship between purchasers and providers was to be based upon the service level agreements or contracts.

A system based on market principles was thus introduced into community care (see Chapter 4, for a discussion of market principles). Local authorities became the purchasers of care from a selection of providers. Competition was introduced into the social care market and it was believed by policy makers that this would increase quality and standards. Service users and their care managers would make choices on the basis of quality and appropriateness of services. In practice, the ability to make choices was limited by the funds available to care managers to purchase care and the lack of a thriving private sector in many areas.

The role of local authorities thus changed. Many councils transferred their care homes to the independent sector and they ceased to be direct service providers. It was also anticipated that local authorities would develop needs led services not just on the basis of individual care plans, but that the accumulation of knowledge about individuals would lead to community-based needs planning and the production of a Community Care Plan. In developing services and in planning for the future, local authorities were expected to involve their partner health authorities in joint working arrangements. The policy-making approach to the development of partnerships up to and including this period has been described as 'optimistic' in that it was based on the assumption that health and social care organizations would work together when exhorted to by government because it was in the best interests of patients or service users to do so (Hudson 1999: 198).

In developing a mixed economy, the provision of care was redistributed across the formal health and social care sectors, to the independent or private, and voluntary sectors. Conservative governments of the 1980s and 1990s introduced changes in the way services were funded, planned and delivered to clients and service users. The legislation that underpinned the reforms – based on the two separate 1989 White Papers – maintained the distinctions between health and social care and thus had only limited success in achieving their stated objectives of collaboration and partnership. Indeed the NHS and Community Care Act sustained divisions between health and social care and lacked clarity over the responsibilities of each sector to service users. The Act in extending the number of sectors engaged in service delivery inevitably made coordination more problematic. It exacerbated the historic fragmentation of service responsibilities for patients and service users between:

- Local Government (social services, housing, environmental health, regulation and inspection units)
- Health sectors (primary, secondary, community and public health)
- Voluntary sector agencies
- Private and independent providers.

As to the role of nursing in community care, the White Paper for health, *Working for Patients* (DoH 1989b), paid scant attention to nursing's role in community care. On the other hand, *Caring for People* (DoH 1989a), referred to the importance of the role of health practitioners including district nurses and health visitors in the multidisciplinary assessment of needs and the provision of care or support. Local government social services' departments were given lead responsibility for coordinating the activities of multidisciplinary teams of social workers, nurses and professions allied to medicine.

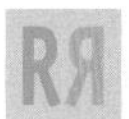

REFLECTION POINT

Consider the ways in which the following case study of the 'social bath' may illuminate our understanding of the nature of nursing work.

Case study

The health and social care divide and the concept of the 'social bath'

This section discusses the concept of the 'social bath', originally conceptualized by Twigg (1997) to analyse the boundary between medicine and social care, and used by Griffiths (1998) to develop the concept in the context of district nursing.

From a community nursing perspective, one of the most significant outcomes of the NHS and Community Care Act was the way in which the Act confirmed changes in the work of district nurses that had been set in motion years earlier. The task of bathing patients at home had devolved from district nurses to nursing assistants or auxiliaries. Following the Act, personal care could be administered by unqualified but trained care assistants and bathing became 'a symbol for the uneasy divide between nursing and social care' (Griffiths 1998: 237). Nursing assistants could help bathe a patient with 'medical' or 'nursing' needs and care assistants helped bathe clients for hygiene or 'social' reasons. In practice, as Griffiths' study indicates, distinguishing between a 'nursing' and a 'social' bath was based on a curious blend of subjective decision-making and interpretations of local authority eligibility criteria. Some district nurses continued to bathe patients at risk of developing, or who had, pressures sores, whereas in other cases the patient's hygiene needs would be attended to by social services' carers and a nurse would visit to manage the patient's pressure area. Some nurses, but not all, continued to manage catheterized patients as this extract from one of Griffiths' respondents illustrates:

'Is it a medical problem or is it social? A very fine line. Yes that man with a catheter can go to social care because he never has any bother with it, but this one we have bother with all the time and he gets sore sometimes: much more ours. Social care for the other one probably'. (Griffiths 1998: 237)

Decision-making about the category of bath required was further complicated because 'health baths' are provided free to the patient; but social baths are subject to a means tested charge. Social care is seen as care for which the individual bears personal responsibility compared to collective responsibility for meeting the costs of healthcare. For most nurses the distinction between health and social care was 'hopelessly blurred' (Griffiths 1998: 239).

New Labour's community care policies

The legacy for the Blair government after 20 years of Conservative rule was confusion, conflict and competition at the boundaries of health and social care, as Hudson (2000) argues. Local authority social services departments could not require other agencies to cooperate in assessments of individuals or in care management arrangements. The lack of a single budget made it difficult to plan integrated care packages for clients. Responsibilities for continuing care of older people with complex needs remained unclear and complex and concerns were growing about gaps in services for vulnerable individuals. At the same time, the development of performance indicators within the NHS meant that hospitals came under increasing pressure to increase throughput of patients with the result that 'bed blocking' by patients who had no safe alternative to a hospital bed became a problem. The pejorative term 'bed blocker' has been used to describe individuals who occupy a hospital bed but no longer require consultant-led care; more recently the less contentious 'Delayed transfer of care' has been used as an alternative. We drew attention to the impact of pejorative labels on patients in Chapter 8. Latimer (2000) in her ethnographic study of medical nursing discusses the ways in which nurses are expected to act as 'conductors' of care. She describes the ways in which nurses are responsible for 'pulling' patients through their hospital journey in order to facilitate throughput and the sometimes negative consequences for patients (see also Chapter 9).

The reforms led to mutual interdependence rather than collaboration between health and social care (Glendinning 2002). For example, local authority social services departments required the agreement of primary care to provide district nurses for patients who otherwise would have needed residential care. Conversely, if the NHS was to achieve its targets to facilitate hospital discharge and prevent unnecessary admissions, then it required local government to develop community care. The Labour party set out to achieve more effective cooperation, if not full integration of health and social care services. The 1997 White Paper for Health *The New NHS Modern, Dependable* (DoH 1997) set out a modernization agenda that continues into the next decade. The NHS Plans for England (DoH 2000) and Wales (National Assembly for Wales 2001) proposed a major redistribution of resources away from the hospital sector and to community and primary care and structural reorganization. Some elements of the old system have been retained such as the purchaser and provider split in health and social care. England has seen the development of Primary Care Trusts (PCTs) with responsibilities for providing community health and social services, for example, for people with mental health problems. In Wales and Scotland, the pace of change towards integration of purchaser and provider functions for community based services has been slower.

Partnership working and the 'Third Way'

Collaboration between health and social care organizations and their staff is seen as the key to the provision of effective, responsive services to patients and service users. Directives such as National Service Frameworks for Mental Health (DoH 1999a, Welsh Assembly Government 2002a) address the need for collaboration and partnership between care sectors. Partnerships extend beyond health and social care organizations and should embrace patients and service users. By involving community representation in policy planning, the process of decision-making should become more inclusive and transparent to all partners. The Blair government's 'Third Way' claims to be a system based on partnership between statutory bodies, communities and individuals (DoH 1997: 10). Partnerships were given legal backing when the Health Act (1999) introduced a statutory duty of partnership between health and local authorities to work together. Strategic plans developed by local councils and health bodies must show evidence that they were drawn up in partnership with relevant health or social care bodies. The 1999 Act removed obstacles to joint working by allowing the use of:

- Pooled funds – a single dedicated budget containing contributions from health bodies and local authorities to fund a wide range of care services
- Lead commissioning – the commissioning of a range of services from a single point for a client group where either the health organization or the local authority takes the lead in commissioning services on behalf of both bodies
- Integrated provision – health organization and local authorities merge their services to deliver one stop packages of care and to employ different professionals under one management structure.

The so-called 'Increased Flexibilities' introduced by the 1999 Act allow for the development of community-based joint initiatives at a micro level through to full unification of services into a single Primary Care Trust at the macro level. Locality-based initiatives include, for example, the use of pooled funds to establish 'rapid response teams' consisting of community nurses, physiotherapists, occupational therapists and social workers. Such teams may respond quickly in a crisis to avoid inappropriate hospital admissions when a person's caring arrangements have broken down, or their needs change but fall short of the requirement for consultant led services in hospital. With 'rapid' or 'first' response of this type in place, the objective is to relieve pressure on the acute sector by avoiding unnecessary admissions and enabling older people to return home from hospital to the community. The overall thrust of reforms is to develop a 'whole systems' health and social care focused approach to commissioning and providing flexible, responsive patient-centred services. Future evaluation of these schemes will reveal whether these aspirations have been achieved.

INGREDIENTS OF SUCCESSFUL PARTNERSHIPS

Research has identified principles and features of successful interagency and interprofessional partnerships. Foremost among these are shared vision and trust. Hardy et al (2000) set out six principles in their Partnership Assessment Tool for health and social care agencies. These include

- Acknowledging the need for partnership
- Developing a clear statement of purpose
- Maintaining trust
- Robust partnership arrangements
- Monitoring, measuring and learning.

Resources to finance the objectives of joint working are also essential (Powell et al 2001). Power should be shared between partners and based upon knowledge and expertise and not title or role (Henneman et al 1995). A study of an interdisciplinary community team supporting stroke patients at home identified three themes for successful interprofessional team working including the commitment and personal qualities of staff; effective communication within the team and opportunities for team members to develop creative working methods (Molyneux 2001).

BARRIERS TO PARTNERSHIP WORKING

In practise, partnerships have proved difficult to establish. The pace of change in recent years coupled with the necessity to keep services running can pose significant problems. Barriers remain in that different accountability and performance management mechanisms, such as Best Value in local government and clinical governance in the NHS, mean that planners have been reluctant to lose control of projects because of different auditing and governance arrangements. Separate funding streams, discrete organizational structures and different statutory responsibilities have long been seen as major barriers to collaborative working (Glendinning & Coleman 2000, Linck et al 2002). Conflicting priorities and agendas, such as the culture of business and the culture of care, and differences in planning and decision-making cycles, add to these difficulties. A study of hospital discharge arrangements uncovered quite different data collection systems to record the point at which a patient was ready to be discharged, with the result that one local authority emerged as the best in Wales for minimizing delayed transfers of care but their partner hospital trust appeared to be one of the worst (Phillips et al 2000). A study by Hardy et al 1992 categorized barriers to effective joint working between organizations as:

- Structural where there is fragmentation of service responsibility for client groups; procedural where there are differences in planning cycles and horizons
- Financial where there may be difference in resource inputs
- Professional divergence in values and ideology
- Organizational legitimacy or status differences, for example, between an NHS Trust and a small charitable organization.

Following the implementation of the 1999 Act, a survey of the first partnerships to be formed found that some structural barriers to partnership had been removed but other challenges remained (Glendinning 2002). Major service reorganization destabilized the local workforce and reduced the morale and motivation of key staff. Local managers were unable to change the terms and conditions of service of local authority or health staff and professional staff – nurses, general practitioners or social workers – could resist changes and thus threaten the development of new initiatives. The reforms continued to underestimate the difficulty in influencing relationships from the top down (Glendinning & Coleman 2000). Nevertheless, the wave of reforms has continued and, as Powell et al (2001: 39) argue, health and social care organizations and their staff are expected to 'play the game of partnership without being fully informed of the rules'.

PARTNERSHIPS WITH SERVICE USERS – ASSESSMENT AND CARE MANAGEMENT

The NHS Plans of England (DoH 2000) and Wales (National Assembly for Wales 2001) reminded health and social care providers once again that standardized, high quality assessment and care management of older people and other vulnerable service users and patients were essential if seamless care was to be achieved. The Single Assessment Process (DoH 2002a), Unified Assessment Process (Welsh Assembly Government 2002b) and Shared Assessment Process (Scottish Executive 2002) reinforce this key message. The core feature of single, unified and shared assessment processes is effective information sharing between care professionals so that the person being assessed gives information about their circumstances once. A systematic approach to care management incorporates the follow seven main elements:

- A public information strategy including for example directories of service providers
- A system to deal with inquiries about how to access
- Assessment tools and scales
- Eligibility criteria
- Care planning
- Monitoring
- Review
- Performance management.

The single assessment process applies to older people and other adults with disabilities or mental health problems and specifies that all assessments should be person-centred and begin with service user and carer perspectives. Twelve domains of assessment covering basic personal information, user and carer perspectives, activities of daily living (e.g. washing and dressing) and instrumental activities of daily living (e.g. meal preparation) and immediate environment (where the person lived) are identified. Four types of assessment are specified including contact, overview, specialist/in depth and comprehensive. The category of assessment to be undertaken depends on the individual's needs at any given time. Information should be given once and assessment data built up in a layered way. Contact assessment may be the first meeting between an individual and care professional and it should establish the nature of the presenting problem and whether potential wider health or social care needs exist. Basic personal information is collected at this stage. An overview assessment explores all or most of the domains of assessment and may trigger the need for a specialist or in depth assessment by a physiotherapist or other care professional. A comprehensive assessment is undertaken where all domains are triggers and explored through an assessment, for example, a geriatrician. Assessment information should be evaluated against four factors which determine independence including autonomy over personal circumstances, risk to health and safety, ability to manage daily routines and degree of involvement in family and social networks.

The purpose of eligibility criteria set out in Fair Access to Care (DoH 2002b, Welsh Assembly Government 2002b) was to ensure equity across England and Wales so that people in the same circumstances but living in different localities would have access to similar services and achieve broadly similar outcomes. The eligibility framework covers low, moderate, substantial and critical risk to independence and the implicit aim of the government is that at risk individuals would receive support services before crisis point was reached. However, there is little evidence to date that this aspiration has been achieved. Care plans should be individually tailored and begin with a statement of the objectives and outcomes of the care to be organized. Service users care packages should be monitored and reviewed at regular intervals and any amendments put in place as appropriate when needs change.

Informal care

Contemporary policy developments such as the Single Assessment Process extend the concept of partnership to those people who provide informal care including parents, spouses, daughters and sons, or friends and neighbours (see Chapter 2 for a further discussion of informal care). Informal care provided by relatives and friends have been enshrined in UK welfare policy as Elizabeth Wilson (1977) pointed out:

> *'Thus, the welfare state is not just a set of services, it is also a set of ideas about society, about the family, and – not least important – about women, who have a centrally important role within the family, as its linchpin' (Wilson 1977: 9)*

Informal care was a 'taken for granted' feature of policy life until it was brought into 'political limelight' during the 1990s (Malin et al 2002: 119). For governments and the general public unpaid carers were resources to be used as sole providers of care working in collaboration with the statutory or voluntary sectors (Twigg & Aitken 1994). The NHS and Community Care Act acknowledged the role of carers but was weak in terms of the support that it offered to them. This shortcoming was partially remedied by the Carers (Recognition & Services) Act 1995 which set out a requirement for a carers' needs to be assessed once 'the person being cared for' had been assessed and found to be in need of more formal care. At the time, the Act was heralded as a milestone in the identification of the role of carers but subsequent research has indicated systematic failures. The Act lacked sanctions with the results that carers' assessments were not always undertaken and even where they were carried out there was no guarantee that services would follow (Perry & Felce 2001).

The National Strategy for Carers (DoH 1999b) laid out a rationale for a legislative framework for direct provision of practical support for carers. The Strategy acknowledged three key principles. Carers should be offered help and support when required, be in a position to decide whether or not to provide care and thirdly, provide care and support without compromising their own physical, psychological or economic health. However, the reality for many carers is that they have little choice but to take on a supportive role when the health and well-being of a close relative is compromised through frailty, illness or disability. A clearer recognition of carers' needs was set out in the Carers and Disabled Children Act 2000. The Act gave carers the right to ask for an assessment of their needs. The National Service Framework for Mental Health (DoH 1999a) incorporates a standard focused upon carers' needs and the role of carers is also acknowledged in the English and Welsh National Service Frameworks for Older People (DoH 2001).

The experience of unpaid caring is grounded in the understandings that qualitative feminist research has provided. Research undertaken in the 1980s highlighted inequality on gender lines (Finch & Groves 1983, Ungerson 1987). Further studies detailed the nature of carework and offered a fuller picture to be revealed (Merrell et al 2005, Phillips 1994, Phillips et al 2002, Twigg & Aitken 1994). Carers are a heterogeneous group of people in terms of their age, faith, ethnicity, paid work status, disability, gender and sexual orientation. The experiences of caring are highly varied and subject to change. Caring may be carried out during the whole of one individual's life-course as responsibility for one generation is supplanted by the growing dependency of another. Carers may form substantial partnerships over considerable periods of time with the nurses, social workers and or other care staff who provide formal care. For others, caring may be a brief and intense experience at the end of a life of a loved friend or relative.

In addition to research findings, the development of carers' lobby groups such as Carers UK (formerly Carers National Association, CNA) added weight to the need to consider the circumstances of carers. The CNA evolved as the umbrella organization for locally based carers' support groups into an advocacy group that participates in major policy developments and evaluations. Carers UK continues to represent the interests of individual carers in national policy making and research initiatives. However although the influence of carers (and service users) in the policy arena nationally and locally has grown, they continue to remain relatively powerless when set within the context of the combined forces of statutory, private and voluntary agency provision. Thus, the extent of their partnership with service providers continues to be limited (Chambers & Phillips 2005).

RR REFLECTION POINT

Consider the nurse's role in supporting informal carers.

Discussion points

1. How can nurses improve interprofessional relationships?
2. What are the best ways for nurses to highlight their contribution to partnerships?

CHAPTER SUMMARY

Since the late 1990s, England and Wales have seen the development of a more 'realistic' model of policy making with partnerships being encouraged through the intro of additional funding streams as well as statutory obligations and additional funding (Hudson 1999: 200). Policy developments have affected interorganizational partnerships as well as relationships between practitioners and service users or patients. Clear agendas for collaboration have been set out by governments in order to improve the quality of care for service users and carers. Progress has been made in recognizing the centrality of service user and carer perspectives at mainstream policy levels but evaluation of existing policies is needed. To date much remains to be achieved if partnerships with care professionals are to be fully achieved.

FURTHER READING

Carnwell R, Buchanan J, eds 2005 Effective practice in health and social care: A partnership approach. Open University Press, Maidenhead.

This edited collection considers collaboration between different professions, service users and voluntary groups. Case examples are provided to highlight the challenges of partnership working where coordination is essential for good practice.

Means R, Richards S, Smith R 2004 Community care policy and practice. Palgrave, Basingstoke.

This book analyses developments in the delivery of care and support to individuals who are vulnerable because of old age, disability or mental health problems since the nineteenth century. Contemporary developments since the creation of the welfare state are explored in detail and the 2004 edition has been updated to include developments since the Blair government came to power.

Twigg J 1997 Deconstructing the social bath: Help with bathing at home for older and disabled people. Journal of Social Policy 26(2):211–232

In this paper, Julia Twigg challenges conceptualizations of community care with an in-depth discussion of assistance with bathing. She examines the social meaning of bathing, the ways in which the health and social care boundary is constructed and contrasts the nature of power in the private sphere of the home with the public spaces of a hospital ward.

REFERENCES

Audit Commission 1992 Community care: Managing the cascade of change. HMSO, London

Carers (Recognition & Services) Act 1995. HMSO, London

Carers and Disabled Children Act 2000. The Stationery Office, London

Chambers P, Phillips J 2005 Working across the interface of formal and informal care of older people. In: Carnwell R, Buchanan J (eds) Effective practice in health and social care: A partnership approach. Open University Press, Buckingham, p 228–242

Department of Health and Social Security 1981 Care in action. HMSO, London

Department of Health 1989a Caring for people. HMSO, London

Department of Health 1989b Working for patients. HMSO, London

Department of Health 1997 The new NHS modern dependable. The Stationery Office, London

Department of Health 1999a National service framework for mental health. The Stationery Office, London

Department of Health 1999b The national strategy for carers. The Stationery Office, London

Department of Health 2000 The NHS plan. The Stationery Office, London

Department of Health 2001 National service framework for older people. The Stationery Office, London

Department of Health 2002a Single assessment process. The Stationery Office, London

Department of Health 2002b Fair access to care. The Stationery Office, London

Dingwall R, Rafferty A, Webster C 1988 An introduction to the social history of nursing. Routledge, London

Finch J, Groves D 1983 A labour of love: Women work and caring. Routledge and Kegan Paul, London

Glendinning C 2002 Breaking down barriers: integrating health and care services for older people in England. Health Policy 65:139–151

Glendinning C, Coleman A 2000 Taking your partners. Developing relationships between primary care groups and local authorities. Research Policy and Planning 18(3):25–33.

Goffman E 1961 Asylums: Essays on the social situation of mental patients and other inmates. Penguin, Harmondsworth

Griffiths J 1998 Meeting personal hygiene needs in the community. Health and Social Care in the Community 6(4):234–240

Hardy B, Turrell A, Wistow, G 1992 Innovations in community care management. Aldershot, Avebury

Hardy B, Hudson B, Waddington E 2000 What makes a good partnership? A partnership tool. Nuffield Institute for Health, Leeds

Health Act 1999. The Stationery Office, London

Henneman EA, Lee JL, Cohen JI 1995 Collaboration: a concept analysis. Journal of Advanced Nursing 21:103–109.

Hudson B, Exworthy M, Peckham S 1998 The integration of localised and collaborative purchasing: A review of the literature and framework for analysis. Nuffield Institute for Health, University of Leeds/Institute for Health Policy Studies, University of Southampton, Leeds

Hudson B 1999 Dismantling the Berlin Wall: developments at the health-social care interface. In:

Dean H, Woods R (eds) Social policy review 11. Social Policy Association, London, p 187–204

Hudson B 2000 Inter agency collaboration – a sceptical view. In: Brechin A et al Critical practice in health and social care. Open University, Milton Keynes, p 253–274.

Latimer J 2000 The conduct of care. Blackwell, Oxford

Lewis J, Glennerster H 1996 Implementing the new community care. Open University, Buckingham

Linck P, Ellison P, Miles L, et al 2002 The Inter-agency working capabilities of local health groups (Final Report to the Wales Office of Research and Development for Health and Social Care). Institute for Medical and Social Care Research, University of Wales, Bangor

Malin N, Wilmot S, Manthorpe J 2002 Key concepts and debates in health and social policy. Open University Press, Buckingham

Martin J 1984 Hospitals in trouble. Blackwell, Oxford

Mental Health Act 1983. HMSO, London

Merrell J, Kinsella F, Murphy, F et al 2005 Hidden carers: Exploring the support needs of carers of dependent adults from a Bangladeshi Community. Journal of Advanced Nursing 51(6):549–557

Molyneux J 2001 Interprofessional teamworking: what makes teams work well? Journal of Interprofessional Care 15(1):29–35

Morris P 1969 Put away: A sociological study of institutions for the mentally retarded. Routledge, London

National Assembly for Wales 2001 Improving health in Wales: A plan for the NHS with its partners. National Assembly for Wales, Cardiff

NHS and Community Care Act 1990. HMSO, London

Perry J, Todd S, Felce D et al 2001 A study of current activity to support carers in Wales. Health and Social Care Research Support Unit for South East Wales, University of Wales College of Medicine, Cardiff

Phillips C J, Lambert S, Griffiths L et al 2000 Partnerships, policies and protocols: hospital discharge arrangements in Wales. University of Wales Swansea, Swansea

Phillips J 1994 The employment consequences of caring for older people. Health and Social Care in the Community 2:143–152

Phillips J, Bernard M, Chittenden M 2002 Juggling work and care: The experiences of working carers of older adults. Policy Press, Bristol

Powell M, Exworthy M, Berney L 2001 Playing the game of partnership. In: Sykes R, Bochel C, Ellison N (eds) Social Policy Review 13. Social Policy Association, London, p 39–61

Robb B 1967 Sans everything: A case to answer. Allen & Unwin, London

Scottish Executive 2002 Shared assessment process. Scottish Executive, Edinburgh

Scull A 1977 Decarceration. Prentice Hall, NJ

Timmins N 2001 The five giants: A biography of the welfare state. Harper Collins, London

Titmuss R 1968 Commitment to welfare. Allen and Unwin, London.

Townsend P 1962 The last refuge: A survey of Residential Institutions and Homes for the Aged in England and Wales. Routledge, London

Twigg J 1997 Deconstructing the social bath: Help with bathing at home for older and disabled people. Journal of Social Policy 26(2):211–232

Twigg J, Aitken K 1994 Carers perceived: Policy and practice in informal care. Open University Press, Buckingham

Ungerson C 1987 Policy is personal: Sex, gender and informal care. Tavistock, London

Welsh Assembly Government 2002a National Service Framework for Mental Health. Welsh Assembly Government, Cardiff

Welsh Assembly Government 2002b Creating a Unified and Fair Care Management System. Welsh Assembly Government, Cardiff

Williams R 1976 Keywords: A vocabulary of culture and society. Fontana, London

Wilson E 1977 Women and the welfare state. Tavistock, London

PART

3

The experience of illness

CHAPTER 11

Understandings of health, illness, risk and bodies

Susan Philpin

KEY CONCEPTS

- Health professional perspectives of health and illness
- Lay concepts of health and illness causation
- Social constructionism in relation to health and illness
- The sociology of the body: social meanings attached to the body

Introduction

This chapter will explore the ways in which sociology can contribute to our understanding of the ways in which people – both lay and professional – make sense of health and illness causation. It will start by outlining what is meant by lay and professional understandings of health, illness and risk, including their origins, similarities and differences. This chapter will also introduce the concept of social constructionism – the idea that interactions between individuals and groups construct what we perceive as reality. In addition, and related to this concept, the particular genre of sociology, the 'sociology of the body' will be explored through the analysis of Jocalyn Lawler's study of the ways in which nurses deal with bodies.

Lay and professional perspectives

When discussing ideas about health, the term 'lay', referring to people without a professional qualification, is usually used to differentiate between the 'official' or professional understanding of health and people's everyday understanding.

As this section will show, lay people's understandings of health and illness are complex and influenced by their particular social environment – their social class, gender, education and cultural identity – as well as by aspects of their personal biography, such as their age and health history. Health professionals' understandings of health and illness causation are rooted in the *biomedical model* (see Box 11.1), which stems from scientific knowledge. On the other hand, as will be shown in a later section of this chapter, it has been argued that this scientific knowledge is itself *socially constructed.*

However, it would be a mistake to think that there are clear demarcation lines between lay and health professional perspectives; as this

Box 11-1 The biomedical model

- The mind and body can be treated separately – known as *mind–body dualism*
- The body can be repaired like a machine – medicine adopts a *mechanical metaphor*
- The merits of technological intervention are sometimes overplayed – medicine adopts a *technological imperative*
- Biomedicine is *reductionist* in that explanations of disease focus on biological changes to the relative neglect of social and psychological factors
- Every disease is caused by a specific, identifiable agent, namely a 'disease entity' (such as a parasite, virus or bacterium) *the doctrine of specific aetiology*

(Adapted from Nettleton 2006: 2).

chapter will illustrate, there is often a blurring of the boundaries between these two groups and an intermingling of ideas. For example many lay people will have considerable health-related knowledge gleaned from their formal education, official health promotion campaigns and the media in all its forms, including the internet. Moreover, as a study by Helman (1978) shows, medically qualified people are still repositories of lay knowledge, which may well influence their practice and their perceptions of illness. The knowledge boundaries are further blurred by the fact that many of those who work in paid employment providing health care, including nursing care, for patients are unqualified and as such may be working with lay definitions of health.

DISEASE AND ILLNESS

A further dimension to the differing perceptions of professionals and the laity arises from a distinction that is sometimes made between disease and illness, inasmuch as the former is sometimes seen as the professional perspective, whereas illness refers to the subjective experience of patients. Although the two words are often used interchangeably, Eisenberg (1977: 11) differentiates between them as follows: '... patients suffer "illnesses", physicians diagnose and treat "diseases" '. Thus in this sense, illness refers to people's subjective experiences, while disease refers to abnormalities of bodily organs detected, by health professionals, through objective scientific examination. The distinction between felt experience and objective abnormality is summed up succinctly by Cassell (1976: 42) as 'Disease, then, is something an organ has; illness is something a man *sic* has'.

PROFESSIONAL PERSPECTIVES ON HEALTH AND ILLNESS CAUSATION

One 'official' definition of health is the following much-quoted and all-encompassing definition, which explains health in a *positive* way as 'a state of complete physical, mental and social well-being, and not merely the absence of disease or infirmity' (WHO 1948: 1). In contrast, despite the current rhetoric promoting 'holistic' care, Western medicine's conception of health often appears instead to be disease-oriented, with less concern for its social and psychological dimensions than the WHO definition would suggest. Western medicine's understanding of health is premised on the biomedical model of health which Nettleton (2006) describes as having the five defining characteristics listed in Box 11.1.

LAY CONCEPTS OF HEALTH AND ILLNESS CAUSATION

A sociological understanding of lay concepts of health and illness causation contributes to nursing practice in a number of ways. First, an appreciation that people have different ideas about the meaning of health and about which particular aspects of health are deemed to be important, facilitates understanding of the patients' and carers' standpoints, thus improving communication. In particular, when health professionals recognize that lay perspectives on health, while possibly different from the professional perspective, have a logic and rationale to them, as opposed to being simply incorrect, it engenders respect for a different point of view.

Second, understanding of the lay perspective is a necessary starting point for planning patient care, including health education and promotion. For instance, Prior et al's (2000) study of health beliefs in two Chinese communities in England found that there were frequent references to happiness and inner contentment in their respondents' perceptions of health. However, as Prior et al note, this focus on happiness and inner contentment, by implication also meant that:

> '... *it did not really matter how you behaved in relation to what professionals might consider unhealthy activities. If smoking cigarettes made one happy then it was acceptable to smoke. If eating fatty foods led to contentment then that was acceptable also – all in the name of happiness*'. (Prior et al 2000: 833)

Thus, nurses advising lifestyle changes would need to consider and attempt to work with these different priorities of what comprises good health. That is to argue that acceptance or resistance of professional advice is linked to lay people's understandings of what it means to be healthy. In addition, acceptance or resistance of health advice is connected to ideas about responsibility for one's own health. As we shall see later, sociological research indicates that perceptions of responsibility for one's own health are variable and influenced by a number of factors.

WHAT DOES IT MEAN TO BE HEALTHY?

The term 'health' carries different meanings for different people and it has been the subject of a considerable amount of sociological research, providing a complex picture of people's everyday understandings of it. Broadly speaking, the studies indicate that ideas of health are influenced by people's socioeconomic status, culture, religion, age, gender and previous health experience. The studies also indicate that while there are often discrepancies between expert medical conceptions of health and lay conceptions there are similarities in the ways these conceptions are arrived at, which hints again at the complexity of lay understandings. For instance, Blaxter (1983), whose studies of Scottish working class women are described below, argues that although the women's explanations for illness causation were often scientifically wrong in their detail, by virtue of the fact that their explanations were 'painstakingly derived from their experience as they saw it', their methods of forming their explanations were 'not in principle unscientific' (Blaxter 1983: 68). That is, they were arguably using the same methods to make sense of illness as medical science uses.

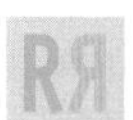

REFLECTION POINT

What does it mean to be healthy – and what factors have influenced your answer?

SOCIOLOGICAL RESEARCH INTO LAY CONCEPTS ABOUT HEALTH AND ILLNESS CAUSATION

The now classic sociological research into lay concepts of health and illness in the later decades of the last century conveys both the complexity of people's ideas and, as will be shown, the ways in which the research methods used influence people's articulation of their ideas. As a starting point, it is useful to note that the research indicates that although people's understandings are their own personal thoughts and ideas, these ideas are intrinsically connected to their wider social milieux. That is the research findings make clear the link between what Mills (1959) termed private 'troubles' and public 'issues' inasmuch as people's understandings are interwoven into their surrounding social structures. The influence of these social structures on lay understandings will now be considered.

The research indicates that **socioeconomic status** (see Chapter 6) influences people's understanding of health and illness causation, particularly in relation to responsibility for one's own health and also positive or negative conceptions of health. For example, Blaxter (1983) interviewed a sample of middle-aged, working class women in a Scottish city about the causes of 'disease' (see distinction between illness and disease above). The most commonly cited cause was infection, followed by heredity, then by environmental hazards, then a variety of other things such as the secondary effects of other diseases, stress and childbearing. It was rare for the women to see diseases as being the result of their own behaviour. A similar study, exploring lay beliefs about personal responsibility for health, was carried out in South Wales by Pill and Stott (1982), this time looking at working class women in their early 30s. As with Blaxter's study, infection or germs were the most commonly-cited causes of disease, followed by lifestyle, heredity and stress. However, about half the women in Pill and Stott's study employed concepts of cause that involved *choice* over behaving in one way or another and also a degree of individual responsibility for illness. These women were more likely to be home-owners and to have had more education than the women in Blaxter's sample and their feeling of greater control over their lives may account for the different emphasis.

Blaxter (1983) also found that the women in her study had low *expectations* of health, accepting poor health as a normal part of the ageing process. Moreover, despite only being in their late 40s or 50s, they saw themselves as older than their years, a situation which Blaxter puts down to the harshness of their earlier lives. A similar study of socially disadvantaged women in Scotland by Blaxter and Paterson (1982) again identified low expectations of good health, with health being perceived in a *functional* way in terms of being able to carry on with normal activities such as going to work or school; there was a lack of a positive conception of health. This is a significant finding for health professionals in that people holding low expectations of health may be less likely to seek help early or to attend preventative clinics.

A study carried out by Calnan (1987) in roughly the same period, comparing social class differences in health beliefs of women in England found only a slight difference between the two groups in terms of positive and negative definitions of health. He did however find that working class women's definitions were more likely to be 'uni-dimensional', or a functional definition, that is, 'getting through the day, whereas their professional counterparts more frequently operated with multi-dimensional definitions that incorporated a wider range of elements that included being fit, being active, and the and the absence of illness' (Calnan 1987: 35). However, Calnan also notes that this difference may reflect the social context of the interview rather than differences in ideas; that is 'the more elaborate definition given by the professional women may only reflect their greater familiarity with circumstances where they are asked to give their views about abstract concepts, as well as the relative ease with which they are able to give articulate responses to a middle class interviewer'. Blaxter (1990: 15) also comments on the fact that in qualitative studies of lay concepts, if poorly-educated respondents are given time to elaborate on their ideas they 'can express very fluent ideas on this topic', which might not be elicited from a more superficial survey.

A further intriguing finding from Calnan's (1987) study was that working class women were less likely than their middle class counterparts to accept the influence of economic circumstances on their health. For instance, when told of the findings of the recent (at that time) Black Report (see Chapter 6), Calnan (1987: 79) notes that: 'A large group of women, almost entirely from social classes IV and V, did not believe it or did not agree with the findings'. This finding is also echoed in Blaxter's (1993) paper, which draws on data from an earlier study.

In addition to these qualitative studies, Blaxter (1990) carried out a large national survey of the population of England, Wales and Scotland, encompassing 9000 respondents – the 'Health and Lifestyle Survey'. This survey questioned respondents about their own health and lifestyles and their opinions and attitudes towards health and health-related behaviour. A further component of this study was a set of physiological measurements (by a nurse) to assess respondents' fitness.

Lifestyle is a much used term, usually describing people's behavioural 'choices'. However, Blaxter (1990) points out that these choices are significantly influenced by people's social and economic circumstances (see Chapter 6).

The study identified differences in conceptions of health **over the life course** and also **gender** differences. For instance, younger men tended to speak of physical strength and fitness and younger women favoured 'ideas of energy, vitality and ability to cope' (Blaxter 1990: 30). She found that older people, particularly men, were likely to describe health in terms of *functional* ability. Gender differences were also apparent in the responses to the questions: she notes that women's answers tended to be more expansive than men's and also that 'many women, but few men, include social relationships in their definition of health'. Blaxter's (1990) study also indicates that people described aspects of health, such things as contentment or happiness, within themselves even in the presence of illness.

A number of writers have also identified a *moral* dimension to lay understandings of health and illness causation. For instance, in the earlier mentioned study of working class women in Scotland, Blaxter and Paterson (1982) observed that health was perceived as a 'good' quality and few of the women described themselves as unhealthy. They also note that 'Even more, they would not wish to say that their families were unhealthy, for this might reflect on their mothering competence' (Blaxter & Paterson 1982: 32). Similarly, Pill and Stott (1982) identified a moral dimension to illness in that people were deemed culpable if they failed to look after each other or took unnecessary risks. Blaxter's (1990) survey also identified moral elements in relation to health beliefs about a healthy lifestyle and also in terms of responding appropriately to illness (Links between good health and virtue are also discussed in Chapter 3).

Finally, further insight into lay perceptions of illness causation may be found in a study by Davison et al (1991) who explored lay perceptions of the causes of heart disease in relation to lifestyle in a context of a public health campaign to reduce heart disease by 'Heartbeat Wales', a division of the Welsh Health Promotion Authority, as it was then.

Davison et al (1991) coined the term 'lay epidemiology' (see also Chapter 12) to refer to the ways in which people make sense of illness episodes, usually within the family or community. Lay epidemiology includes the notion of 'candidacy' with regard to heart disease – that is respondents in the study indicated who they thought would be a likely candidate for this condition. In similar vein to the ways in which scientific epidemiologists study patterns of illness, the respondents would link particular instances of heart disease to the circumstances surrounding the event. From this information certain patterns were noted, which fed into respondents' views of likely candidates for heart disease.

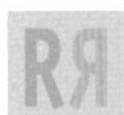

REFLECTION POINT

Consider the differences between lay epidemiology and professional epidemiology. How might an understanding of lay epidemiology help nurses in planning health education?

However, the respondents in this study also recognized their system of candidacy as being fallible in that not all candidates had heart disease and some non-candidates did develop the illness. This was explained by the fact that candidacy only increased the risk of heart disease; it also reinforced the view that heart disease strikes randomly and in some cases, it is all down to 'chance'. Clearly, ideas about fate and luck exist alongside more rational influences on knowledge of disease causation.

Davison et al's (1991) study is a good example of the ways in which people's ideas about disease causation stem from many different sources and also that the development of these ideas is a collective, rather than individual activity. They note that:

> *'The mass media and official bodies are the sources of much processed scientific data; reports of illness and death are available from family, friends, work colleagues and neighbours; celebrities such as politicians and sports people suffer and die in the public gaze; individuals make their own observations of themselves and of those around them'. (Davison et al 1991: 7)*

In making sense of, or trying to explain, illness causation, it appears that the lay population of this study have assimilated the messages from various sources with their own observations of illness episodes; however, they still see fate and luck as part of the explanatory framework. Davison et al's (1991) study also illustrates the ways in which lay and professional people assess *risk*, and it is to this that we shall turn next.

THE CONCEPT OF RISK – INSIGHTS FROM SOCIOLOGY AND ANTHROPOLOGY

The concept of 'risk', from both lay and professional perspectives, is an important theme in the sociology of health illness; it also permeates nursing practice and education. It is embraced by the Nursing and Midwifery Code of Professional Conduct (NMC 2004, 8) and a risk assessment is a preliminary for many nursing activities. In addition, the ability to assess and manage risk is a stated expected competency for student nurses to acquire. The environment in which nursing care is accomplished is perceived as risky for patients and also for nurses, who may fear personal injury and/or litigation. Why is this and why are some hazards identified as risks and other not? Useful insights into our understandings of risk may be gained from sociological and anthropological literature in this area.

The German sociologist Ulrich Beck (1992) describes contemporary western society as a 'risk society', which refers to both the particular hazards of modern society and also to people's heightened awareness of these hazards. Beck notes that, unlike in earlier periods, risks today (particularly environmental risks) are perceived as arising from human activities, such as industrial and scientific development. In addition, he argues that the extent and nature of these modern day risks are not easily calculable and that there are disagreements among experts about the extent and nature of particular threats. He suggests that consequently scientists have lost their authority and credibility in relation to risk assessment. This loss of public trust in scientists has been exemplified recently in the conflicts over the suspected (by some scientists) link between the MMR vaccine and autism.

In similar vein, the British sociologist Anthony Giddens (1991) also describes contemporary society as a 'risk culture', but notes that this is not to suggest that life is more risky than in previous times. 'Rather, the concept of risk becomes fundamental to the way both lay actors and technical specialists organize the social world' (Giddens 1991: 3). As with Beck, Giddens (1991) refers to a decline of trust in 'experts' to calculate risks or provide solutions, which serves to heighten levels of anxiety (see also Chapter 12).

Both Beck and Giddens refer to the reflexive nature of contemporary society in relation to risks. Beck notes that risk awareness prompts society to critically examine its actions. While Giddens argues that in order to manage risks and avert hazards 'the future is continually drawn into the present by means of the reflexive organization of knowledge environments' (1991: 3). This is exemplified by the need for assessment of possible future risks in many activities, including nursing practice.

The anthropologist Mary Douglas has made a number of significant contributions to our understanding of risk by exploring the relationship between a society's culture and its identification of and responses to perceived dangers.

Douglas (1992) reminds us that the concept of risk originally emerged in the context of calculations of probability and was neutral, whereas the idea of risk has evolved to now be associated with dangerousness. Indeed, she observes that the word risk 'now means danger; *high* risk means a lot of danger' (Douglas 1992: 24). However, she argues that what is perceived as risky is itself culturally constructed, reflecting the wider concerns of cultural groups. She notes that when individuals are required to estimate the probability and credibility of particular risks 'they come already primed with culturally learned assumptions and weightings' (Douglas 1992: 58). Hence, some hazards are deemed to be dangerous while others are ignored.

Taking a cross-cultural example, Douglas and Wildavsky (1982: 6–7) describe the Lele people of Zaire as suffering 'all the usual devastating tropical ills – fever, gastroenteritis, tuberculosis, leprosy, ulcers, barrenness, and pneumonia'. And yet, they note that from this selection of hazards, the Lele focused mainly on being struck by lightning, afflicted with barrenness and bronchitis. Moreover, they note that the Lele mainly attributed such misfortune to specific types of immorality, where the victim was usually seen as innocent and some powerful leader or village elder would be blamed.

This links with another aspect of Douglas's work on risk – the ways in which cultural groups attribute blame. Again, writing with Wildavsky in 1982, they argue that in addition to focusing concern on particular dangers 'the type of society generates the type of accountability' (Douglas & Wildavsky 1982: 7). In her later work, Douglas (1992) explores notions of blame in relation to risk in modern industrial society, noting the idea of someone being at fault when misfortune occurs. She describes contemporary society's readiness to almost 'treat every death as chargeable to someone's account, every accident as caused by someone's criminal negligence, every sickness a threatened prosecution' (Douglas 1992: 15).

Later in this chapter, we look at another key aspect of Douglas's (1966) theorizing on risk, her analysis of the ways in which people avoid pollution; she suggests that 'our pollution behaviour is the reaction which condemns any object or idea likely to confuse or contradict cherished classifications' (Douglas 1966: 35); that is, the idea that 'matter out of place' is an anomaly requiring pollution avoidance strategies.

In addition, Douglas analogizes the body to society where the boundaries and margins of the body are similar to the boundaries of society – leaking boundaries are considered as threats (because of their creation of anomalies) to order and stability. Risk, in this case may be understood in terms of transgressing boundaries.

A further contribution from Douglas's theorizing on risk attempts to explain how people's perceptions of risk are influenced by the extent to which they are integrated into and regulated by their social group, using the 'grid/group model' of social organization (Douglas 1992). Briefly, in this model 'grid' represents the extent to which individuals' perceptions are regulated by their society, and 'group' represents the extent to which their perceptions are influenced by their integration into society.

In an earlier work, Douglas and Wildavsky (1982: 138) explain 'group' as the 'outside boundary that people have erected between themselves and the outside world'. A high group rating would indicate strong cohesion among group members and strong distinctions between members and non-members of the group. They explain 'grid' as 'all the other social distinctions and delegations of authority that they use to limit how people behave to one another'. Douglas (1992) applies her grid/group theory in relation to risk perceptions in relation to AIDS. More recently, Godin et al (2007) have applied the model to explore the ways in which the culture of a particular social group – a forensic mental health care unit – is shaped by its staff and also shapes the staff's risk thinking and actions.

These insights from sociology and anthropology help us to locate people's understanding of risk in its sociocultural context. However, although there is considerable research into people's experiences and understandings of health and illness (see also Chapter 13), there is little research into people's experiences and understandings of actually being 'at risk' of illness. With the advancement of knowledge in the field of genetic testing and screening, apparently healthy people are finding themselves identified as at risk of potentially serious illness. In Chapter 12, Lindsay Prior reports on a study which explores the ways in which both health professionals and lay people make sense of being genetically at risk of breast cancer.

REFLECTION POINT

In nursing, which hazards are deemed to be particularly dangerous and why? Which hazards are ignored or played down?

Social constructionism in relation to health and illness

Social constructionism is a theoretical approach which argues that what people perceive as 'reality' is itself 'socially constructed' inasmuch as it is a creation of the interaction of individuals and groups (Berger & Luckmann 1967). Such an approach encourages the questioning of what are often 'taken for granted' aspects of issues by problematizing accepted wisdom, in that all knowledge is seen as an expression of particular social interests and contexts. There are a number of different perspectives under the broad umbrella of social constructionism – Bury (1986) provides a useful overview of the various arguments.

In relation to health and illness, the social constructionist approach argues that ideas about what constitutes both health and illness are social constructs inasmuch as they recognize the social interactions involved in the construction of medical and lay knowledge. Earlier parts of this chapter have explored the ways in which lay knowledge of health and illness arises out of various social interactions; the social constructionist approach also explores the social interactions involved in constructing medical knowledge. This is not to suggest that this approach denies the reality of disease, rather, it argues that both medical and lay knowledge are shaped by particular sociocultural contexts and also, as will be shown later, shifting **paradigms** of thought.

Paradigm is a term used by Thomas Kuhn (1972: 93), which refers to a model or set of rules defining scientific enquiry in a particular historical period. Kuhn notes that the particular paradigm informs scientists 'of the questions that may legitimately be asked about nature and of the techniques that can properly be used in search for answers to them'.

Morgan et al (1985: 29) argue that from the social constructionist perspective, concepts of disease 'have no necessary, transhistorical, universal shape, and reflect a particular way of viewing the world'. Indeed, the approach is probably best illustrated through exploring a particular historical example as set out in a paper by Peitzman (1989) – 'From Dropsy to

Bright's Disease to End-stage Renal Disease', which outlines the changing conceptualization of kidney disease from the late eighteenth century to the present day. In so doing, he is able to show the ways in which physicians' understandings of disease signs and symptoms moved through a series of different paradigms and disease classifications.

In the late eighteenth century, 'dropsy' referred to a distressing disease characterized by bodily swelling through fluid retention – oedema in today's parlance – which reflected the old **humoral** theory of health and illness. Peitzman uses the celebrated eighteenth century author, Samuel Johnson, as an example of an early sufferer of dropsy, drawing on one of Johnson's letters to his friend Boswell:

> *'A dropsy gains ground upon me; my legs and thighs are very much swollen with water, which I should be very content if I could keep it there, but I am afraid it will soon be higher'. (cited in Peitzman 1989: 18)*

The **humoral** theory of health and illness, which dates back to the time of Hippocrates in the fifth century BC, perceived the human body as a microcosm of the universe. The body was thought to be composed of four *humours*: hot, dry, wet and cold, which were equivalent to what were thought to be the four elements of the universe: fire, earth, water and air. Illness was understood as an imbalance between the humours and hence treatment consisted of correcting the balance (see the anthropologist Helman's (2000) accounts of the application of this theory in different cultures).

Although dropsy meant something very specific to physicians in the late eighteenth century, their knowledge framework and clinical skills at that time did not allow them to differentiate between oedema caused by different disease processes – such as cardiac failure. By the early nineteenth century, through developments in anatomy and chemical analysis of urine, physicians began to understand these symptoms in a different way, and Richard Bright of Guy's Hospital, distinguished a particular category of oedema caused by kidney disease. Bright was able to construct a disease entity out of the association between patients' signs and symptoms during life, post-mortem lesions of the kidney and chemical changes in the urine. Later in the century, clinicians redefined and refined the characteristics of what had come to be known as 'Bright's Disease', using such techniques as microscopic examination of tissue and urinary sediment.

Bright's disease was understood as a way of 'getting sick through your kidneys' (Peitzman 1989: 21). However for twentieth-century physicians, this same 'getting sick through your kidneys' category came to be occupied by more than one disease and physicians looked to *physiology* – involving renal function tests – rather than the old lesion-based, anatomical approach to the problem to differentiate between them. Peitzman's paper then focuses on a particular sub-category of kidney disease – end-stage renal disease – a disease requiring dialysis and/or renal transplantation. He notes that modern-day physicians rarely see 'dropsical' patients now in that their oedema is controlled through dialysis and they also rarely see post-mortems of people with diseased kidneys because it is no longer necessary for diagnosis.

Peitzman's paper demonstrates the ways in which a basic clinical picture – oedema – is defined and redefined over time using a series of differently-focused ways of explaining things. Importantly, it is not simply that different names are applied to the same condition, rather that the whole conceptual scheme changes. The shift between dropsy and end-stage renal disease is extraordinary in terms of both physician and patient experience. Today's physicians, as noted above, employ different methods of diagnosis and are able to contain the disease through dialysis. While for patients with end-stage renal disease, Peitzman (1989: 28) notes that rather than experiencing oedema and other symptoms of kidney failure, their experience is:

'mainly the illness of dialysis. The treatment becomes the sickness. When renal patients talk about their experiences – and a fair number of them do – they write about being a dialysis patient, *about the hours on the machine, about their remarkable ability to cope and prevail'.*

(See also the example of patient experience of dialysis in Chapter 13.)

A social constructionist approach to health and illness is useful in that it encourages the exploration of the 'taken for granted' aspects of knowledge about health and illness. In so doing it also indicates the ways in which scientific 'facts' are socially produced and may alter over time. (There are links here with Chapters 4, 5 and 7, where the ways in which ideas change in response to their social context are discussed.)

The sociology of the body: social meanings attached to the body

INTRODUCTION

Sociological enquiry, as we have seen, is concerned with social structures and interactions and has not, until relatively recent times, focused on the *physical* body. However, as much nursing work is fundamentally concerned with caring for bodies and nurses use their own bodies in the accomplishment of their work, sociological investigation into this area makes a considerable contribution to nursing knowledge. In this section, we will first explore the concept of *embodiment* and then examine the work of a number of key writers who contribute to our understandings of the sociology of the body. Finally, an important and innovative sociological study of the ways in which nurses manage bodies which was undertaken by the Australian nurse, Jocalyn Lawler (1991), will be used as a framework to exemplify sociological understandings of the body in relation to nursing (see also Chapter 8).

EMBODIMENT AND BODYWORK

Cregan (2006: 3) explains embodiment as encompassing the 'physical and mental experience of existence'. Indeed, Nettleton and Watson (1998: 1) claim that:

> *'Everything we do we do with our bodies – when we think, speak, listen, eat, sleep, walk, relax, work and play we 'use' our bodies. Every aspect of our lives is therefore embodied'.*

Attention to the concept of embodiment facilitates understanding of the ways in which people experience physical and emotional pain and chronic illness and disability addressed in later chapters. In addition, Savage (1997: 238) notes the embodied nature of nurses' relationships with patients and other staff. That is, in her study she observed the nurses' 'use of the body helped make tangible or endorsed their values and beliefs about nursing . . .' .

This management of their own bodies by nurses in their interactions with patients and others has been described as 'bodywork' (Shakespeare 2003). The term bodywork is also used to describe the management of patients' bodies by nurses and other caregivers (Lawler 1991, Ray & Street 2006, Twigg (2000, 2006)). This bodywork includes washing, feeding and dealing with excreta and, as indicated in Lawler's analysis, in the next section is often perceived as 'dirty' work (Hughes 1984: 46), which she notes nurses conceal 'by doing much of their dirty jobs behind closed doors'.

Twigg (2000, 2006) describes an ambivalence within nursing in relation to bodywork. On the one hand, within the nursing hierarchy bodywork is usually performed by lower status staff, while on the other nursing values bodywork, using it a marker of difference between itself and medicine.

Foucault

Any discussion of the sociology of the body requires some attention to the work of the French philosopher **Michel Foucault** (1926–1984) in that our understanding has been significantly influenced by his writing. Of particular importance is *The Birth of the Clinic* (1973), where Foucault introduces the concept of the medical 'gaze'. The medical gaze refers to the ways in which the development of anatomy coupled with new methods of accessing the inner workings of the body enabled clinicians to see and know the body in different ways. Doctors were able to move on from surface appearances and patients' subjective descriptions of their symptoms to objective measurements; in this way, the body was objectified. Foucault argued that this penetrating (literally) 'gaze' was the source of medicine's power (see Chapter 8 for further development of Foucault's understanding of the relationship between knowledge and power). Moreover, Foucault argued that this new way of seeing and knowing the body represented a paradigm shift, the clinical gaze represented a new way of seeing and understanding the body.

Jocalyn Lawler – 'behind the screens'

An important contribution to our understanding of the body in relation to nursing work comes from a study by Lawler (1991). Lawler used fieldwork observations followed up by interviews with nurses to explore the ways in which nurses manage the contradictions and taboos bound up in body care. The findings from her study are situated within the broader field of sociological and anthropological enquiries into the body.

First, Lawler's study of nurses' body care is informed by the work of the German sociologist **Norbert Elias** (1897–1990) whose book, *The Civilizing Process* (1978) contends that since around the period of the Middle Ages there has been a major attitudinal change in Western Europe toward the body and its functions. He describes a 'civilizing process' whereby bodily functions such as urination, expectoration and defecation, became increasingly viewed as shameful and requiring to be hidden from public view. Lawler argues that this process has influenced the ways in which the body is managed in society. That is, she argues that the civilizing process or, as she prefers to call it, the 'privatizing process' with regard to bodily functions, leads to contradictions for nurses in their role as providers of bodily care in that they are required to deal with functions which are essentially private, embarrassing and shaming (see also discussions of 'too posh to wash' in Chapter 9).

Second, Lawler draws upon the work of the British anthropologist Mary Douglas (1966) who argues that dirt avoidance is common in all cultures inasmuch as dirt is regarded as 'matter out of place' – an anomaly (in an anthropological sense) that is potentially dangerous and polluting. In her classic analysis of our ideas about dirt as matter out of place, Douglas explains that:

> *'Shoes are not dirty in themselves, but it is dirty to place them on the dining-table; food is not dirty in itself, but it is dirty to leave cooking utensils in the bedroom, or food bespattered on clothing ... In short, our pollution behaviour is the reaction which condemns any object or idea likely to confuse or contradict cherished classifications'. (Douglas 1966: 37)*

Developing on Douglas's analysis, Lawler notes the body's potential for dirt, especially at its margins or openings into the body. In all cultures, matter issuing from these margins – such as excrement, pus or menstrual blood – is regarded as an anomaly, matter-out-of-place, which requires careful 'pollution avoidance' strategies to resolve the anomaly.

In relation to bodily fluids and boundaries, it is useful at this stage to consider the work of a later writer – the French feminist philosopher and literary critic, Julia Kristeva (1982), who uses the notion of 'abjection' to explain why bodily excretions produce an involuntary revulsion in us. In a similar vein to Douglas's (1966) ideas of 'matter out of place', although taking a psychoanalytical perspective, Kristeva describes a body substance as 'abject' when it crosses bodily boundaries and in so doing 'disturbs identity, system, order' (Kristeva 1982: 4). However, in addition to the dangers of anomaly inherent in matter out of place, for Kristeva abjection also has an 'engulfing' quality. That is when bodily fluids have penetrated their containing boundaries they threaten to also permeate our own bodily boundaries. 'Abject. It is something rejected from which one does not part, from which one does not protect oneself ... it beckons to us and ends up engulfing us'.

A number of writers have commented on the feelings of repellence that leaking body boundaries may engender in those caring for them. For example, Lawton (1998) uses the concept of the 'unbounded body' to describe patients who, as a result of their physical deterioration are suffering from conditions such as incontinence, decay or disfigurement and are thus unable to maintain the *boundaries* of their bodies. With regard to the hospice patients in her study, she notes that:

> '... *what most of the symptoms requiring control shared in common was that they caused the patient's body to rupture and break down. As a consequence, fluids and matter normally contained within the patient's body were leaked and emitted to the outside, often in an uncontrolled and* ad hoc *fashion'. (Lawton 1998: 127)*

Lawton argues that such patients' bodily unboundedness led them to be 'sequestrated' away from the rest of society into private secluded places such as a hospice to end their days. She notes that their carers:

> *'were not explicitly concerned about the fact that the patient was dying, rather, the primary reason they suggested for wanting the patient to be admitted [to the hospice] was because they felt repelled by the patient being incontinent, vomiting, and/or emitting other bodily fluids within their homes'. (Lawton 1998: 132)*

Abjection, in the form of uncontrollable drooling is described in Ray and Street's (2006) study of people's experiences of caring for individuals with motor neurone disease. As one caregiver explains:

> *'Caregiver 4: [When I am helping him to eat] the slime, oh, it nearly makes me sick!'*

Somology

'Somology' is a term coined by Lawler referring, as its name suggests, to knowledge of the body. The knowledge to which she refers is an understanding of the complex nature of the physical body in that is simultaneously 'an object, a means of experience, a means of expression, a manner of presence among other people, and a part of one's personal identity' (Lawler 1991: 29). She notes that nurses care for the object (material) body and also what she calls the 'lived body' or the body as it is experienced by people; and that nursing care involves integrating the objective body with the lived body. In similar vein, Savage (1995) describes the knowledge underlying nurses' interactions with patients as 'embodied knowledge' which involves both intuition and experience. However, for Savage this knowledge also includes an 'integration of the nurse's object body and lived body in relation to others' (Savage 1995: 68).

Lawler argues that for nurses to perform their body care in the light of the earlier mentioned taboos and contradictions, they must learn, through their practice experience, what she calls four basic 'somological' rules (Box 11.2). Interestingly, the first three of these rules set out below, actually apply to the nurses' expectations of patient behaviour rather than actual nurse behaviour. That is to argue that 'appropriate' patient behaviour is a necessary pre-requisite for nursing work in this delicate area – it is a two-way process.

In addition, Lawler also describes five 'specific contextors' (things which set the context) needed to create an environment where body care is possible – that is to argue that these contextors are essential in that they define particular situations

Box 11–2 'Somological' rules

- *The compliance and control rule*: an understanding that the patient will comply with what the nurse wants them to do
- *The dependency rule*: the patient is completely (or almost completely) dependent on the nurse for body care
- *The modesty rule*: the patient is expected to be neither too modest or embarrassed, nor too free to expose him/herself
- *The protection rule*: the nurse will protect the patient's privacy (Lawler 1991: 147–151, abridged).

and events as constituting nursing practice. The first two contextors are part of the nurse's persona – her/his uniform and manner. The nurses in Lawler's study felt that the uniform was of paramount importance in the performance of their role, in 'defining the situation', as exemplified in the following interview data extract:

> *'Oh no! [I couldn't cope without my uniform.] Take that off and that would be ... a different situation. [Laughter] I wouldn't be too sure what I was doing! I wouldn't know what I was doing'. (Lawler 1991: 151)*

The meanings attached to nurses' uniforms are interesting from a sociological and anthropological perspective (*cf* Bashford 1998, Littlewood 1991, Wolf 1988). In addition to helping to define the situation, uniforms are associated with cleanliness and purity – both useful attributes when dealing with bodies. Savage (1995) suggests that nurses' uniforms serve in managing intimacy by transforming their wearers into 'representations' rather than individuals as exemplified in the following comment from a nurse in her study:

> *'you put on your uniform as a nurse and that gives you access to, you know, things that you just wouldn't do ... it's outrageous really but a nurse's uniform, a nurse's title, gives you ... like a passport to do all these things ...'. (Savage 1995: 65)*

The nurses in Lawler's study also felt that acting in an appropriate 'professional' or 'matter-of-fact' *manner* was important in establishing order in potentially embarrassing situations. There are clear links here with a classic study by Henslin and Briggs' (1971), which analysed the roles adopted by doctors, nurses and patients during the various stages of a gynaecological examination. Henslin and Briggs used a 'dramaturgical' model (Goffman 1969) which likens social encounters to roles performed by actors on a stage, to explore the particular roles adopted by all the participants in this potentially embarrassing procedure.

The remaining three contextors, namely 'minifisms'; asking relatives and visitors to leave; and discourse privatizations, are 'deliberate nursing acts which confer a protective and private social atmosphere on the situation' (Lawler 1991: 151). Lawler uses the term 'minifisms' to refer to either verbal or behavioural strategies which *minimize* the severity of a situation in order to limit their patient's embarrassment. For instance, when confronted with disturbing amounts of vomit, blood or faeces in the patient's bed (matter out of place) they would comment that 'you've made a *bit* of a mess'. The nurses would also ask relatives and visitors to leave the area before assisting with body care, thus protecting the patient's privacy. Lastly, Lawler describes the nurses' use of 'discourse privatizations', by which she means creating a private context in which to discuss matters to do with normally private bodily functions. This private context would be created by lowering of the nurse's voice or moving to an area out of other's ear-shot.

Lawler's study also indicates that in addition to the taboos surrounding private bodily functions, nurses also need to manage the *sexuality* inherent in naked bodies. The female nurses in her study reported experiencing anxiety and embarrassment when they were required to wash male patients. In these situations, as in Henslin and Briggs' (1971) study, it was deemed to be particularly important that the aforementioned 'rules' were adhered to.

To conclude this section, Lawler's study had many insights to offer nurses. She draws attention to the ways in which the physical body is often excluded from academic study in that academic disciplines are organized into discrete bounded subject areas (such as biology, chemistry, sociology), which render it inaccessible to inquiry. She also makes the pertinent observation that certain theoretical developments in nursing may also exclude the body. For example, the notion of 'holistic' care may also be a way of hiding the body in that body care is subsumed into 'nurse-identified needs', again the body is scientized and sanitized. In similar vein, Bjørk (1995) argues that as a result of changes in the theoretical discourse underpinning nursing and nurse education, with its increased emphasis on the 'psychosocial' elements of care, 'the patient's body has moved out of focus in nursing' (Bjørk 1995: 6). She suggests that this shift in focus has led to a devaluing of physical care and its relegation to auxiliary workers. This devaluation of body care and its relegation to unqualified carers is also noted by Twigg (2000) who comments that although holistic approaches are attractive, the introduction of skill-mix in practice ensures that 'basic bed and bodywork is confined to the lowest skill, one which may not indeed require a trained nurse' (Twigg 2000: 138).

Lawler's study also shows that nursing work as body work is often denigrated and regarded as dirty and menial work; however, her research identifies the complexity and sophistication at the heart of the ways in which nurses manage the bodies of others.

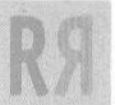

REFLECTION POINT

Reflect on your own experiences of 'bodywork' with patients and the embodied nature of your care.

Discussion points

1. How do you think patients' understandings of health and illness could influence your planning and implementation of nursing care?
2. How might insights from sociology and anthropology help us to understand the perceived 'riskiness' inherent in nursing practice?
3. Social constructionism argues that all knowledge is socially produced – consider the ways in which nursing knowledge may be socially produced.

CHAPTER SUMMARY

This chapter has drawn on sociological insights to illuminate the ways in which people – both the laity and healthcare professionals – come to understand health, illness and risk. The blurring of boundaries between lay and health professional perspectives has been highlighted and attention has been drawn to the socially constructed nature both types of understandings. It is clear from this account that nurses need to be able understand the origins and rationale of both perspectives in the planning and implementation of their care.

In addition, this chapter has introduced a key genre in sociology – the sociology of the body – exploring it in relation to nursing work. Jocalyn Lawler's cogent analysis of the ways in which nurses manage their patients' bodies in the accomplishment of nursing work has provided a useful and relevant framework in exemplifying the sociology of the body in relation to nursing. Further insights into the ways in which nurses manage the hidden and 'dirty' aspects of their care have been provided from key anthropological studies.

FURTHER READING

Godin P 2007, ed. Risk and nursing practice. Palgrave Macmillan, Basingstoke

Lupton D 1999 Risk. Routledge, London.

REFERENCES

Bashford A 1998 Purity and pollution: Gender, embodiment and Victorian medicine. Macmillan, Basingstoke

Beck U 1992 Risk society: Towards a new modernity. Sage, London

Berger P, Luckmann T 1967 The social construction of everyday life: A treatise in the sociology of knowledge. Penguin, Harmondsworth

Blaxter M 1983 The causes of disease: Women talking. Social Science and Medicine 17(2):59–69

Blaxter M 1990 Health and lifestyles. Routledge, London

Blaxter M 1993 Why do victims blame themselves? In: Radley A (ed.) Worlds of illness: Biographical and cultural perspectives on health and disease. Routledge, London

Blaxter M, Paterson E (1982) Mothers and daughters: A three-generational study of health attitudes and behaviour. Heinemann, London

Bury M 1986 Social constructionism and the development of medical sociology. Sociology of Health and Illness 8:137–169

Bjørk I T 1995 Neglected conflicts in the discipline of nursing: perceptions of the importance and value of practical skill. Journal of Advanced Nursing 22:6–12

Calnan M 1987 Health and illness: The lay perspective. Tavistock, London

Cassell F J 1976 The healer's art: A new approach to the doctor-patient relationship. Penguin, Harmondsworth

Cregan K 2006 The sociology of the body. Sage, London

Davison C, Davey-Smith G, Frankel S 1991 Lay epidemiology and the prevention paradox: the implications of coronary candidacy for health education. Sociology of Health and Illness 13:1–19

Douglas M 1966 Purity and danger. Routledge, London

Douglas M 1992 Risk and blame: Essays in cultural theory. Routledge, New York

Douglas M, Wildavsky 1982 A risk and culture. University of California Press, Berkeley

Eisenberg L 1977 Disease and illness: Distinctions between professional and popular ideas of sickness. Culture, Medicine and Psychiatry 1:9–23

Elias N 1978 The civilizing process: The history of manners and state formation and civilization. Blackwell, Oxford (translated by E. Jephcott)

Foucault M 1973 The birth of the clinic: An archaeology of medical perception. Tavistock, London

Giddens A 1991 Modernity and self identity: Self and society in the late modern age. Polity, Cambridge

Godin P, Davies J, Heyman B 2007 Different understandings of risk within a forensic mental health unit: a cultural approach. In: Godin P (ed.) Risk and nursing practice. Palgrave Macmillan, Basingstoke

Goffman E 1969 The presentation of self in everyday life. Penguin, Harmondsworth

Helman C 1978 Feed a cold, starve a fever; folk models of infection in an English suburban community and their relation to medical treatment. Culture, Medicine and Society 2:107–137

Helman C 2000 Culture, health and illness. Butterworth-Heinemann, Oxford

Henslin J, Briggs M 1971 Dramaturgical desexualization: The sociology of the vaginal examination. In: Henslin J (ed.) Studies in the sociology of sex. Appleton-Century-Crofts, New York

Hughes EC 1984 The sociological eye. Transaction Books, New Brunswick

Kristeva J 1982 Powers of horror: An essay on abjection. Columbia University Press, New York (translated by L. Roudiez)

Kuhn T 1972 Scientific paradigms. In: Barnes B (ed.) Sociology of science. Penguin, Harmondsworth

Lawler J 1991 Behind the screens: Nursing, somology and the problem of the body. Churchill Livingstone, London

Lawton J 1998 Contemporary hospice care: the sequestration of the unbounded body and 'dirty dying'. Sociology of Health and Illness 20(2):121–143

Littlewood J 1991 Care and ambiguity: Towards a concept of nursing. In: Holden P, Littlewood J (eds) Anthropology and nursing. Routledge, London, p 170–189

Mills C W 1959 The sociological imagination. Oxford University Press, New York,

Morgan M, Calnan M, Manning N 1985 Sociological approaches to health and medicine. Croom Helm, London

Nettleton S, Watson J 1998 The body in everyday life. Routledge, London,

Nettleton S 2006 The sociology of health and illness, 2nd edn. Polity, Cambridge

Nursing and Midwifery Council (NMC) 2004 The NMC code of professional conduct: standards for conduct, performance and ethics. Nursing & Midwifery Council, London

Peitzman S 1989 From dropsy to Bright's disease to end-stage renal disease. The Milbank Quarterly 67(Suppl 1):16–32

Pill R, Stott N 1982 Concepts of illness causation and responsibility: Some preliminary data from a sample of working class mothers. Social Science and Medicine 16:43–52

Prior L, Chun PL, Huat SB 2000 Beliefs and accounts of illness. Views from two Cantonese-speaking communities in England. Sociology of Health and Illness 22(6):815–839

Ray R A, Street A F 2006 Caregiver bodywork: family members' experience of caring for a person with motor neurone disease. Journal of Advanced Nursing 56(1):35–43

Savage J 1995 Nursing intimacy: An ethnographic approach to nurse-patient interaction. Scutari, London

Savage J 1997 Gestures of resistance: the nurse's body in contested space. Nursing Inquiry 4:237–245

Shakespeare P 2003 Nurses' bodywork: is there a body of work?. Nursing Inquiry 10:47–56

Twigg J 2000 The body in community care. Routledge, London

Twigg J 2006 The body in health and social care. Palgrave Macmillan, Basingstoke

Wolf ZR 1988 Nurse's work, the sacred and the profane. University of Pennsylvania Press, Philadelphia

World Health Organization 1948 Constitution of the World Health Organization. WHO, Geneva

CHAPTER 12

Lay understandings of health and risk: a changing picture

Lindsay Prior

KEY CONCEPTS

- The changing status of lay understandings of health and risk
- Being-at-risk of a 'cancer gene'
- Normalizing genetic risk
- The implications of this for healthcare

The changing status of lay understandings of health and risk

It seems reasonably clear that during the later stages of twentieth century, and the earliest part of the twenty-first century, health professionals have been required to be more clearly and openly accountable to lay assessment, and more sensitive to patient viewpoints than had previously been the case. There are, of course, various reasons for growing significance accorded to lay assessments of health and illness. On the one hand, there can be little doubt that it is related to declining legitimacy of professional dominance (*cf* Freidson 1970, see also Chapter 4). On the other hand, it is evidently connected to the desire on behalf of policymakers to activate the role of the laity in aspects of self-care and illness management (see Chapter 10). Whatever the reasons, the growing importance of lay participation emerges through both policy formulations of western governments and through current accounts of medical practice. Hence in the UK, for example, the Department of Health Circulars (such as DoH 1999), speak routinely of the need for patient involvement and partnership in matters of care and treatment. While in medical practice there is an increased concern to develop what has been called patient-centred medicine (Stewart et al 1995), and to instigate a pattern of shared-decision making (Elwyn et al 2000), as well as patient friendly forms of communicative practice as a whole. Practices that have recently been referred to by some as forming a 'new medical conversation' between practitioner and patient (Mazur 2002).

CHALLENGE TO PROFESSIONAL EXPERTISE

These trends are undoubtedly related to the operation of other, wider, forces that have led to a challenge on the expertise of professionals. Thus medicine as a profession – as with so many other forms of professional activity – has been confronted by something of a legitimation crisis during the late twentieth century. Whether or

BIO GRA PHY

Jürgen Habermas (1929–present)

It would do Habermas (a German Social Theorist) a grave disservice to attempt to summarize his work in an explanatory box; however, in order to illuminate this chapter's reference to this theorist, it is useful to elaborate briefly on his *Theory of Communicative Action*, which was published in two volumes, 1984 and 1987. Habermas places great emphasis on *communication*, arguing that in a free integrated society, freedom depends on undistorted communication between its members. He argues that modern capitalist societies are in 'crisis' in that this ability to communicate has been undermined with the result that people no longer trust and/or feel loyalty towards the institutions within which they live (see also other critical theorists mentioned in Chapter 5; a very useful and readable account of Habermas's work in relation to medicine and nursing may be found in Porter 1998).

not such a crisis was and is linked (as Habermas would have it) to the extended interests of the state in the generalized sphere of 'welfare', is not perhaps for us to judge. It is enough to note its presence. It has certainly led to a negative evaluation of expertise. Habermas (1987) had argued that the notion of an expert culture whether in medicine or any other sphere of activity, was essentially anti-democratic in itself, and this position is strongly echoed in the work of other social theorists (Beck 1992).

At the professional level, the response to the legitimation crisis has been to encourage participation in decision-making and a democratization of decision-making procedures. This, in itself, has led to various expressions of a desire to activate the patient in matters of illness management. I have already mentioned trends toward shared decision-making (Mazur 2002), and to these we can easily add mention of the rising influence of the Expert Patients Movement as developed, for example, by Kate Lorig.

At the level of intellectual debate, there has been a wider trend to argue for what might be called a democratization of knowledge (Turner 2001). In medical sociology, this democratizing trend has tended to express itself in two ways. The first has been an increased interest in what lay people have to offer by way of knowledge of health and illness. The second has been a tendency to argue that lay knowledge can be every bit as valuable as professional knowledge. The two trends often come together in discussions of that 1990s hybrid, the 'lay expert'. However, before we examine the hybrid it will serve us well to note how the trends of which I speak have rippled through the sociology of health and illness.

We need to note, first of all, that direct attacks upon the privileged position of medical knowledge and practice have been rare. The attacks that have arisen have been linked, in the main, to the intellectual influence of Michel Foucault (see Chapter 8). So, for example, Armstrong (1985) – a devotee of Foucault – has consistently argued that 'modern medicine occupies no privileged epistemological position' (1985: 111) (see Chapter 11). That is to say, all knowledge forms are equal. What is more, and as Bury (1986) indicated, Foucault and his followers were not the only advocates for the democratic evaluation of knowledge forms. Indeed, Bury pointed toward an amorphous though influential group of scholars whom he bagged together as 'social constructionists' (see Chapter 11). To Bury, the latter had variously argued against the privileging of scientific (and by implication, medical) knowledge over other forms of understanding. One of his most cogent complaints against them being that they left us with 'No way of judging one account of reality as better than another' (1986: 165).

Confronting issues of epistemology head on has not, of course, been at the forefront of sociology of health and illness. More common has been an examination of the use and expression of knowledge in particular contexts and circumstances. In this regard, it is the study of patient 'perspectives', patient 'viewpoints', and lay health beliefs that has preoccupied medical sociologists (Calnan & Williams 1992, Emslie et al 2001, Parsons & Atkinson 1992, Pinder 1992, Prior et al 2000 and Chapter 11). In many cases, these authors were originally concerned with lay beliefs rather than lay knowledge, but as the years have passed, it seems that the concept of knowledge has gained the upper hand. Thus Williams, for example, had opened his 1984 paper with the statement that he was about to demonstrate how 'people's *beliefs* about ... aetiology' need to be understood (1984: 175, my emphasis). This is in direct contrast to later papers where lay knowledge was the term that was used (see, for example Popay et al 1998). In a parallel manner, it is of interest to note how an earlier concern with lay concepts of aetiology and disease causation (Blaxter 1983) was, by 1991, turned into a focus on 'lay epidemiology'. The paper of Davison et al (1991) was seemingly the first time that this concept had appeared in print (although Brown (1987) had been using the term 'popular epidemiology' for some time).

CHANGES IN LANGUAGE

One might be tempted to argue that we are dealing with roses by any other name. However, my feeling is that the change of language indicates the emergence of an entirely new object. Epidemiology, after all, is a form of highly skilled practice and quite different from having some (untested) ideas about what may or may not cause a disease. In a similar way, the concept of belief has a far less sturdy status than the concept of knowledge. (One may believe in unicorns, but it would be difficult to claim knowledge of them.) In any event, it seems clear that as the 1990s developed a concern with belief had been transposed into a concern with knowledge (Busby et al 1997) and that lay people had metamorphosed into multi-skilled and knowledgeable individuals; epidemiologists even. It is not so surprising, then, that around the same period one sees a new hybrid emerge – namely, the lay expert. This expert has since acquired the skills relating to diagnosis (Sarangi 2001), and pharmacology (Monaghan 1999), and has appeared as an expert in the medication of minor illness (Hibbert et al 2002).

Despite all of this, the origins of the term 'lay expert' are not entirely clear. However, it is clear that a concept of expertness among the lay population had been circulating through medical sociology for some time (Tuckett et al 1985). It is certainly true that researchers in the sociology of science from the late 1980s onward had tended to argue that lay people often possessed expert knowledge about complex causal relationships in the physical world (Wynne 1989, 1996). In medical sociology, the initial claims are somewhat tentative. Thus, Tuckett et al (1985: 217) used parentheses when they referred to patients as 'experts', and recognized that any expertise that did exist in the patient world was limited to aspects of self-care. However, such limitations were far from evident during the 1990s. For example, during that period, Arksey was advancing a series of claims. First, that 'in health matters, patients may themselves be experts' (1994: 464). Second, that it was possible to blur 'the differences traditionally assumed to exist between science and non-science, and by extension the distinction between expert and lay systems of knowledge' (Arksey 1998: 9). It is a blurring that is characteristic of those who choose to talk of patients as lay experts (Willems 1992). In a parallel manner, Epstein (1996) had spoken of hierarchies of expertise and claimed that there was now a problem in understanding the distinction between a lay person and an expert (1996: 3). Since that point, it has been a claim echoed by numerous authors (Sarangi 2001).

As to how lay people become expert, this is a matter of some difference. For some authors lay people are experts by virtue of having experiential knowledge of a condition (Busby et al 1997, Monaghan 1999). In other cases, lay experts seem to be on a par with those who have scientific training (Arksey 1998, Epstein

1996, Wynne 1996). In yet other cases, the expertise of lay people appears as an emergent property of social groups that contain scientifically trained experts – where qualified scientists serve as translators for lay concerns (Brown 1987). Whatever the case, it seems clear that those who argue for the usefulness of the concept of lay expertise have yet to specify more precisely what lay people are (and can be) expert in. They also have need to clarify how such expertise may differ from that brought to the table by, say, nurses, and other health professionals. In what follows, and by way of example, I am going to highlight some contrast between the ways in which health professionals and lay people understand some of the detail of inheriting mutations for breast cancer. The data upon which I draw was gained from a recent ESRC funded study into the use of 'risk' in a cancer genetics clinic. Among other things, my example should serve to illustrate how this debate relates to the role of nurses in a modern healthcare system and how that role might be defined.

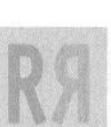
REFLECTION POINT

Consider the extent to which patients may be 'experts' about their own conditions. How might this influence your nursing care for them?

Being-at-risk of a 'cancer gene'

Despite enormous advances in medical knowledge and technology, cancer remains one of the greatest threats to our physical health. It has been estimated that this disease causes a quarter of all deaths in the UK, with one in three people being affected at some point in their lives (Cancer Research UK 2003). The most common types of cancer are those of the breast, lung, large bowel (colorectal) and prostate gland, which account for more than 50% of new cases and a significant proportion of the budget available for healthcare services. Recently, the advancement of genetic knowledge has been heralded as offering the most promising breakthrough for cancer detection and treatment. In particular, the development of genetic testing and screening technologies has enabled clinicians to make visible an individual's risk of disease well before it becomes manifest (Prior et al 2002). Insofar as genetic risk assessment promises to increase our ability to predict, detect and intervene so as to ameliorate the effects of such a serious disease, this might be seen as the latest attack in the long running 'war on cancer' (Proctor 1995). Insofar as cancer genetics focuses on being-at-risk, it positions itself at the very centre of current health practice – especially so since risk and risk assessment have become increasingly pivotal to the exercise of medical discourse and health practice in the contemporary world (Skolbekken 1995, see also Chapter 11).

The shift in focus from the actual to the potential presence of disease that is evident in clinical cancer genetics is, then, part of a much wider movement. Indeed, as Lupton (1995) argues, the discourses of public health and health promotion in general, have tended to redefine illness as a danger that threatens us all and demands that we devise strategies of self-protection. So, in the modern world, each and everyone is 'at-risk' of something or other and the category of 'being-at-risk' may be said to constitute a new source of social identity. The consequent extension of 'surveillance medicine' (Armstrong 1995) into the routines of our everyday lives has been well documented as a factor responsible for changes in diet, lifestyle and self-regulation in the population at large (Hughes 2000). In most cases, of course, our status of being-at-risk is acquired by little more than membership of a population group – older people, cigarette smokers, people with diabetes. In other cases, the status is acquired by evident possession of some particular, and personal, quality – as with HIV and AIDS. And it is into this latter group that genetic mutation carriers fall. So that, for such individuals, to be 'at-risk' is to feel well, be asymptomatic, yet always to be aware of the potential for becoming otherwise. Such 'being-at-risk' must consequently confront the possibility of their future self as suffering from a bodily pathology that is probable rather than actual, and to incorporate this tentative knowledge into their 'life-world' and 'life-plans'.

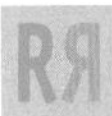

REFLECTION POINT

How might a diagnosis of being-at-risk genetically of developing cancer impact on a person's sense of identity and life-plan? Consider this diagnosis in terms of Bury's (1982) concept of 'biographical disruption', outlined in Chapter 14.

It is well known that the communication of risk assessments between doctors, nurses and patients raises important and fundamental issues about the nature of medical consultations. This not least because the numerical and statistical data from population risk estimates have to be translated into terms that are meaningful to the patient and communicated effectively (Lloyd 2001; Edwards et al 2002; Alaszewski & Horlick-Jones 2003). In the case of cancer risks, communication of risk status can lead to adverse psychological outcomes (Rees et al 2001). In fact, much of the early work on genetic risk assessment tended to highlight the negative, 'troubled', consequences of receiving genetic risk information (see the essays in Marteau & Richards 1996). Partly in response to this, clinical genetics has tended to engage with various forms of 'counselling' so as to mollify adverse consequences of risk assessment and communication procedures. And health psychologists have subsequently commented on the positive effects of genetic counselling, in terms of reducing patients' levels of stress and anxiety (Meiser & Halliday 2002, Randall et al 2001) and making them feel more optimistic about avoiding the development of a heritable disease (Shaw & Bassi 2001). Genetic counselling, it has also been argued, increases an individual's sense of self-efficacy, empowering them to make autonomous decisions about treatment (McConkie-Rosell & Sullivan 1999) as well as increasing their willingness to engage in 'preventative' behaviours such as breast self-examination (Lloyd et al 1996).

Beyond psychology, it has further been recognized that patients strive to make meaningful sense of their genetic risk estimates in terms of their social worlds – everyday lives, biographical experiences and family backgrounds – as well as in spheres of personal psychology (Hallowell 1999). In this respect, it is important to recall that medical sociologists and anthropologists, in particular, have long been concerned with locating illness in such wider social and cultural frameworks, and especially with understanding the subjective experience of illness (see Eisenberg 1977, Kleinman 1978 and Chapter 11). Yet, such concern has rarely extended to a study of those 'at-risk'. Similarly, with respect to the study of chronic illness, the focus on such features as biographical disruption (Bury 1982; Charmaz 1983), and narrative reconstruction (Williams 1984), has not been extended to cover the 'at-risk' populations. Yet, as we have already noted, it is clear that the risk assessments can be significantly disruptive (Cox & McKellan 1999) – at least at the level of personal psychology.

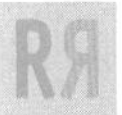

REFLECTION POINTS

People have their own ways of making sense of information and relating it in meaningful ways to their own life experiences. How can nurses help people make sense of information about their genetic risks?

What I wish to emphasize here is that where clinical risk assessments are available to individuals, such individuals are commonly faced with the necessity of carrying out repair work. Such repair work as is necessary to reconcile medical information with what they already 'know' as lay actors. This is so because 'being-at-risk' restructures not only clinical and psychological identity, but also the social position of the patient-client in their kinship network. So, for example, an individual may be repositioned as the pivotal point in a lineage of heritable disease or as the carrier of potential danger to future generations. In fact, it is not only the individual, but also their family that is redefined in terms of genetic risk. Consequently, the patient–client may perceive a moral responsibility to manage the implications of their own risk assessment for significant others as well as for themselves (Cox & McKellan 1999, Hallowell 1999). In patients' accounts of this process, therefore, we may find not only their understandings of genetic knowledge but also a defensive recourse to a body of family-centred, socially grounded beliefs that seek to contextualize risk in a familiar world.

Very often, there is a marked discrepancy between lay and professional understandings of risk. This, not least because health risks tend to be perceived by patients in highly social, emotive and symbolic terms (Joffe 2003). Indeed, lay risk estimates tend to be formulated on a different basis from those of health professionals. And as Parsons and Atkinson (1992) explain, information that is as potentially inaccessible as a genetic risk estimate (which is often constructed in mathematical, statistical terms) has to be translated by the patient–client into descriptive, 'recipe knowledge' that is personally meaningful. People may then draw upon shared stocks of background knowledge that abound in their family nexus, reinterpreting the clinical information – both retrospectively and prospectively – in terms of their effects upon decisions about reproduction, career paths and so on. Indeed, it has been argued that lay ideas about inheritance tend to reflect perceptions of the social relatedness of family members rather than any 'objective' medical risk estimates (Richards 1997). One issue that might arise out of such analyses is a need to consider the role that genetic (nurse) counsellors might have in mediating between these two spheres of knowledge.

REFLECTION POINT

Can you think of examples of differences in lay and professional understandings of risk? How might nurses help to bridge this divide?

Normalizing genetic risk

While patients in the ESRC study were generally prepared to trust in the scientific expertise of the medical profession, many remained sceptical about the extent to which genetics could account for their personal or family circumstances. As anthropologists of other cultures have occasionally indicated, a key question that people may ask themselves in the face of misfortune or sickness is often 'why me and why now?' (see also Chapters 3 and 11). Perhaps in order to answer such questions some patients felt moved to reconcile the information received from the clinical service with their knowledge of their personal social worlds. This was partly achieved by translating the rather abstract medical knowledge into literally 'familiar' terms that were personally meaningful and resonated with the life-world. Routine procedures such as completing the family history questionnaire and discussing the pedigree were important in this respect, as these 'boundary objects' helped to bridge the gap between the domains of lay and professional discourse (Atkinson et al 2001). Genetic risk was, in the main, *normalized* as just one of many aspects of family life that might affect health, and as something that must be understood in relation to one's everyday experiences.

Such a strategy of normalization was often reflected in the patients' beliefs about the role of genes in causing cancer. Many believed that while a 'cancer gene' might run in the family, they would only develop the illness if the gene were 'triggered' by knocks and bumps to the body or other distressing life events. There was a sense perhaps that, in some circumstances, one could take steps to ameliorate any 'bad-hand' that fate might have dealt out to one. Thus, patient–client '24' referred to a highly stressful job, a violent relationship and a car accident as possible factors that might have damaged her body and left her more vulnerable to genetic disease; while patient–client '28' said quite simply, 'if I have got the genes I don't want anything to trigger them'. Others used this idea of an interaction between genetic and environmental factors to increase their sense of control over their future health. Thus, many people accounted for the steps they had taken to modify their lifestyle and gather information that might prevent them from triggering a predisposition to cancer. As patient–client '16' explained:

> *'You may have the gene but provided you are educated you may be able to prevent that gene from developing into anything. And that I think is what the key is, that you have that knowledge ... I just think you are taking control of things as opposed to sweeping it under the carpet, and don't talk about it ... At least you are informed and you are taking precautions'. (P16: Clinical assessment = moderate risk, breast cancer)*

Meanwhile, some of the respondents had begun to think about inheritance as a wider issue than one of genetics alone, identifying aspects of their family backgrounds that suggested links between the generations. Patient–client '12' referred to her family history of cancer to estimate the crude probability of her own risk level, confessing that she was 'a bit concerned because of the number of people with cancer in my family. My mother died of breast cancer [and] I've got 4 sisters who have had mastectomies'. Meanwhile, patient–client '31' had consulted with other family members to devise a lay theory of who was at most risk of cancer, drawing on various non-genetic factors:

> P31: *'Well because of family history. I am bound to be at a bigger risk. I mean possibly I am not carrying the gene, but I know I am more at-risk maybe than I would normally be'.*
>
> FW: *'So irrespective of whether you have the gene or not, you think you might be at a higher risk?'*
>
> *'Yeah. I think in the back of my mind. Although that doesn't make sense because you have got to be having the gene to be at-risk, don't you? But I think it is always there in the back of my mind. And my cousin and I go through all sorts because as I say she is in on the risk. And she says 'well we will both be all right because we smoke and none of the others smoked.' And we have read now that there is a link there. She found something on that. 'We will be all right because we smoke' [laughs] And we have passed 40 so we are OK'. (P31: Clinical assessment = high risk, ovarian/breast cancer)*

Another of the most commonly cited lay theories, also reported by Richards (1997), was that there must be a close link between **genotype** and **phenotype**.

> **Genotype** refers to the genetic code inherited by each individual.
> **Phenotype** refers to inherited appearance.

That is, many people said that they believed themselves to be at high risk of cancer because they physically resembled a relative who had been affected by it, which in turn was related to observations about that person's social position in the family. Thus, patient–client '10' reported that her grandmother, her mother and her seven maternal aunts shared many of the same physical features; she accounted for one aunt's refusal to have mammograms in terms of the woman's eccentricities and health problems that marked her out as 'different' from others in the family:

> *'So my auntie, the youngest one who won't have the screening, she is a bit of an odd bod really, she has got lots of her ways, [although from] lots of features about her you can tell she is part of the family. But she never had any children. Well she had a miscarriage and that was it; it frightened her ... she is very much like my mother and two of her sisters. To look at, size and their shapes. We are all the same shape. As you have seen my shape, you have seen all my aunties. We have all got big hips and bottoms and little boobs. And there are strong features throughout the family. And it isn't until you do something like this and you look at all the family on one photograph that you start picking out all these things, you realize that they are really strong in your family'. (P10: Clinical assessment = high risk, breast cancer)*

The conceptual organization of the family as divided into maternal and paternal 'sides' has been identified by Davison (1997) as a common way in which British people talk about kinship and inheritance, along with the belief that individuals 'take after' older relatives. This was also reflected in the ESRC data. Patient–client '33' believed that cancer had affected her family through '[my] mother's side. With my father's side it was all heart and stroke'. Similarly, patient–client '16' had until recently, thought that she was protected from a genetic risk that ran down the male side of the family; all of the women in the family had lived to a 'ripe old age'. She was highly surprised when her mother developed breast cancer, and had had to adjust her beliefs to accommodate the new question of risk.

> *'... the eldest son of the eldest son of the eldest son has died for four generations. Completely unrelated. I do know that the women lived to ripe old ages. So I thought about this and I don't see anything there. My mother's mother, her mother lived until 86 years of age. I think she died of old age ... She didn't have any full sisters, she had two half sisters, they both lived to ripe old ages. So there is nothing there. That's why before ... when it was just my mum I wasn't thinking along the lines of genetic ...'(P16: Clinical assessment = moderate risk, breast cancer)*

In other cases, the patients observed from their family history that cancer had occurred variously *between* rather than *within* each generation. They accounted for this in terms of the belief that cancer 'skips a generation', a popular lay theory also identified by Richards (1997). This is to an extent supported by the biomedical notion of non-penetrance: those who inherit a faulty gene have only a 30–40% of actually developing cancer, and so it is possible for them to remain well and pass on the gene to a less fortunate son or daughter. Uppermost in the patients' minds, however, was simply an awareness of cancer occurring sporadically in their families and posing a threat to their family members. For example, patient–client '13' had agreed to take part in a research project about breast cancer because her mother had died of the disease and she feared for her own daughter's health:

> *'Yes, in all honesty when I was in my 30s I can't say I was paranoid about it but it was on my mind a lot. The reason I agreed to take part in the research in all honesty*

was because any study I felt would help, perhaps if it would skip my generation it would reappear perhaps in my daughter's generation. And any research could help her and my grand-daughter, is the real reason that I agreed to take part in it … I think for my age now I think you have put [my risk status] higher than I would'. (P13: Clinical assessment = moderate risk, breast cancer)

Patient–client '13' was unusual in underestimating her own risk level, for it was much more common for patients to overestimate relative to the genetic risk assessment (*cf* Hallowell et al 1998). However, this apparent difference can in fact be traced back to the same underlying factor: whatever version of reality had become established as 'truth' within the person's everyday life-world would shape their perceptions of risk. Thus patient–client '19', who was at moderate risk of developing colorectal cancer, overestimated her own risk as around 50% because she had compared her family history with information she had absorbed from the media in order to make a more meaningful, individualized estimate:

'I mean I sort of, you know you read magazines and on the TV and they talk about 1 in 3 or 1 in 5 people in the population. And then you do a quick calculation in your head and there is my mum, my uncle and my auntie. And so that really puts me higher than 1 in 3. So I reckon I have got about 50:50 chance'. (P19: Clinical assessment = moderate risk, colorectal)

The implications of this for healthcare

In this chapter, I have pointed out how a concern within medical sociology and anthropology with lay belief gradually metamorphosed into a concern with lay knowledge and thereafter with lay expertise. The concern with patients as experts has emerged both in intellectual discourse and in healthcare practice. In terms of practice, the rise of the lay expert is very closely bound up with the emphasis placed in modern healthcare systems on self-care. It is, after all, in the arena of self-care that the expert patient movement developed.

In the first section of the chapter, I attempted to pinpoint the origins of a concern with patients as experts. While in the second part of the chapter, as an example, I looked at how lay and medical knowledge about the genetics of breast cancer might differ. Above all, we saw that lay knowledge about risk and inheritance and the onset of illness tends to be anchored in the realm of personal experience. What happens to 'me' and to members of 'my' immediate family becomes the touchstone of evidence and practice. This, of course, is all very well and there is no doubt that health professionals need always to start their interactions with patients on the basis of personal experience. It is also the case that nurses and others need to understand the world as seen from the point of view of the laity so as to be capable of translating the concerns of professionals into the language of the patient and vice versa. However, I also hope to have demonstrated that there are profound and very real limitations to lay expertise. In particular, I would suggest, that the focus on personal and family experience as the touchstone of evidence often leads lay people astray as regards their understanding of the aetiology of medical conditions, the nature of medical conditions, and the ways in which such conditions ought to be managed. In the case of cancer genetics, these misunderstandings (and they are misunderstandings rather than alternative understandings) can give rise to unfounded anxieties on behalf of patients and unrealistic demands for medical intervention. Indeed, many of those in the ESRC study who were categorized as being at low risk by health professionals often expressed a sense of abandonment and a desire to be screened for inherited conditions of which they were simply not at-risk (Scott et al 2005). This was partly because they viewed the onset and distribution of disease as random, capricious and often illogical.

One of the great virtues of sociology and of the sciences in general, is to illustrate how the great evils of the world such as famine, poverty, want and disease are subject to patterns and structures. In almost all cases, those patterns and structures are the product of human interactions – not of 'natural', inevitable or even random events. The demonstration that such problems arise out of human activity is based essentially on the study of large numbers, many cases and big populations. One of the limitations of what is referred to as lay knowledge and lay expertise is that it so often eschews the study of big numbers and of many cases in favour of what happens to me and my family. Indeed, I would argue that the rejection of 'big number' evidence is often a hallmark of the lay viewpoint. A focus on one's immediate world can, naturally enough, have strengths. However, for an understanding of illness and disease it can also lead people astray (as it seemingly does with claims about MMR vaccine and autism). One task of medical sociology and medical sociologists is to study the basis and limitations of knowledge and that often means questioning what 'everyone knows'. In the world of nurses, it implies questioning one's own (professional) assumptions and evidence. However, it also implies that one should remain sceptical about the degree to which patients can be 'expert' in the understanding the causes, nature and management of disease and illness – and, consequently, of the degree to which they can undertake appropriate self-care without the assistance of health professionals.

Discussion points

1. How might the focus on personal and family experiences mislead people in understanding both the causes of particular illnesses and the risks for them of their development?
2. Discuss the particular care needs of people and families who carry an identified cancer gene.

CHAPTER SUMMARY

The first part of this chapter charted the changing status of lay people's understanding of health and illness, exemplified in the change of language in the medical sociology literature from lay beliefs to lay knowledge and finally lay expertise. The second part explored, through a particular research study, the ways in which medical and lay knowledge of genetic risk of cancer might differ. This study made clear that the limitations to lay knowledge (or indeed expertise) lie in its grounding in personal or family experience rather than larger population studies.

REFERENCES

Alaszewski A, Horlick-Jones T 2003 How can doctors communicate information about risk more effectively? British Medical Journal 327:728–731

Arksey H 1994 Expert and lay participation in the construction of medical knowledge. Sociology of Health and Illness 16(4):448–468

Arksey H 1998 RSI and the experts. UCL Press, London

Armstrong D 1985 The subject and the social in medicine: an appreciation of Michel Foucault. Sociology of Health and Illness 7(1):108–117

Armstrong D 1995 The rise of surveillance medicine. Sociology of Health and Illness 17(3):393–404

Atkinson P, Parsons E, Featherstone K 2001 Professional constructions of family and kinship in medical genetics. New Genetics and Society 20(1): 5–24

Beck U 1992 Risk Society: Towards a new modernity. Sage, London

Blaxter M 1983 The causes of disease. Women talking. Social Science and Medicine 17(2):59–69

Brown P 1987 Popular epidemiology: Community response to toxic waste-induced disease in Woburn, Massachusetts. Science, Technology and Human Values 12(3–4):78–85

Bury M 1982 Chronic illness as biographical disruption. Sociology of Health and Illness 4:167–182

Bury M 1986 Social constructionism and the development of medical sociology. Sociology of Health and Illness 8(2):137–169

Busby H, Williams G, Rogers A 1997 Bodies of knowledge: lay and biomedical understandings of musculoskeletal disorders. In: Elston M A (ed.) The sociology of medical science and technology. Blackwell, Oxford, p 79–99

Calnan M, Williams S 1992 Images of scientific medicine. Sociology of Health and Illness 14(2): 232–254

Cancer Research UK 2003 Scientific yearbook 2002/03. Cancer Research UK, London

Charmaz K 1983 Loss of self: a fundamental form of suffering in the chronically ill. Sociology of Health and Illness 5:168–195

Cox S M, McKellan W 1999 There's this thing in our family: predictive testing and the construction of risk for Huntingdon Disease. Sociology of Health and Illness 21(5):622–646

Davison C, Davey-Smith G, Frankel S 1991 Lay epidemiology and the prevention paradox. Sociology of Health and Illness 13(1):1–19

Davison C 1997 Everyday ideas of inheritance and health in Britain: implications for predictive genetic testing. In: Clarke A, Parsons E (eds) Culture, kinship and genes. St Martin's Press, New York, p 167–174

DoH Department of Health 1999 Patient and public involvement in the new NHS. HSC 1999/210 Department of Health, London

Edwards A, Elwyn G, Mulley A 2002 Explaining risks: turning numerical data into meaningful pictures. British Medical Journal 324:827–830

Eisenberg L 1977 Disease and illness. Distinctions between professional and popular ideas of sickness. Culture, Medicine and Psychiatry 1:9–23

Emslie C, Hunt K, Watt G 2001 Invisible Women? The importance of gender in lay beliefs about heart problems. Sociology of Health and Illness 23(2): 203–233

Elwyn G, Edwards A, Kinnersley P et al 2000 Shared decision-making and the concept of equipoise: Defining the 'competencies' of involving patients in healthcare choices. British Journal of General Practice 50:892–899

Epstein S 1996 Impure Science. Aids, activism and the politics of knowledge. University of California Press, Berkeley

Freidson E 1970 Professional dominance: the social structure of medical care. Atherton, New York

Habermas J 1987 The theory of communicative action. Vol. 2. Beacon, Boston (translated by Thomas McCarthy)

Hallowell N 1999 Doing the right thing: genetic risk and responsibility. Sociology of Health and Illness 21(5):597–621

Hallowell N, Statham H, Murton F 1998 Women's understanding of their risk of developing breast/ovarian cancer before and after genetic counselling. Journal of Genetic Counselling 7(4):345–364

Hibbert D, Bissell P, Ward P R 2002 Consumerism and professional work in the community pharmacy. Sociology of Health and Illness 24(1):46–65

Hughes B 2000 Medicalized bodies. In: Hancock P, Hughes B, Jagger E et al (eds) The body, culture and society. Open University Press, Milton Keynes, p 12–28

Joffe H 2003 Risk: from perception to social representation. British Journal of Social Psychology 42(1):55–73

Kleinman A 1978 Concepts and a model for the comparison of medical systems as cultural systems. Social Science and Medicine 12:85–93

Lloyd A J 2001 The extent of patients' understanding of the risk of treatments. Quality in Healthcare 10(1): 114–118

Lloyd S, Watson M, Waites B et al 1996 Familial breast cancer: a controlled study of risk perception, psychological morbidity and health beliefs in women attending for genetic counselling. British Journal of Cancer 74:482–487

Lupton D 1995 The imperative of health: Public health and the regulated body. Sage, London

Marteau T, Richards M (eds) (1996) The troubled helix. Social and psychological implications of the new human genetics. Cambridge University Press, Cambridge

Mazur D 2002 The new medical conversation. Rowman and Littlefield, Boulder

McConkie-Rosell A, Sullivan J A 1999 Genetic counselling – stress, coping and the empowerment perspective. Journal of Genetic Counselling 8(6): 345–357

Meiser B, Halliday J L 2002 What is the impact of genetic counselling in women at increased risk of developing hereditary breast cancer? A meta-analytic review. Social Science and Medicine 54:1463–1470

Monaghan L 1999 Challenging medicine? Body building, drugs and risk. Sociology of Health and Illness 21(6):707–734

Parsons E, Atkinson P 1992 Lay construction of genetic risk. Sociology of Health and Illness 14(4): 437–455

Pinder R 1992 Coherence and incoherence: doctors' and patients' perspectives on the diagnosis of Parkinson's disease. Sociology of Health and Illness 14:1–22

Popay J, Williams G, Thomas C et al 1998 Theorising inequalities in health. The place of lay knowledge. Sociology of Health and Illness 20(5): 619–644

Porter S 1998 Social theory and nursing practice. London, Macmillan

Prior L, Pang L C 2000 Beliefs and accounts of illness. Views from two Cantonese-speaking communities in England. Sociology of Health and Illness 22(6): 815–839

Prior L, Wood F, Gray J et al 2002 Making risk visible: the role of images in the assessment of genetic risk. Health, Risk and Society 4(3):242–258

Proctor R 1995 Cancer wars: How politics shapes what we know and don't know about cancer. Basic Books, New York

Randall J, Butow P, Kirk J et al 2001 Psychological impact of genetic counselling and testing in women previously diagnosed with breast cancer. Internal Medical Journal 31(7):397–405

Rees G, Fry A, Cull A 2001 A family history of breast cancer. Women's experiences from a theoretical perspective. Social Science and Medicine 52:1433–1440

Richards M 1997 It runs in the family: lay knowledge about inheritance. In: Clarke A, Parsons E (eds) Culture, kinship and genes. St Martin's Press, New York, p 175–194

Sarangi S 2001 Editorial. On demarcating the space between 'lay expertise' and 'expert laity'. Text 21 (1/2):3–11

Scott S, Prior L, Wood F et al 2005 Re-positioning the patient. The implications of being-at-risk. Social Science and Medicine 60:1869–1879

Shaw J S, Bassi K L 2001 Lay attitudes toward genetic testing for susceptibility to inherited diseases. Journal of Health Psychology 6(4):405–423

Skolbekken J-A 1995 The risk epidemic in medical journals. Social Science and Medicine 40:291–305

Stewart M, Brown J B, Weston W et al 1995 Patient-centred medicine. Transforming the clinical method. Sage, Thousand Oaks

Tuckett D, Boulton M, Olson C et al 1985 Meetings between experts. An approach to sharing ideas in medical consultations. Tavistock, London

Turner S 2001 What's the problem with experts? Social Studies of Science 31(1):123–149

Willems D 1992 Susan's breathlessness. The construction of professionals and laypersons. In: Lachmund J, Stollberg G (eds) The social construction of illness. Franz Steiner, Stuttgart, p 105–114

Williams G 1984 The genesis of chronic illness. Narrative re-construction. Sociology of Health and Illness 6(2):175–200

Wynne B 1989 Sheep farming after Chernobyl: A case study in communicating scientific information. Environment 31(2):10–15, 33–39

Wynne B 1996 May the sheep safely graze? A reflexive view of the expert-lay knowledge divide. In: Lash S, Szerszynski B, Wynne B (eds) Risk, environment and modernity. Towards a new ecology. London, Sage, p 44–83

CHAPTER 13

Experiencing ill-health

Susan Philpin

KEY CONCEPTS

- Talcott Parsons and the sick role
- The experience of chronic illness
- Strauss's framework of problems of chronic illness
- Coping actions required by patients
- The experience of pain

Introduction

This chapter will explore how sociology may contribute to our understanding of the ways in which people experience ill-health. Its focus is on the patient's perspective of this experience, that is, the ways in which patients make sense of their illness – what the illness *means* to them. Hence, the research studies underpinning this chapter are predominantly from the interpretive paradigm, including such methodologies as symbolic interactionism; phenomenology; ethnography and narrative analysis.

Useful sociological insights into people's experience of illness may be gained from a wide variety of sources, including a number of 'classic' sociological studies and more recent research accounts including nursing studies which have used a sociological framework. Further understanding of the meaning of illness experiences may also be gained from more 'general' literature, where people write their own accounts of their illness experiences; some examples of these accounts are listed at the end of this chapter. However, it must be borne in mind that these autobiographical accounts, illuminating though they are, serve different purposes than specific research studies (Bury 2001).

Talcott Parsons and the sick role

Although the meaning of illness from the sufferers' perspective is best explored from an interpretive perspective, the first classic study to be considered in this section is, in fact, not based on this approach and arguably is more concerned with society's (rather than the patient's) understanding of what it means to be ill. However, as will be shown, the patient's experience of illness is very much influenced by society's perception of just what counts as illness and how that illness is to be dealt with.

Talcott Parsons was one of the earliest writers to consider the social dimensions of illness and to some extent, his writing reflects a particular culture and era – North America in the 1950s. His work is grounded in a theoretical perspective known as *functionalism*, which argues that social actions are explained in terms of their functions towards the continuity of a society (see Chapter 2). His concept of the sick role to explain the illness experience is premised on the following key points:

- To be ill (or 'sick' in North American parlance) is to deviate from normal social behaviour inasmuch as the sick person is unable to fulfil her/his normal social roles, which interferes with important social functions. The concept of deviance is examined in Chapter 13
- Such deviance needs to be contained and controlled in order to maintain a functioning society
- Doctors play a key role in controlling deviance by defining and legitimating sickness.

As befits the functionalist perspective, the patient role 'functions' in accordance with the doctor's role; there is a symbiotic link between the two roles. Hence, the elements of the sick role are best understood in terms of the relationship between the specific rights and obligations inherent in both the doctor and patient roles.

Parsons (1951) describes four elements of the sick role for the patient – two 'rights' and two 'obligations'. The rights are that first, the patient will be exempted from normal social role responsibilities and second, the patient will also be exempted from responsibility for her/his condition. The obligations are that first, the patient must want to get well and, second will seek competent help and cooperate with that help. Parsons notes the ways in which the patient role and the doctor role *complement* each other in that the doctor is required to legitimate the patient's entry into the sick role and also that the patient is required to cooperate with the doctor. Thus in this way, the sick role functions to control the threat that illness poses to the individual and to the social order. This is set out diagrammatically in the Box 13.1.

This typology makes it clear that the 'sick role' is not just about the sick person's conception of their role, rather, it consists of a set of expectations about what it takes to be counted as really sick and what can and cannot be expected of sick people. In her diaries, Virginia Woolf recounts the particular pleasures of being absolved from social responsibilities when ill. She comments that while in health, people are required to keep up a 'genial pretence' to communicate with others and fulfil their various responsibilities, but notes that:

Box 13–1 The roles of the patient and doctor

Patient role

Rights

- Exempted from normal social role responsibilities where this is authorized by the appropriate agents
- Not seen as responsible for illness and not able to get better by an act of will

Obligations

- Must see illness as undesirable and want to get better
- Must seek technically competent help (usually from a physician) and comply with treatment

Doctor role

Rights

- Granted privileged access to physically and emotionally examine patients
- Granted autonomy in professional practice
- Granted authority over the patient

Obligations

- To apply technical competence to patient's illness
- To be altruistically orientated towards the patient's welfare rather than own self-interest
- To maintain affective neutrality, i.e. should avoid judging patient's behaviour in terms of personal value system or becoming emotionally involved with patients.

'In illness this make-believe ceases. Directly the bed is called for, or, sunk deep among pillows in one chair ... we cease to be soldiers in the army of the upright; we become deserters. They march to battle'. (Woolf [1926] 1994: 321)

CRITIQUES OF PARSONS' SICK ROLE

In spite of its influence and utility in explaining illness behaviour, Parsons' sick role has, not surprisingly, provoked considerable criticism and debate. Some of this criticism stems from criticism of the functionalist perspective upon which the theory is based inasmuch as this perspective treats social relationships, including doctor–patient relationships, as being essentially *consensual,* that is to argue that this approach tends to discount conflict (see Chapter 8).

Moreover, there would appear to be a plethora of conditions to which the sick role does not apply. These include minor illness conditions where recourse to the sick role is not necessary and also pregnancy, which, although sometimes grants exemption from normal roles is not usually viewed as an abnormal condition. The issue of not being responsible for one's condition is also problematic in relation to so called 'self-inflicted' conditions, such as alcoholism, sexually transmitted diseases and smoking-related diseases, where people could be deemed to be responsible for their illness.

However, it is in relation to chronic illnesses (which we will explore in the next section) that the application of the sick role is particularly problematic, for a number of reasons. First, in many cases, people are unable to absolve themselves from their usual responsibilities and tasks in the long term; second, people with chronic illness may never return to complete functional levels despite seeking competent help and cooperating with treatment. In response to this last point, Parsons (1975) pointed out that although complete recovery from some conditions may not be possible, these conditions may be 'managed' to enable the patient to lead a relatively normal life (e.g. diabetes).

In spite of these criticisms, the concept of the sick role made an important contribution to understanding health and illness, in that it moved on from focusing on physical and mental symptoms to include exploration of the *social* processes involved in becoming ill; that is that other people play a part in defining and legitimating illness. The concept is best suited to acute illnesses where the patient is the passive recipient of medical skills. For example, in one of the few sociological studies of the experience of acute, critical illness, a medical sociologist, Rier (2000) documents and analyses his own experiences of being a patient in an Israeli intensive care unit where he was admitted in acute respiratory and renal failure following viral pneumonia. Rier makes the point that in the acute stage of his illness, he was content to take the passive patient role and had no desire to have medical information shared with him or to be involved in decision making. Indeed, he argues that in the critical phase of illness it makes therapeutic sense for the doctor to take the paternalistic (Parsonian) role, concealing frightening information from patients (although not from their families) in order to instil confidence.

In addition, Parsons' concept of the sick role contributes to our understanding of the ways in which certain categories of patients (and illnesses) may be regarded as socially unacceptable and treated differently by healthcare workers. For example, people who self-harm in various ways – be it through smoking, drinking, abusing substances or cutting themselves – may be seen as responsible for their own conditions and therefore less deserving of care. That is to argue that their legitimate access to the sick role is denied.

RR REFLECTION POINT

Consider the ways in which Parsons' concept of the sick role helps you to understand patient and nurse behaviour in particular illness conditions from your practice.

The experience of chronic illness

Much, though not all (see for instance Frank 2002, Richman 2000, Rier 2000) of the sociological studies concerning the experience of illness focus on the experience of *chronic* illness, reflecting the nature of illness and indeed much nursing work, at the start of the twenty-first century. Chronic illness can only be *controlled* rather than *cured* and thus, as its name suggests, refers to a long-term condition. However, the boundary between acute and chronic illness is not necessarily clear-cut. For instance in the case of spinal cord injury, the initial trauma would be an acute problem but the consequences of the injury are also long-term disability. Given that any system of the body may be affected by this type of illness, the term encompasses a wide range of physical and mental conditions which many areas of nursing work, in both hospital and community, will deal with on a regular basis. Chronic obstructive pulmonary disease, diabetes, congestive cardiac failure, stroke, asthma, rheumatoid arthritis, leg ulcers, schizophrenia are all examples of chronic illness.

In addition, many forms of cancer have, in recent years, become perceived as chronic conditions since the treatment may control the spread of the disease in the long term without necessarily curing it. Thus, people may be symptom free, so not 'ill', yet not cured of this disease. Sufferers of other chronic illnesses may also have periods of relative 'wellness' when their symptoms are in remission, while by no means being cured; thus, there is a blurring of boundaries between illness and health. Frank (1995) describes people who are well but not cured as the 'remission society' which include people who have had:

> '... *almost any cancer, those living in cardiac recovery, diabetics, those whose allergies and environmental sensitivities require dietary and other self-monitoring. Those with prostheses and mechanical body regulators, the chronically ill* ...'. *(Frank 1995: 8)*

Similarly, Verbrugge and Jette (1994) note that most people with chronic illness 'live with rather than die from' their condition. Many chronic illnesses are of course also associated with varying degrees of **disability**, which will be considered in depth in Chapter 14.

Chronic illness has become increasingly prevalent in the last few decades, partly as a result of the ageing population (the incidence increases with age) and partly as a result of the effective prevention and treatment of infectious diseases. Chronic illness is usually measured by the amount of 'limiting long-standing illness' in a particular area. In Great Britain, the Department of Health reports that '17.5 million people may be living with a chronic disease' and that 'it is likely that three-quarters of those over 75 years are suffering form chronic disease, and this figure continues to rise' (Department of Health 2004). More than half of pensioners living alone have a limiting long-term illness (52.8%). In pensioner–family households, 60.4% contains someone with a limiting long-term illness (Census 2001).

Within the literature pertaining to the experience of chronic illness, there are a number of classic and more recent sociological studies, patients' narrative accounts (some of which are first-person accounts) and also a burgeoning nursing literature, which draws on sociological methods to explore the experience of chronic illness. This range of studies indicates that while different chronic illnesses present with different physical and mental symptoms for sufferers and carers to manage, there are also certain *commonalities* to chronic illnesses, an understanding of which helps healthcare workers plan and implement holistic care which will address patients' complex needs. Of particular relevance for health workers is the fact that the research reveals that patients often feel distanced socially and *emotionally* from their professional carers at a time when they are most vulnerable (see Chapter 8). In the absence of a cure for their conditions and the possibly limited efficacy of medical interventions, social support plays a vital role in coping with chronic illness and nurses are in a position to improve their patients' experiences by listening to them, providing emotional support and helping them to adapt to their changing symptoms (Frank 2002).

POTENTIAL PROBLEMS ASSOCIATED WITH LIVING WITH CHRONIC ILLNESS

A framework that is still useful in considering the impact of chronic illness on the daily lives of patients and their families is one that was developed by the North American sociologists Strauss and Glaser in the 1970s. Strauss et al (1984) outline eight key potential problems – listed in Box 13.2 – that people with chronic illness may have to deal with. Although developed over thirty years ago, many studies of chronic illness draw on this framework and the rest of this section will also utilize its main points, developing them further where appropriate.

Box 13–2 Impacts of chronic illness

1. The prevention of *medical* crises and their management once they occur
2. The control of *symptoms*
3. The carrying out of prescribed *regimens* and the management of problems attendant on carrying out the regimens
4. The prevention of, or living with, *social isolation* caused by lessened contact with others
5. The adjustment to changes in the *course of disease*, whether it moves downwards or has remissions
6. The attempts at *normalizing* both interaction with others and style of life
7. *Funding* – finding the necessary money – to pay for treatments or to survive despite partial or complete loss of employment
8. Confronting attendant *psychological, marital* and *familial* problems

(Strauss et al 1984: 16)

To avoid repetition, the final point in their framework – 'confronting attendant *psychological, marital,* and *familial* problems' – will be included where appropriate within the other problems rather than addressed as a separate issue.

Medical crises, symptoms and regimens

Strauss et al (1984) argue that these problems intrude into people's everyday lives and require great effort and hard work from patients and their families to learn how to deal with them. Although the first three of these problems may appear to be more medical than social, as Strauss et al point out, dealing with them often involves social strategies in terms of altering lifestyles and enlisting the help of others.

For instance, people (and/or their families) with type II diabetes need to learn to recognize the signs of either hypoglycaemia or hyperglycaemia and ensure that glucose or insulin is always available to manage either of these medical crises. The special diet prescribed may require adjustments to family meals and to social arrangements such as going out for meals or drinks with friends. In addition, with diabetes, the patient (or family) must learn how to inject insulin and monitor glucose levels in blood and urine and recognize and deal with side-effects of injecting. People who need to inject outside the home need to find safe and private places to do this and also to find safe and acceptable ways of disposing of needles possibly in the workplace or in school in the case of children.

In many cases, the drug therapy necessary to relieve chronic illness symptoms produces unwanted side effects and patients have to attempt to strike a balance between symptom control and unwanted side-effects. This is illustrated by Pinder's (1988) study, based on **symbolic interactionism,** of people with Parkinson's disease. This study also indicated the *intrusiveness* of medication regimes for some people with this condition, requiring timetabling and scheduling other activities around pill-taking.

Symbolic interactionism refers to a theoretical approach which focuses on the ways in which people communicate with each other using *symbols*. 'Symbol' in this sense denotes something which *stands* for or represents something else, such as language, clothing and demeanour. In particular, this approach focuses on the ways in which people interpret the *meaning* of experiences and actions through the symbols which convey this meaning.

Many studies refer to the time-consuming nature of treatment regimens. For example, Jobling's (1988) participant observation and interview study of people with psoriasis describes the ways in which the 'ointment-based treatment regimens for psoriasis ... generate an arduous demand, every day for weeks on end and hours of work, sometimes with little obvious reward' (Jobling 1988: 233). Similarly, Hagren et al's (2005: 296) study of Swedish patients undergoing maintenance haemodialysis, necessary for their survival, highlights the ways in which the dialysis procedure encroaches on patients' lives:

> *'I have five hours of it, so I'm the first to come and the last to leave. We lie there for four hours ... But honestly, I have to say that often when I come here, it seems more grey and dismal each time. Actually even before I get here, you know. But when you get here, you do it anyway. Still five hours is a long time. So I'll leave home at around ten past six and get home again at two, or half past two'.*

Pain is also often a significant symptom needing to be managed in chronic illness and is addressed in a later section.

Social isolation

An important issue for healthcare workers to consider in relation to people with chronic illness is their vulnerability to social isolation, which Pinder (1988) describes as 'perhaps one of the most distressing features of chronic illness' (Pinder 1988: 78). Strauss et al (1984) note the difficulties of maintaining social relationships, which:

> *'are disrupted or falter and disintegrate under the impact of lessened energy, impairment of mobility or speech, hearing impairment, body disfigurement, time spent on regimens and symptom control, and efforts made to keep secret so much about the disease and its management'. (Strauss et al 1984: 75)*

The social isolation may result from withdrawal by the patient, possibly through the **stigmatizing** (addressed in Chapter 14) nature of their illness, or from avoidance from other people. Social isolation may be psychologically harmful and links very closely with damage to the self and self identity, which is explored later in this Chapter. Lawton's (2000) study of the isolation of a woman dying with distressing symptoms is explored in Chapters 8 and 15. Walshe's (1995: 1096) **phenomenological** study of patients' experiences of venous leg ulcers similarly illustrates the social difficulties engendered by malodorous and leaking wounds:

> *'Because I thought, if I can smell it how do other people feel, and that, it made me really sick inside, the smell was so strong'.*

Phenomenological methods in qualitative health research are used to capture and describe people's experience of illness.

Carers of people with chronic illness are also vulnerable to social isolation, as Pinder's (1988: 78) study makes clear, exemplified in the following comments from the spouse of a man with Parkinson's disease:

> *'Friends, they don't* come *here very often. They phone me and tell me this and tell me that. But they don't actually* visit *here any more. They don't know how to behave towards him, I suppose'.*

Changes in the course of the disease

People with a chronic illness experience changes (sometimes unpredictable changes) over time, which may involve worsening or improvement in their condition. In relation to the changes in the course of the disease, Strauss et al (1984: 630) have introduced the concept of an 'illness trajectory', which they argue is different from the course of an illness in that it 'refers not only to the physiological unfolding of a sick person's disease but also to the *total organization* of work done over that course, plus the *impact* on those involved with that work and its organization'. That is, they suggest that the illness trajectory also encompasses the experiences and problems of people with chronic illness and their carers.

Many chronic illnesses are characterized by uncertainty in that people experience periods of remission and exacerbation, making it difficult for people to plan for the future. For example, Weiner's (1984) study of people with rheumatoid arthritis describes the unpredictability of the disease, in that: 'Most cases are marked by flare-up and remission. Even in the most hopeful case, bad flare-ups may suddenly occur, just as the most severe case may suddenly and inexplicably become arrested' (Weiner's 1984: 89). Similarly, in Barnett's phenomenological study of patients' experiences of chronic obstructive pulmonary disease, a patient commented:

> *'I can't plan anything. It depends on what sort of night I've had. I avoid early mornings because I can't do it. That can be frustrating sometimes. I wish I could put my coat on and go. I'd like to go on holiday with my family and go shopping'. (Barnett 2005: 810)*

Our understanding of illness trajectories and uncertainty is further illuminated through a classic study by Bury (1982), which introduces the concept of 'biographical disruption' and explains the ways in which the onset of chronic illness disrupts a person's *biography* or life story. In his study of people with rheumatoid arthritis, Bury illustrates the ways in which the onset of such illnesses disrupts the structures and relationships of everyday life, necessitating re-thinking of past events, dealing with current problems and readjusting plans and expectations for future life in the light of this altered state.

Normalizing interactions with others and style of life

Much of the research literature on chronic illness indicates chronically ill people's desire to lead as normal a life as possible. Strauss et al (1984) note that for chronically ill persons, their chief business is 'not just to stay alive or keep their symptoms under control, but to live as normally as possible despite the symptoms and the disease' (Strauss et al 1984: 79). Attempts to normalize interactions with other people will be affected by the visibility and/or intrusiveness of symptoms and often involve strategies of 'passing' as normal, which links with issues of stigma discussed in the next chapter. An important aspect of normalizing interactions with others concerns maintenance of the patient's sense of self, in that social interactions and a person's sense of identity are intrinsically linked to a 'normally' functioning body.

Impact of chronic illness on self-identity

Before we consider the ways in which chronic illness impacts on a person's self-identity it is useful to briefly look at what we mean by 'self' and 'self-identity' drawing on the work of the early symbolic interactionist writers, George Herbert Mead (1934) and Charles Cooley (1962, 1964).

George Herbert Mead (1863–1931) was an American philosopher and social psychologist and a founder of symbolic interactionism; his major contribution was the nature of the human 'self'. In *Mind, Self and Society* (1934), which was published posthumously, Mead explored the nature of the human self. He argued that our sense of our self is not something that we are born with, but arises out of symbolic exchanges with other people, especially through exchange of language. Mead also explored ideas of 'reflexivity' or the ability to reflect (through inner conversation) on our own thoughts and actions, arguing that this ability is what distinguishes human beings from animals.

Similarly, Cooley, a colleague of Mead, argued that our sense of self can only develop through interactions with other people; thus, the self and society are inextricably linked, or as Cooley put it 'self and society are twin-born' (1962: 5). He noted that we learn who we are, from early infancy and throughout life, by observing the responses of other people towards us, what Cooley (1964: 184) called the reflected or '*looking glass self*'. Mead argued that interactions with '*significant others*', people with whom we have significant and lasting relationships, were particularly important for identity formation. Thus, social relations play a crucial role in the development and maintenance of self identity.

Drawing on these insights from symbolic interactionism, Charmaz's (1983) classic study examined the ways in which the experience of chronic illness influenced a person's sense of self. In particular, she noted that the restricted lives and social isolation which are often a consequence of chronic illness, are damaging to the self inasmuch as they deny people the opportunities of meaningful social interactions. Charmaz describes this losing of self identity as a 'fundamental form of suffering' for people with chronic illness as they experience a 'crumbling away of their former self-images without simultaneous development of equally valued new ones' (Charmaz 1983: 168).

Asbring's (2001) study of women suffering from either chronic fatigue syndrome or fibromyalgia similarly describes profound loss of identity, particularly in relation to loss of work and withdrawal from social roles. However, Asbring's study also describes the women as eventually coming to terms with their changed identity, transforming their old identity into their new situation. Indeed, in many instances the women described positive aspects of this identity transformation, claiming that it had allowed deeper understanding of themselves and others.

Another classic exploration of the effects of chronic illness on people's self-image is a study by Gareth Williams (1984) which used **narrative analysis** (Box 13.3). This study focussed on long-term consequences of chronic illness in that respondents had been diagnosed with rheumatoid arthritis for at least 5 years.

Williams (1984) introduces the notion of 'narrative reconstruction', which means the ways in which his respondents' accounts (and understandings) of how and why their illness started were constructed as a means of helping them to make sense of their disrupted lives. In the absence of a satisfactory medical explanation for the devastating changes in their bodies, they sought explanations from within relationships in their wider society. That is, in the construction and telling of their stories of their illness causation, they were able to bring a sense of order and coherence to their lives, helping to preserve their sense of self. As Williams succinctly explains, their reconstruction of their illness story or narrative is 'an attempt to reconstitute and repair ruptures

Box 13–3 Narrative analysis

Narrative analysis refers to the analysis of illness narratives – the 'stories' or accounts that people give of their illness experience. In similar vein to literary analysis, analysis of an illness narrative attempts to tease out its 'plot', including the social context of the account. Bury (2001) notes that narrative analysis differs from other forms of qualitative analysis in 'the way in which lay people's accounts or stories are dealt with. In much content analysis of interview data, various themes are identified and then illustrated with quotes from across the interview data set . . . In narrative analysis the interview or story is taken as a whole, and set in the context in which it has been generated or told' (Bury 2001: 281).

between body, self and world by linking-up and interpreting different aspects of biography in order to realign present and past and self with society' (Williams 1984: 197).

The medical anthropologist, Arthur Kleinman (1988) also describes a need to report and 'witness' people's suffering experiences, in addition to imposing some sort of order and control on such suffering (we discussed religious and cultural approaches to the meaning of suffering in Chapter 3). Kleinman argues that such witnessing and ordering of their illness experience has therapeutic value for the sufferer.

A more recent study by Kelly (1992a), based on symbolic interactionism, calls attention to the ways in which changes to the body's appearance and functioning, such as following radical surgery (in this case total colectomy and formation of ileostomy) impact on the sense of self and identity. Kelly's respondents voiced their concerns that their changed bodies made them different from their previous selves and from other people; they also found these bodily changes as 'undesirable in themselves and likely to be appraised as undesirable in others' (Kelly 1992b: 397). Significantly for healthcare workers, Kelly's study indicates that these concerns over bodily changes were more salient when the person was in pain (from the surgery) or suffering emotional trauma from such things as the sight of the scar and stoma and also from the need to defecate through a stoma. Thus, this study clearly brings the relationship between the appearance and functioning of the body and the sense of self identity to the fore.

RR REFLECTION POINT

Reflect on people you have cared for in practice and consider the impact of their chronic illness on their sense of self and identity.

Funding

Loss of income through inability to continue working may lead to financial hardship for both patients and their carers. In addition, although healthcare is free in the UK, chronic illness may entail extra costs for heating, dietary requirements, prescription charges and adaptations to the home. Anderson and Bury (1988), in the conclusion of their now classic collection of patients' experiences of chronic illness, refer to the substantial financial disadvantage stemming from the experience of chronic illness and also contributing to it (Anderson & Bury 1988: 248). The impact of chronic illness on material circumstances is, of course, influenced by patients' (or their families') previous income and socioeconomic status as we saw in Chapter 6.

The experience of pain and suffering

Healthcare work frequently involves helping people to deal with the pain that may accompany illness. This section will explore the ways in which, in addition to the neuro-physiological elements of pain, people's experiences of and responses to pain are also influenced by the sociocultural context of that experience. As with other aspects of the illness experience, the experience of pain is entirely subjective – health professionals can only assess and understand this experience through their interpretations of people's responses. As McCaffery's (1968: 95) now classic statement on pain makes clear 'Pain is whatever the experiencing person says it is, existing whenever he (sic) says it does'.

THE SOCIOCULTURAL CONTEXT OF PAIN EXPERIENCE AND RESPONSE

The medical anthropologist, Helman (2000: 128) usefully outlines the following propositions in relation to the sociocultural nature of pain experience and response:

1. Not all social or cultural groups may respond to pain in exactly the same way.
2. How people perceive and respond to pain, both in themselves and others, can be influenced by their cultural and social background.
3. How, and whether, people communicate their pain to health professionals and to others can also be influenced by social and cultural factors.

Helman (2000) distinguishes between 'private' or 'public' pain, noting that pain only becomes public when the sufferer signals it in some way. Helman is concerned here with the *voluntary* and deliberate public expression of pain, obviously pain may also be expressed involuntarily and/or be observable through physiological changes such as pallor or sweating. He suggests that the decision to translate private pain into publicly expressed pain is influenced by sociocultural factors including whether or not the pain is perceived as 'normal' or 'abnormal' or not. Societies that values stoicism or view certain painful conditions as normal may be more inclined to keep pain private.

Classic and much quoted studies by two American sociologists Zborowski (1952) and Zola (1966) in relation to cultural influences on the experience and reporting of pain are useful in considering cultural differences in response to pain. Both studies describe the ways in which patients of different ethnic backgrounds perceive and report the intensity of their pain. Briefly, Zborowski (1952) found that patients of Italian-American and Jewish-American ethnic backgrounds tended to be more expressive about their pain and to seek public sympathy, while those of 'Old American' background displayed more stoical behaviour, tending to withdraw from the company of others. Similarly, Zola's (1966) study found that Italian-Americans responded to pain by over expressing it, while the Irish-Americans tended to ignore or play down their symptoms.

However, caution must be exercised to avoid stereotyping of particular ethnic group's responses to pain. Indeed, there have been a number of studies where nurses and midwives have been influenced in their responses to patients' complaints of pain by their preconceived notions of the behaviour of particular ethnic groups. Bowler's (1993) ethnographic study of South Asian descent women's maternity experiences in a British hospital indicates negative stereotyping of these women by their midwives – similar to other forms of negative social judgements which we discussed in Chapter 8. The midwives interviewed in the study characterized Asian women as 'attention seeking'; making too much noise and 'unnecessary fuss' during labour because of 'low pain thresholds' (Bowler 1993: 166). Bowler notes that all the labour ward midwives interviewed mentioned the issue of noise during labour and low pain thresholds in relation to Asian women. Bowler also suggests the possibility of Asian women being disadvantaged in terms of pain control because of the midwives' assumptions.

Bowler's study is also suggesting that the culture of the healthcare provider influences the ways in which providers respond to their patients' pain. This has also been strongly indicated in a study by Bates et al (1997) which compared healthcarers' responses to pain in a New England and a Puerto Ricans clinic. Among other findings, these authors indicated that when Puerto Ricans (referred to as 'Latinos') were cared for by staff in the New England centre (Anglo-Americans), the staff tended to view the Latino response to pain as inappropriate and to react negatively towards them, as indicated in the following interview excerpt:

> *'He starts to yell when I apply the alcohol swab – even before I put the needle in (for the IV). He looks so macho but he acts like a baby'. (Bates et al 1997: 1437)*

In contrast, when Latinos were cared for by Puerto Rican staff, their expression of pain was viewed as appropriate and as an indication that they were in serious pain that needed prompt treatment. Bates et al (1997) comment on the need for nurse (and physician) education, in addition to exploring ethnic variations in patients, should also encourage understanding of the healthcare providers' own culture. That is:

> *'Healthcare providers (physicians, specialists and nurses) should be cognizant that their own cultural backgrounds are comprised of their individual experiences and the norms, beliefs and practices intrinsic to their professional training; that the culture of 'medicine' and their own cultural background affect their communications, perceptions and interactions with pain patients, and ultimately, the care and treatment they provide'. (Bates et al 1997: 1444)*

It is also important to distinguish between the *experience* of pain and public *expressions* of pain. As Mumford (1993: 237) notes, with reference to the ethnic differences in the ways in which people describe their physical symptoms (including symptoms of pain), these differences 'may have more to do with complaint behaviour than with differences in symptom perception'. That is to argue that 'complaint behaviour' or the public expression of pain is bound by cultural norms and expectations. This is classically exemplified in the Case study below, abridged from Wall (1999), of Grantley Dick-Read's study of pain in childbirth.

Case study

In the 1930s, Grantley Dick-Read was a colonial doctor in the Tulkarm region of northern Kenya. He wrote of witnessing childbirth in local women who were quiet, calm, dignified and conversing with their tribal neighbours. He was inspired by this and wrote the book *Childbirth Without Fear,* which was to have a revolutionary effect on antenatal training classes and the education of mothers-to-be in the West. For him, the Kenyans showed that pain did not occur in the absence of fear, anxiety, tension and ignorance. He set about showing that a mother who was transported by herself and others into a 'natural' setting benefited greatly.

Fifty years later a female anthropologist who could speak Tulkarm witnessed a similar scene to that which so changed Dick-Read and the nature of antenatal training. She asked the woman after the delivery whether it had hurt. The woman answered that the pain had been great. She was then asked why she had not said so, and was told: 'That is not the custom of my people'. There really should be no surprise at this answer. The women in labour rooms in Oslo do not shout out, not because they are not in pain, but because it is not the custom of their people. At the other end of Europe, in Naples, women in labour do shout very loudly, not because they are in more pain than the Norwegians, but because those around them would be worried if they did not shout.

(Wall 1999: 71, abridged).

As with culture, the relationship between gender and pain is similarly complex. Bendelow's (1993) study of the role of gender in the development of beliefs about pain identified two key gender differences in pain perception. First, she notes that men were more reluctant than women to consider emotional pain as 'real' pain. Second, she found that both men and women expressed the view that 'the combination of female biology and the reproductive role served to equip girls and women with a "natural" capacity to endure pain, both physically and emotionally' (Bendelow's 1993: 286). In addition, her study indicates that 'male socialization is seen to actively discourage males from being allowed to express pain, either physical or emotional, so it is seen as a state of "abnormality", in contrast to the "natural" expectations of females' (Bendelow's (1993: 289).

The language of pain

Frank (2002: 29–30) comments that although there are many words to describe specific pains:

'sharp, throbbing, piercing, burning, even dull ... these words do not describe the experience of pain. We lack terms to express what it means to live "in" such pain'. In similar vein, Virginia Woolf notes that if we should want to express other life experiences, there is an abundance of literature to call on, but nothing in literature to give meaning to pain – 'let a sufferer try to describe a pain in head to a doctor and language at once runs dry' (Woolf [1926] 1994: 318).

The language used by health professionals is also influential in terms of how they perceive their patients' pain. McCaffery and Pasero (1999) note that in describing their patients' reports of pain, it is common for doctors and nurses to use the phrase 'complains of pain', arguing that this suggests a 'much more negative evaluation of the patient than does saying that the patient reports pain' (McCaffery and Pasero 1999: 42).

Discussion points

1. Apply Strauss et al's (1984) framework to explore particular chronic illness conditions you have encountered in your practice.
2. Consider the ways in which chronic illness may bring about 'biographical disruption' in relation to people you have cared for.
3. What sort of factors may influence the ways in which nurses respond to people's expression of pain?

CHAPTER SUMMARY

This chapter has attempted to explore the complexities of the experience of illness through a sociological perspective in order to inform nursing practice. A particular area of focus has been on the *meanings* attached to this experience for patients and their families. Almost 20 years ago, Anderson and Bury (1988: 256) concluded their collection of accounts of patients' illness experiences with the call for a response from professionals that 'places the experiences of patients and their families at the centre of the caring process', – advice that is still relevant today. Another underlying thread running through this chapter is that an important element of the illness experience is the response of other people; accordingly in Chapter 14 the *social response* to illness will be further explored.

FURTHER READING

McCrum R 1998 My year off: Rediscovering life after a stroke. Picador, London.

A powerful and moving personal account of Robert McCrum's (literary editor of The Observer) *experience of suffering a stroke at the age of 42.*

Reissman CK 1993 Narrative analysis. Sage, California.

An accessible introduction to narrative analysis

REFERENCES

Anderson R, Bury M 1988 (eds) Living with chronic illness: The experience of patients and their families. Unwin Hyman, London

Asbring P 2001 Chronic illness – a disruption in life: identity transformation among women with chronic fatigue syndrome and fibromyalgia. Journal of Advanced Nursing 34(3):312–319

Barnett M 2005 Chronic obstructive pulmonary disease: a phenomenological study of patients' experiences. Journal of Clinical Nursing 14:805–812

Bates M, Rankin-Hill L, Sanchez-Ayendez M 1997 The effects of the cultural context of health care on treatment of and response to chronic pain and illness. Social Science & Medicine 45(9):1433–1447

Bendelow G 1993 Pain perceptions, emotions and gender. Sociology of Health and Illness 15(3):273–294

Bowler I 1993 'They're not the same as us': midwives' stereotypes of South Asian descent maternity patients. Sociology of Health and Illness 15(2): 157–178

Bury M 1982 Chronic illness as biographical disruption. Sociology of Health and Illness 4(2): 167–162

Bury M 2001 Illness narratives; fact or fiction? Sociology of Health and Illness 23(3):263–285

Census 2001 Office for Population Census and Surveys, Great Britain 2001 Census. Available at www.statistics.gov.uk

Charmaz K 1983 Loss of self: a fundamental form of suffering in the chronically ill. Sociology of Health and Illness 5(2):168–195

Cooley C 1962 Social organization. Schocken Books, New York

Cooley C 1964 Human nature and the social order. Schocken, New York
Department of Health 2004 Improving chronic disease management. HMSO, London
Frank A W 2002 At the will of the body: Reflections on illness. Houghton Mifflin, Boston
Frank A W 1995 The wounded storyteller: Body, illness and ethics. University of Chicago Press, London
Hagren B, Pettersen I, Severinsson E, et al 2005 Maintenance haemodialysis: patients' experiences of their life situation. Journal of Clinical Nursing 14, 294–300
Helman C G 2000 Culture, health and illness, 4th edn. Butterworth-Heinemann, London
Jobling R 1988 The experience of psoriasis under treatment. In: Anderson R, Bury M (eds) Living with chronic illness: The experience of patients and their families. Unwin Hyman, London, p 225–244
Kelly M 1992a Colitis. Routledge, London
Kelly M 1992b Self, identity and radical surgery. Sociology of Health and Illness 14(3):390–415
Kleinman A 1988 The illness narratives: Suffering, healing and the human condition. Basic Books, New York
Lawton J 2000 The dying process: patients' experiences of palliative care. Routledge, London
McCaffery M 1968 Nursing practice theories related to cognition, bodily pain, and man-environment interactions. University of California at Los Angeles, Students' Store, Los Angeles
McCaffery M, Pasero C 1999 Pain: Clinical Manual 2nd edn. Mosby, St Louis
Mead G H 1934 Mind, self and society: from the standpoint of a social behaviorist. University of Chicago Press, Chicago
Mumford D B 1993 Somatization: a transcultural perspective. International Review of Psychiatry 5:231–242
Parsons T 1951 The social system. Routledge and Kegan Paul Ltd, London
Parsons T 1975 The sick role of the physician reconsidered. Millbank Memorial Fund Quarterly: Health and Society 53:257–278
Pinder R 1988 Living with Parkinson's disease. In: Anderson R, Bury M (eds) Living with chronic illness: The experience of patients and their families. Unwin Hyman, London, p 67–88
Richman J 2000 Coming out of intensive care crazy: Dreams of affliction. Qualitative Health Research 10(1):84–102
Rier D A 2000 The missing voice of the critically ill: a medical sociologist's first-person account. Sociology of Health and Illness 22(1):68–93
Strauss AL, Glaser BG 1975 Chronic illness and the quality of life, 1st edn. Mosby, St Louis
Strauss A L, Corbin J, Fagerhaugh S et al 1984 Chronic illness and the quality of life, 2nd edn. Mosby, St Louis
Verbrugge LM, Jette AM 1994 The disablement process. Social Science and Medicine 38(1):1–14
Wall P 1999 Pain: The science of suffering. Weidenfeld and Nicholson, London
Walshe C 1995 Living with a venous leg ulcer: a descriptive study of patients' experiences. Journal of Advanced Nursing 22:1092–1100
Weiner C 1984 The burden of rheumatoid arthritis. In: Strauss A L, Corbin J, Fagerhaugh S et al, 2nd edn. Chronic illness and the quality of life. Mosby, St Louis, p 71–80
Williams G 1984 The genesis of chronic illness: Narrative reconstruction. Sociology of health and illness 6:175–200
Woolf V [1926] 1994 On being ill. In: McNeillie A (ed.) The essays of Virginia Woolf. Hogarth, London
Zola IK 1966 Culture and symptoms: an analysis of patients' presenting complaints. American Sociological Review 31:615–630
Zborowski M 1952 Cultural components in responses to pain. Journal of Social Issues 8:16–30

CHAPTER

14 Social responses to illness and disability

Susan Philpin

KEY CONCEPTS

- Deviance and labelling perspectives
- The application of labelling perspectives to mental illness
- Stigma
- Moral panics
- Disability – concepts, definitions and models
- Disabling barriers – physical and attitudinal
- Language in relation to disability – including anti-discriminatory language
- Anti-discriminatory practice

Introduction

Chapter 13's focus was on people's experience of illness; this chapter will turn our attention to the ways in which society responds to illness, although of course people's experience of illness is inextricably linked to society's reaction to it. Social reaction to illness and disability profoundly affects the ways in which people think about themselves and their levels of self-esteem; for instance, as this chapter will demonstrate, society's reaction to disability influences the extent to which 'disabling' barriers are a feature. In order to explore social reaction to illness, this chapter will draw on insights from sociological studies of the closely related concepts of deviance, labelling perspectives and stigma. In particular, labelling perspectives in relation to *mental* illness will be explored inasmuch as this is an area where there has been considerable controversy and debate. In addition, given that disability has often been presented as a form of social deviance, different aspects of social responses to disability will be examined.

Much of the research concerning social reaction to illness and disability draws on the methods described in the previous chapter concerning the experience of illness – qualitative interpretive studies. In relation to people with disabilities however, disabled people such as Oliver (1997) and Priestley (1997) argue for an *emancipatory* research paradigm based on the social model of disability, which is outlined later in the chapter. As its name suggests, this paradigm is concerned with emancipating socially oppressed people through the research process. Oliver (1997) argues that what made this type of research a new paradigm was 'the changing of the social relations of research production – the placing of control in the hands of the researched, not the researcher' (Oliver 1997: 17). (See Chapters 5 and 12 for accounts of critical theory.)

The key principles of the emancipatory research paradigm are set out by Priestley (1997: 92) as follows:

1. The adoption of a social model of disability as the **ontological** and **epistemological** basis for research production.
2. The surrender of falsely-premised claims to objectivity through overt political commitment to the struggles of disabled people for self-emancipation.
3. The willingness only to undertake research where it will be of some practical benefit to the self-empowerment of disabled people and/or the removal of disabling barriers.
4. The devolution of control over research production to ensure full accountability to disabled people and their organizations.
5. The ability to give voice to the personal while endeavouring to collectivize the commonality of disabling experiences and barriers.
6. The willingness to adopt a plurality of methods of data collection and analysis in response to the changing needs of disabled people.

The emancipatory research paradigm continues to raise questions and debate about the importance of objectivity and neutrality in research and also about how realistic it is to expect research to emancipate oppressed people. However, approaches based on this paradigm, such as 'Participatory Action Research' are now being used in many areas of nursing research in order to elicit patient perspectives and address perceived needs.

Ontology refers to the study of the nature of reality
Epistemology refers to the study of the nature of knowledge

Deviance and labelling perspectives

The word 'deviate' is commonly used to mean to depart from the usual path, and sociological understandings of deviance and deviant behaviour develop this idea of actions that depart from the norms, rules and expectations of a particular social group. In relation to health and illness, illness may be perceived as deviant inasmuch as it also departs from social norms and expectations. As we saw in Chapter 13, Parsons' (1951) concept of the *sick role* is premised on the idea that sickness is deviant (in that sick people may be unable to fulfil their expected roles) and needs to be controlled in some way.

The intellectual roots of sociological studies of deviance, labelling and stigma stem from **symbolic interactionism**, which (see Chapter 13) attempts to explain social actions and interactions in terms of the *meanings* of those actions to the people involved. Within this theoretical approach, reality is socially constructed and open to negotiation and different interpretations, rather than there being one absolute social reality. Deviance and labelling perspectives are also products of a particular point in time – the 1960s – a period marked by the growth of radical movements and challenges to authority and ideas of absolute knowledge in various parts of the Western world. With respect to *mental* illness, which the labelling perspective has been applied to, this period also saw the growth of the 'anti-psychiatry' movement, where there was opposition to contemporary psychiatric diagnoses and treatments.

LABELLING PERSPECTIVES

Edwin Lemert (1961), one of the earliest proponents of the labelling perspective, proposed the following three-stage model of the relationship between deviant behaviour and society's reaction to it:

1. Primary deviation – initial rule-breaking event

2. Social reaction to the event
3. Secondary deviation – the response of the individual to society's reaction.

Lemert is essentially arguing that the initial rule-breaking event only becomes important when its perpetrator has been identified and labelled as a rule breaker. Secondary deviation occurs as a result of society's disapproval and subsequent treatment of the individual. For example,

> *'the primary deviance of the armed bank robber is the robbing of the bank, the societal reaction is his arrest, conviction and jailing, and his secondary deviance resides in him identifying with other bank robbers and prisoners, committing further crimes and fulfilling the expectations of his custodians and others'. (Bowers 1998: 2)*

Kelly (1992) elaborates the idea of secondary deviation in a slightly more complex way in relation to someone who has undergone surgery resulting in an ileostomy. Kelly argues that the ileostomy operation initially produces secondary deviation in that 'the whole life of the person revolves around the operation and its sequelae' (Kelly 1992: 94). However, he goes on to argue that gradually, *provided* the ileostomy 'can be managed, concealed, and kept out of the gaze of the world at large, and the person goes back to leading a life of functioning ordinarily, then he or she is in a situation of primary deviance: his or her difference makes no difference' (Kelly 1992: 94).

The following classic definition of deviance by Becker (1963) makes clear its link with society's reaction to and labelling of behaviour but also takes Lemert's ideas further by arguing that it is actually the making of social rules that creates deviance.

> *'Social groups create deviance by making the rules whose infraction constitutes deviance, and by applying those rules to particular people and labelling them as outsiders. From this point of view, deviance is not a quality of the act the person commits, but rather a consequence of the application by others of rules and sanctions to an "offender". The deviant is one to whom that label has successfully been applied; deviant behaviour is behaviour that people so label'. (Becker 1963: 9)*

From this definition, it is clear that people who do not conform to society's expectations of 'normal' behaviour, including people with illness and/or disability, are vulnerable to being labelled as deviant. In relation to people with disabilities, the subject of a later section, Hunt (1966) observes that 'people's shocked reactions to the obvious deviant often reflect their deepest fears and difficulties, their failure to accept themselves as they really are, and the other person simply as "other" (Hunt 1966: 152).

The application of labelling perspectives to mental illness

Although labelling perspectives have been used to illuminate many areas of health and nursing work (see Chapter 8) they have been particularly intriguing and indeed controversial in their application to mental illness. In fact, the North American sociologist Thomas Scheff (1966) went so far as to argue that labelling *caused* mental illness inasmuch as once the label is applied the person fulfils the role of 'being mentally ill'.

Scheff argued that in society there is a 'residue' of odd behaviour, which does not fit into any named category and is not governed by any specific rules but that there are expectations or 'residual rules' concerning this behaviour. He illustrates this by drawing on examples from Erving Goffman's (1963b) accounts of rules of behaviour in public places. Goffman describes the unwritten rule that when we appear in public we should appear to be 'involved' in some way with what is going on rather than wandering around (or 'lolling' as Goffman puts it) doing nothing. He notes that people who appear to be uninvolved in the public arena without a reasonable excuse are perceived as breaking an unwritten (residual) rule and that most symptoms of mental illness come into this category of residual rule-breaking.

Scheff argues that although everyone at times breaks these residual rules, the application of a 'mental illness' label depends on societal reaction to the behaviour. Societal reaction is influenced by such things as the status and power of the rule-breaker, the level of tolerance in the community for the rule-breaking behaviour and whether or not there are other explanations for the behaviour. However, Scheff argues that if the person *is* labelled as mentally ill and treated accordingly this leads to a change in his/her self-image. That is the mental illness label leads to a self conception and behaviour that fits the expectations of the mentally ill role, consequently the label becomes a self-fulfilling prophesy.

Scheff's theory provoked much criticism; in particular in a series of publications by Walter Gove (1970, 1975) where he drew on his empirical studies of people with mental illness to argue that most people who are diagnosed with a mental illness do in fact have a mental disorder rather than simply being guilty of residual rule-breaking. His theory has also been criticized for not explaining the reasons for the original rule-breaking, only society's reactions to it.

Despite these criticisms, an understanding of labelling perspectives in relation to mental health is important for those involved in healthcare in that they encourage a critical questioning approach to the impact of diagnostic and public labelling. Scheff's work indicates the power of labels in becoming self-fulfilling prophecies. When healthcare professionals and the public apply particular labels people can become locked into their deviant roles. In spite of the importance of these insights, it seems that Scheff's theory fell into disrepute as a result of his attempts to over-expand his theory into an explanation of the *causes* of mental illness.

However, the powerfulness of labelling is also suggested by another well-known covert observational study by Rosenhan (1973) involving eight researchers (three women and five men) feigning mental illness and having themselves admitted to psychiatric wards in twelve different hospitals in the USA. In this study, the researchers, after telephoning the hospital for an appointment, presented themselves at the admissions offices claiming to be hearing voices – in all eight cases they were admitted to the hospital, seven with a diagnosis of schizophrenia. Once admitted to the psychiatric ward the researchers (or 'pseudopatients' as Rosenhan calls them) stopped simulating any abnormal symptoms.

The researchers' observations were interesting on a number of levels, including an aid to understanding the kind of care provided in these hospitals. The most significant point emerging from this study however, was what Rosenhan called the 'stickiness of labels'. That is, once the label had been applied by a person in a powerful position, it was almost impossible to shift. 'Having once been labelled schizophrenic, there is nothing the pseudopatient can do to overcome the tag. The tag profoundly colors others' perceptions of him and his behaviour' (Rosenhan 1973: 253). Thus, all the other (quite normal) behaviour was viewed through the lens of this original diagnostic label and interpreted as being abnormal. For instance, all pseudopatients openly made notes of their experience; in three cases, this was perceived as evidence of mental pathology – 'Patient engages in writing behavior' (Rosenhan 1973: 253). The label 'schizophrenic' had assumed what Becker (1963) calls a 'master status', cancelling out any possible other roles and identities.

Rosenhan's covert research has been criticized on ethical grounds for its deception of participants. However, I would suggest that the study is a salutary lesson for health professionals on the power of labelling. It is worth remembering that in some instances, the other (genuine) patients in the hospitals studied detected the researchers' sanity, while the health professionals' perception of, and reaction to the pseudopatients' behaviour was influenced by their diagnostic label.

Studies such as Rosenhan's (1973) also alert us to the disempowering and depersonalizing effects of hospital admission, one of the consequences of which may be the acceptance and internalization of labels. For instance, the following excerpt describing an attempted social exchange between doctor and pseudopatient is a study in depersonalization:

> 'Pseudo-patient: *pardon me, Dr X. Could you tell me when I am eligible for ground privileges?'*
>
> Physician: *'Good morning, Dave. How are you today? (moves off without waiting for a response)'. (Rosenhan 1973: 255, abridged)*

Similarly, Goffman's classic study *Asylums* (1968) describes commonly used admission procedures (at that time) – such as compulsory undressing and washing, removal and listing of personal possessions – that destroy self-identity as 'mortification of the self'. Loss of self-identity may lead people to accept their diagnostic and public labels (see Chapter 4).

REFLECTION POINTS

From your practice, consider instances of when labelling of patients has occurred. How did this influence their subsequent care? Did the status of the person applying the label make any difference to the label's influence or 'stickiness'?

Stigma

The concept of stigma is complex, drawing together the previously discussed ideas of labelling and deviance by focussing on the affects of such negative labelling on social and self-identity. Erving Goffman's (1963a) classic and easily accessible work on stigma – '*Stigma: Notes on the Management of Spoiled Identity* – provides the basis for much of our sociological understanding of people who are not accepted into particular social groups and is particularly relevant to our appreciation of society's reaction to people with chronic illness and disability. For Goffman, stigma refers to a social label or attribute that is 'deeply discrediting', changing both people's perceptions of themselves and the ways in which society regards them. He argues that if someone possesses an attribute that is different and less desirable, he or she is reduced in our minds from an acceptable person to a tainted, discounted one. That is, the attribute – or stigma – constitutes a discrepancy between the desired or 'virtual' identity and the actual social identity, and this discrepancy 'spoils' a person's social and self-identity, cutting them off from social (and self) acceptance.

Goffman classifies stigma into three broad categories:

1. Physical stigma – such as blemishes or deformities
2. Personal/character stigma – such as mental health problems or criminal behaviour
3. Social stigma – such as belonging to a particular ethnic group.

In addition to these categories, Goffman also distinguishes between *discredited* attributes which are clearly visible, and *discreditable* attributes which are invisible and therefore only potentially stigmatizing. For example, facial scarring following a burn would be a discrediting attribute, while the condition of epilepsy, which may be invisible unless a seizure occurs in public, would be discreditable. He argues that people with a discrediting stigma try to use 'impression management' to deal with other people's reactions in order to restore their self-identity. In contrast, people with a discreditable attribute, need to use 'information management' about their attribute in order to preserve their identity.

The medical sociologists Scambler and Hopkins (1986) developed Goffman's ideas of information management in their study of people with epilepsy. They distinguished between *felt* stigma (the fear of being stigmatized) and *enacted* stigma (the actual experience of prejudice and discrimination). Their study indicated that felt stigma in people with epilepsy was so strong that they were predisposed to conceal their condition from others and to attempt to pass as normal. Scambler and Hopkins (1986) found that this felt stigma (fear of enacted stigma) was more disruptive to the lives of people with epilepsy than was enacted stigma, which rarely occurred.

These accounts of 'information management' (Goffman 1963a) and concealment in the case of felt stigma (Scambler & Hopkins 1986) alert nurses to the hard work (extra burden) on the part of patients who already may be dealing with the debilitating effects of their particular symptoms.

STIGMATIZING CONDITIONS

It is evident from these studies so far that some diseases will be more stigmatizing than others, depending on whether or not they are clearly apparent to other people. Thus, more noticeable conditions such as psoriasis, stammering, hair loss from chemotherapy or marked tremor may be stigmatizing, while less apparent conditions such as depression or epilepsy may not be stigmatizing as long as they remain hidden. However, visibility, although significant, is not the only factor to consider, some diseases are stigmatizing in themselves, without necessarily being visible. For instance, the sociologist Arthur Frank (2002) who was diagnosed at different times with both a heart attack and cancer, perceived differences in himself when telling people that he had heart problems and telling them that he had cancer. He notes that while his heart attack was simply bad news, he always thought that his cancer said something about his worth as a person – 'this difference between heart attack and cancer is stigma' (Frank 2002: 91). Echoing Goffman's (1963a) perception of a 'tainted self', Frank found that he 'experienced the visible signs of cancer as defects not just in my experience but in my self' (Frank 2002: 92).

The writer Susan Sontag (1991) also comments that some diseases, such as cancer and tuberculosis become metaphors for evil. The stigma attached to cancer is complex, possibly arising from its perceived connections with death. Healthcare professionals and others often use code names – 'The Big 'C'; 'CA' – shrouding the disease in mystery and fear, implying that it is too awful a disease to even be called by its actual name. Bowel cancer, especially that requiring extensive resection of the affected part and the formation of a colostomy, has been found to be particularly stigmatizing (MacDonald 1988), since in addition to the stigma of cancer it also entails mutilating surgery and faecal matter extruding from the abdomen rather than the anus. Some aspects of cancer treatment are particularly visible, notably the hair loss caused by chemotherapy.

In addition to the stigma experienced by patients with other types of cancer, Chapple et al (2004) found that patients with lung cancer felt particularly stigmatized because of the strong association between this disease and smoking and hence its perception as a self-inflicted disease. Some of the respondents also felt stigmatized because the disease was associated with dirt and a horrible death, graphically described in anti-smoking campaigns. As one patient commented:

> *'I hate those adverts that come on television when they finish it by saying two weeks after this, she died. And one of them said when you've got lung cancer you drowned'. (Chapple et al 2004: 1471)*

Chapple et al's study points to the need for healthcare professionals to exercise care and sensitivity when caring for people with lung cancer and also in the way they present health promotion messages in order not to exacerbate feelings of stigmatization.

Many writers have pointed to the highly stigmatized nature of HIV/AIDS; Angelo and Reynolds (1995) outline the reasons for this:

1. Associated with deviant behaviour
2. Viewed as the responsibility of the individual
3. Tainted by a religious belief as to its immorality and/or thought to be contracted via morally sanctionable behaviour and therefore thought to represent a character blemish
4. Perceived as contagious and threatening to the community
5. Associated with an undesirable and an unaesthetic form of death
6. Not well understood by the lay community and viewed negatively by healthcare providers (Angelo & Reynolds 1995: 305, abridged).

Similarly, Plummer (1988) refers to the triple stigma attached to AIDS in that 'it is connected with stigmatized groups, it is sexually transmitted and it is a terminal disease' (Plummer 1988: 28). Moreover, Plummer comments that people with AIDS may also display physical stigmata – the original meaning of the term – including extreme weight loss, lymphadenopathy and Kaposi's sarcoma.

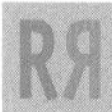

REFLECTION POINTS

Reflect on the illness conditions of patients you have cared for. What is it that made some conditions more stigmatizing than others? Consider how your patients have coped with 'discrediting' and 'discreditable' conditions.

Moral panics

In considering social reaction to illness it is also useful for health professionals to explore another aspect of deviance, labelling and stigma, which arises from the same theoretical and sociopolitical context – the concept of 'moral panics'. Cohen (2002) developed the concept of moral panics in the early 1970s from his observations of the reactions of the media, the general public and the law enforcement agencies to the fights between 'mods' and 'rockers' in Britain in the mid-1960s. Cohen explains the phenomenon of the moral panic as follows:

> *'Societies appear to be subject, every now and then, to periods of moral panic. A condition, episode, person or group of persons emerges to become defined as a threat to societal values and interests; its nature is presented in a stylized and stereotypical fashion by the mass media; the moral barricades are manned by editors, bishops, politicians and other right-thinking people; socially accredited experts pronounce their diagnoses and solutions; ways of coping are evolved or (more often) resorted to; the condition then disappears, submerges or deteriorates and becomes more visible. (Cohen 2002: 1)*

Cohen highlights the crucial role of *the media* in shaping both populist perceptions and political agendas. Thompson (1998: 8) notes that according to Cohen's definition, the following key elements of a moral panic may be identified:

'1 Something or someone is defined as a threat to values or interests.
2. The threat is depicted in an easily recognisable form by the media.
3. There is a rapid build-up of public concern.
4. There is a response from authorities or opinion-makers.
5. The panic recedes or results in social changes'.

Since Cohen's study, there have been frequent media inspired events that appear to fit this description of a moral panic, including many related to health and illness – such as concerns over MRSA and the MMR vaccine. The classic example of a moral health panic is the initial social response to the HIV/AIDS epidemic in the early 1980s, where there was a rapid escalation of hysteria in the tabloid press causing anxiety for the general public. Similarly, with regard to concerns over the ageing population, the media and some politicians and policy-makers have voiced alarm that the younger population will be unable to support this 'burden' of older people. It is important to be aware of the ways in which the media are able to whip up panic about issues which, although requiring serious considered action, are not helped at all by heightened public anxiety and misinformation. (Ideas about moral panic also link with sections on managing risk in Chapters 11 and 12.)

RR **REFLECTION POINT**

Consider examples of current reactions to health issues which may be described as 'moral panics'.

This chapter so far has identified the ways in which the application of 'deviant' labels has negative effects on people's identity and self-esteem, seriously impacting upon their illness experience. People with physical or mental *disabilities* are sometimes presented as a socially deviant group and are particularly vulnerable to the effects of negative labelling; it is to this group that we will now turn.

People with disabilities

The number of disabled people in wealthy industrial societies is high and will continue to rise as the population ages and medical advances prolong life, although the actual figures for the UK vary depending on the ways in which disability is defined and measured (Oliver & Barnes 1998). Thus, an essential part of all branches of nursing work, both in hospitals and in the community, will be to provide care for people with disabling conditions. Moreover, consideration of the complexity surrounding the needs of disabled people, including issues of **anti-discriminatory practice,** needs to be addressed in nurse education, practice and research. It has been argued that disability is a neglected and misunderstood area in nurse education and in nursing texts (Scullion 1999, Nolan & Nolan 1999), and contact between disabled people and nurses and other healthcare professionals has tended to be 'disabling' (Scullion).

CONCEPTUALIZATIONS OF DISABILITY

'Disability' is a highly *contested* term in that different groups have developed different concepts of what disability is and use these differing definitions for different purposes. Definitions confer meaning and, as was outlined in an earlier section, our behaviour towards people, objects and situations stems from the meanings given to them. Thus, definitions both reflect and determine our ideas about disability. For instance, the disabled activist writer Oliver (1990) argues that when disability is conceptualized as a 'tragedy, then disabled people will be treated as if they are the victims of some tragic happening or circumstance' (Oliver 1990: 2). In the case of nursing, Scullion (1999) argues that nurses' conceptions of disability influence the quality of care they provide for disabled people.

Official definitions of disability

In addition, disability needs to be defined in some sort of 'official' way to determine people's eligibility for services and benefits and to frame health and social policies. In the UK, the Disability Discrimination Act (DDA) 1995 defines a disabled person as someone with a:

> *'physical or mental impairment which has a substantial and long-term adverse effect on his* sic *ability to carry out normal day-to-day activities'. (HMSO 1995)*

On an international level, the World Health Organization also provides definitions which are outlined below. However, even official definitions change over time; as we shall see the WHO definition has been recently modified and the DDA definition could also be broadened in the future to include other conditions.

DIFFERENT MODELS OF DISABILITY

Broadly speaking, there are two main models of disability: the individual model which focuses on the disabling conditions itself, and the social model which focuses on the ways in which features of society are disabling.

The individual model of disability

This model emphasizes individual causes of disablement stemming from the malfunctioning or loss of body parts. Some writers refer to this as the medical model in that the focus is on the particular medical impairment and also because the solution to the problem is seen to lie in medical intervention in terms of diagnosing and treating the problem. Thus, within this model, power, control and decision making are attached to the medical professionals rather than with the disabled person. Barnes et al (1999) refer to this as the 'personal tragedy' model of disability in that the disability is presented as a personal problem for the individual and determined by their impairment. The personal tragedy model is a predominantly negative depiction of disabled people and the individual concerned perceived as dependent on others for support and care.

International classification of impairments, disabilities and handicaps

Linked to this individual approach is the International Classification of Impairments, Disabilities and Handicaps (ICIDH), produced by the World Health Organization in 1980 (Box 14.1).

Box 14–1 International classification of impairments, disabilities and handicaps (WHO 1980)

- **Impairment** – refers to any loss or abnormality of psychological, physiological, or anatomical structure or function. This could refer to a loss of a limb, damaged heart muscle or defective mental functioning
- **Disability** – refers to any restriction or lack (resulting from an impairment) of ability to perform an activity in the manner or within the range considered to be normal for a human being
- **Handicap** – refers to the disadvantage for a given individual, resulting from an impairment or a disability, that limits or prevents the fulfilment of a role that is normal (depending on age, sex, social and cultural factors) for that individual.

(Wood 1980: 27–29, abridged)

This model, which has been used until quite recently, was developed in an attempt to include *social* needs in its conceptualization of disability by classifying 'handicap' in terms of social situations rather than the individual. Indeed, Wood (1980: 29) emphasizes that:

> *'[T]he state of being handicapped is relative to other people – hence the importance of existing societal values, which, in turn, are influenced by the institutional arrangements of society'.*

Nevertheless, this model is still described by some writers as the sociomedical model because of its perceived medical orientation.

Critiques of the WHO (1980) model

However, despite the attempts of its authors to include social needs, the WHO schema was rejected by disabled activists, such as Oliver (1990, 1996a) in that it still located the problem for disabled people as stemming from their particular physical or mental impairment. In so doing, it put the onus on the disabled person to adapt and deal with problems rather than addressing the possibility of changing the environment. It is argued that emphasis on dealing with the impairment shifts control away from the individual to the medical profession. Oliver (1990) contends that this focus on the impairment causes the loss of autonomy for disabled people and leads to a perception of them as 'victims' of their impairment. Disabled people also take exception to the use of the word 'handicap' in the WHO schema inasmuch as it is derived from 'cap in hand' – that is the requirement to accept charity (Oliver 1996b). The importance of *language* in conceptualizing disability is addressed in a later section of this chapter.

A social model of disability

In the light of these criticisms, disabled people's organizations and disability studies writers recommend an approach where the disability itself is perceived as socially created – a form of 'social oppression'. From this perspective, rather than disability arising from the particular impairment, it is a result of the ways in which *society responds* to such impairments. This notion of suggesting that the label of 'disability' is not inherent in the individual's condition but is something that is applied to the individual by society resonates with the previously discussed labelling perspectives.

The social model shifts the emphasis from the individual and her/his impairment to society. That is to argue that in this model, people with impairments are disabled by features of their physical and social environment which lead to their social exclusion. Morris (1993c) provides a cogent account of the ways in which the physical environment makes an impairment disabling as follows:

> *'An inability to walk is an impairment, whereas an inability to enter a building because the entrance is up a flight of stairs is a disability. An inability to speak is an impairment but an inability to communicate because appropriate technical aids are not made available is a disability. An inability to move one's body is an impairment but an inability to get out of bed because appropriate physical help is not available is a disability'. (Morris 1993c: x)*

Disabled people's organizations have rejected the WHO (1980) model in favour of the following two-fold classification of disability developed in the 1970s by the Union of the Physically Impaired Against Segregation (UPIAS):

- *Impairment*: lacking part of or all of a limb, or having a defective limb, organism or mechanism of the body
- *Disability*: the disadvantage or restriction of activity caused by a contemporary social organization which takes no or little account of people who have physical impairments and thus excludes them from mainstream or social activities. (UPIAS 1976: 3–4)

Critiques of social model

One of the problems with the social model is that if it is taken to its logical extreme it appears to be dismissing the original bodily impairment. For instance, Oliver (1996b) comments that 'the social model insists disablement is nothing to do with the body. It is a consequence of social oppression' (Oliver 1996b: 35). This way of thinking contradicts ideas concerning the importance of an awareness of the body in our understandings of health and illness. Hughes and Paterson (1997) refer to this as a 'disembodied notion of disability'. In the same way that critics of labelling perspectives argue that these perspectives tend to ignore the primary act of deviance, it could be argued that the social model tends to ignore the primary problem causing the impairment.

Not all disability activists/writers concur with this dismissal of the body. For instance, French (1993), a woman with a visual impairment, although agreeing with the basic tenets of the social model, comments that various profound social problems that she encounters, such as being unable to receive or emit non-verbal cues, are neither socially produced nor amenable to social action; they are as a result of her impairment. Likewise, Morris (1993a) argues that although environmental and attitudinal barriers are disabling, 'to suggest that this is all there is to it is to deny the personal experience of physical or intellectual restrictions, of illness, of the fear of dying' (Morris 1993a: 10). In similar vein, the medical sociologist Michael Bury (1997) cautions that disability theorists' perception of disability as 'social oppression' may have the effect of reducing what are complex individual and social responses to a one-dimensional view; and that focusing on social oppression also ignores the disabling consequences of chronic illness.

In the light of the criticisms of both the medical and social models of disability, an attempt has been made to provide a synthesis of the medical and social models in the following model which takes a 'biopsychosocial' approach:

The International Classification of Functioning, disability and health

This ICF classification differs significantly from the earlier (1980) version in that its focus is on components of health rather than consequences of disease. In this model, people's functioning and disability arise from interaction between their *health conditions* (the disease or disorder) and *contextual factors* (which include environmental and personal factors). This broader 'biopsychosocial' model recognizes the significance of the environment's influence on functioning and health. The ICF is organized into two parts and each part has two components (Box 14.2).

These different conceptualizations of disability provide thought-provoking and challenging ideas, especially for nurses in that they may be familiar with working with the medical model (Scullion 1999). Moreover, nursing's traditional focus on the *individual,* when planning care, may lead to neglect of broader social issues which influence the individual's experience. The social model's insistence on bringing social factors to the fore exemplifies C. Wright Mills' (1959) 'promise' of sociology which is an underlying theme of this book: the relationship between private 'troubles' and public 'issues'. An understanding of this relationship is of particular value to nurses when planning holistic care. The social model highlights the barriers and constraints erected by a disabling society and it is to these disabling barriers that we will now turn.

Box 14–2 International Classification of Functioning, disability and health (ICF)

Part 1: Functioning and disability
Components:

- Body functions and structures
- Activities and participation

Part 2: Contextual factors
Components:

- Environmental factors
- Personal factors

(WHO 2001, abridged)

Disabling barriers

Disabling barriers may be physical or attitudinal or a combination of the two. The built environment may physically exclude people, as in the example below, outlined by disabled writer Jenny Morris – such things as stairs, heavy doors, high shop counters and lack of space for manoeuvring wheelchairs. Physical barriers of course also reflect and convey attitudinal barriers, as Morris (1993a: 26–27) explains:

> *'We receive so many messages from the non-disabled world that we are not wanted, that we are considered less than*

human. For those with restricted mobility or sensory disabilities, the very physical environment tells us we don't belong. It tells us that we aren't wanted in the places that non-disabled people spend their lives – their homes, their schools and colleges, their workplaces, their leisure venues'.

Attitudinal barriers stem from people's prejudice against disabled people, which may be expressed as stares, ridicule, and exclusion; societal reactions which are disabling. The earlier quotation from Morris (1993a) points to her perception that disabled people are 'considered less than human', and her book *Pride against Prejudice* draws on disabled people's experiences of prejudice from non-disabled people and also explores the reasons for dehumanization of people with physical and mental disabilities. Barnes (1992) locates prejudice and stereotyping of disabled people in all the forms that the media take – books, films, television, radio, newspapers and charity advertising. His report (Barnes 1992), although now slightly dated, in that some aspects have changed, is still relevant and thought-provoking. Barnes argues that there is institutionalized prejudice and discrimination against disabled people in Britain, partly because negative stereotypes are constantly reproduced through the communications media (Barnes 1992: part 1).

Language in relation to disability

As we saw earlier with reference to defining disability, definitions are contestable and also change over time; it is important therefore to be aware that any language guidelines provided will be subject to revision. Changes in language over time both reflect and shape current values and meanings; they also often reflect issues concerning power and regulation. Despite frequent attempts in the popular press to ridicule the concept of 'political correctness' there is general agreement that finding more appropriate words for such derogatory terms as 'spastic', 'mongol', 'retard' has been a positive step (Oliver 1996b). Barnes et al (1999) observe in relation to the possibly bewildering changes in terminology 'what is at issue is far more than a choice of words; the debate is about the best way to understand and contest disability and the multiple oppressions that are associated with it' (Barnes et al 1999: 7).

Of particular importance to healthcare workers, are Oliver's (1996b) comments that many disabled people find the language used in much medical discourse distorts their experiences and is offensive:

'In particular the term chronic illness is for many people an unnecessarily negative term, and discussions of suffering in many studies have the effect of casting disabled people in the role of victim and unnecessarily negative – also use of "suffering" and "victim".' (Oliver 1996b: 43)

In relation to nursing practice, Scullion (1999: 654) argues for need to move beyond political correctness and adopt language which is positively acceptable to disabled people themselves.

In addition to this negativity, terminology may be used in such a way that it lumps people together in a way that is both depersonalizing and excluding. To refer to 'the blind', 'the deaf', 'the dumb' or indeed 'the disabled' groups people according to a medical condition with no consideration of personal identity and also segregates these groups from the rest of 'normal' society. It is more acceptable and appropriate to simply refer to 'disabled people'. This kind of depersonalizing and segregating grouping also ignores the heterogeneity of these groups in terms of their members' ethnicity, sexuality, gender, age and social class.

A further important aspect of language concerns the notion of 'normality'. Morris (1993b: 101) notes that the word 'normal' is 'inherently tied up with ideas about what is right, what is desirable and what belongs'. She suggests that able-bodied people assume that disabled people want to be normal, or to be treated as if they were. Similarly, Barnes et al (1999: 25) argue that the notion of 'normality' 'is heavily laden with able-bodied assumptions and prejudices' – not least that everyone else should strive to be 'normal' like them. Oliver (1996b: 44) argues that the Disability Movement is 'rejecting approaches based on the restoration of normality and insisting on approaches based upon the celebration of difference'.

GUIDELINES ON LANGUAGE AND DISABILITY

The following guidelines (Box 14.3), which are not intended to be exhaustive or definitive, are provided by the British Sociological Association (BSA) and are designed to 'challenge disablism ... promote a social rather than individual model of disability and support non-discriminatory practice' (BSA 2004). However, the BSA also point out the changing nature of language and terminology and that 'it must be recognized that the meaning of these terms will be subject to revision and/or change at a faster rate than these or any other guidelines or sources may be issued' (BSA 2004).

Box 14–3 BSA guidelines on language and disability

- Avoid using medical labels as this may promote a view of disabled people as patients. It also implies the medical label is the over-riding characteristic; this is inappropriate
- If it is necessary to refer to a condition, it is better to say, for example, 'a person with epilepsy' not an epileptic, or 's/he has cerebral palsy' not a spastic
- Avoid mental retardation/mentally retarded
- Avoid acronyms when referring to people, e.g. 'the SEN child'
- It may be necessary to place "apostrophes" around terms when referring to historical (and some contemporary) terms
- The word disabled should not be used as a collective noun (e.g. as in 'the disabled').

More specifically, the guidelines in Box 14.4 are recommended:

Box 14–4 Disablist and non-disablist terminology

Disablist	Non-disablist
Handicap	Disability
Invalid	Disabled person
The disabled/the handicapped	Disabled people or people with disabilities
Special needs	Additional needs or needs
Patient	Person
Abnormal	Different or disabled
Victim of	Person who has / person with
Crippled by	Person who has / person with
Suffering from	Person who has / person with
Afflicted by	Person who has / person with
Wheelchair bound	Wheelchair user
The blind	Blind and partially-sighted people or visually-impaired people
The deaf	Deaf or hard of hearing people
Cripple or crippled	Disabled or mobility impaired person
The mentally handicapped	People/person with a learning difficulty or learning disability
Retarded/ backward	Person with a learning disability
Mute or dumb	Person with a speech impairment
Mentally ill or mental patient	Mental health service user
Able-bodied person	Non-disabled person

From: British Sociological Association (BSA) (2004)

The use of appropriate language is an integral part of anti-discriminatory practice, to which we shall now turn.

Anti-discriminatory practice

Thompson (1997) explains anti-discriminatory practice as practice which 'seeks to reduce, undermine or eliminate discrimination and oppression, specifically in terms of challenging sexism, racism, agesim and **disablism**' (Thompson 1997: 33). This requires a sociological understanding of the inequalities associated with structural factors such as gender, age and 'race' as outlined in earlier chapters. It also draws upon knowledge from psychology of prejudice and stereotyping.

Disablism refers to the 'combination of social forces, cultural values and personal prejudices which marginalizes disabled people, portrays them in a negative light and thus oppresses them' (Thompson 1997: 107).

Anti-discriminatory practice (sometimes referred to as anti-oppressive practice) would appear to be enshrined in the Nursing and Midwifery Code of Professional Conduct (NMC 2004a) inasmuch as part 2.2 of the code states registered nurses and midwives are personally accountable for ensuring that they promote and protect:

> '*... the interests and dignity of patients and clients, irrespective of gender, age, race, ability, sexuality, economic status, lifestyle, culture and religious or political beliefs*'. *(NMC 2004a: 5)*

The nursing education curriculum also subscribes to anti-discriminatory practice (NMC 2004b) although Scullion's (1999) study showed little recognition of disability's equal opportunities dimension. Nursing education cannot point to a strong anti-discriminatory philosophy (Scullion 1999: 654), and disability and discrimination appear to be neglected areas in the nursing literature (Northway 1997).

In healthcare, anti-discriminatory practice in relation to disability is promoted through movement away from the individualistic approaches, which as we have already seen locate the problem within the individual, towards the social model which emphasizes the ways in which social barriers contribute to disability. For nurses, again I suggest that C. Wright Mills' (1959) concept of 'private troubles' and 'public issues' is relevant here in that it helps us to understand the relationship between the private trouble, the impairment, and the public issue – the ways in which the larger structures of social life impact upon the experience of disability. Northway (1997: 741–742, abridged) suggests a three-stage framework of awareness, reflection and development, for nurses to engage with anti-oppressive practice:

- Awareness of the nature of disability, including the different models. Nurses should have access to disability equality training and accept responsibility for increasing their personal awareness
- Reflection on current practice, education and research in order to identify area of contribution to (or not challenging of) oppression of disabled people
- Development of nursing practice and research.

At a policy level The Disability Discrimination Act (DDA) (HMSO 1995, 2005) aims to end the discrimination which many disabled people face, giving disabled people rights in the areas of employment, access to goods, facilities and services.

RЯ REFLECTION POINT

Reflect on the ways in which nurses' conceptions of disability may influence the quality of care they provide for people with disabilities.

Discussion points

1. Discuss the factors which may influence society's response to illness.
2. How can nurses promote anti-discriminatory practice in relation to people with disabilities?

CHAPTER SUMMARY

To sum up, this chapter has explored social response to illness and disability indicating the multi-faceted, complex nature of this response. In so doing, it has also called attention to the ways in which societal reaction impacts upon people's experience of illness and/or disability. Key themes in the study of societal reaction – such as labelling, stigma and moral panics – have been introduced and applied to particular health conditions. The chapter has explained concepts, definitions and models of disability and examined physical and attitudinal disabling barriers. In addition to contemporary material, the chapter has drawn upon a number of classic studies pertaining to societal reaction, all of which are accessible and illuminating in their original forms.

FURTHER READING

Gardner F 2006 Blood and sand. Bantam Press, London

Although the chief focus of this book is Gardner's experiences in the Middle East as a BBC journalist; these experiences also include being shot and left partly paralysed by Al-Qaeda gunmen. As such, Gardner's story reveals important insights into the experience of sudden transition from an able-bodied high flying journalist to a man facing up to the rigours of paraplegia.

USEFUL WEBSITES

http://www.leeds.ac.uk/disability-studies/archiveuk/
The Disability Archive UK

http://www.disability.gov.uk
The government disability website

http://www.dipex.org/EXEC
Useful (audio-visual) link to patients' accounts of stigma

REFERENCES

Angelo A A, Reynolds N R 1995 Stigma, HIV and AIDS: An exploration and elaboration of a stigma trajectory. Social Science and Medicine 41 (3):303–315

Barnes C 1992 Disabling imagery and the media. British Council of Organizations of Disabled People and Ryburn Publishing. Online. Available: http://www.leeds.ac.uk/disability-studies/archiveuk/Barnes/disabling%20imagery.pdf 6 Feb 2007

Barnes C, Mercer G, Shakespeare T 1999 (eds) Exploring disability: A sociological introduction. Polity, Cambridge

Becker H 1963 Outsiders: Studies in the sociology of deviance. Free Press, Illinois

Bowers L 1998 The social nature of mental illness. Routledge, London

BSA 2004 British Sociological Association: Disablist terms and non-disablist alternatives, www.britsoc.co.uk

Bury M 1997 Health and illness in a changing society. Routledge, London

Chapple A, Ziebland S, McPherson A 2004 Stigma, shame and blame experienced by patients with cancer: qualitative study. British Medical Journal 328:1470–1473

Cohen S 2002 Folk devils and moral panics: The creation of the Mods and the Rockers, 3rd edn. Routledge, London

Frank A W 2002 At the will of the body: Reflections on illness. Houghton Mifflin, Boston

French S 1993 Disability, impairment, or something in between? In: Swain J, Finkelstein V, French S et al (eds) Disabling barriers – Enabling environment. Sage, London, p 17–25

Goffman E 1963a Stigma: Notes on the management of spoiled identity. Prentice Hall, New Jersey

Goffman E 1963b Behavior in public places. The Free Press, New York

Goffman E 1968 Asylums: Essays on the social situation of mental patients and other inmates. Pelican, Harmondsworth

Gove W 1970 Societal reaction as an explanation of mental illness: an evaluation. American Sociological Review 35:873–884

Gove W 1975 The labelling theory of mental illness: a reply to Scheff. American Sociological Review 40:242–248

Her Majesty's Stationery Office 1995 Disability Discrimination Act. HMSO, Norwich

Her Majesty's Stationery Office 2005 Disability Discrimination Act. HMSO, Norwich

Hughes B, Paterson K 1997 The social model of disability and the disappearing body: towards a sociology of impairment. Disability & Society 12 (3):325–340

Hunt P 1966 Stigma: the experience of disability. Chapman, London

Kelly M 1992 Colitis. Routledge, London

Lemert E 1961 Social pathology. McGraw-Hill, New York

MacDonald L 1988 The experience of stigma: living with rectal cancer. In: Anderson R, Bury M (eds) Living with chronic illness: the experience of patients and their families. Allen and Unwin, London

Mills C W 1959 The sociological imagination. Oxford University Press, New York

Morris J 1993a Pride against prejudice. The Women's Press, London

Morris J 1993b Prejudice. In: Swain J, Finkelstein V, French S et al (eds) Disabling barriers – Enabling environments, 1st edn. Sage, London, p 101–106

Morris J 1993c Independent lives? Community care and disabled people. Macmillan, Basingstoke

Nolan M, Nolan J 1999 Rehabilitation, chronic illness and disability: the missing elements in nurse education. Journal of Advanced Nursing 29 (4):958–966

Northway R 1997 Disability and oppression: some implications for nurses and nursing. Journal of Advanced Nursing 26:736–743

Nursing and Midwifery Council (NMC) 2004a The NMC code of professional conduct: standards for conduct, performance and ethics. Nursing & Midwifery Council, London

Nursing and Midwifery Council (NMC) 2004b Standards of proficiency for preregistration nursing education. Nursing and midwifery Council, London

Oliver M 1990 The politics of disablement. Macmillan, Basingstoke

Oliver M 1996a Understanding disability: from theory to practice. Macmillan, Basingstoke

Oliver M 1996b Defining impairment and disability: issues at stake. In: Barnes C, Mercer G (eds) Exploring the divide: Illness and disability. Disability Press, Leeds, p 29–54

Oliver M 1997 Emancipatory research: realistic goal or impossible dream? In: Barnes C, Mercer G (eds) Doing disability research. The Disability Press, Leeds, p 15–31

Oliver M, Barnes C 1998 Disabled people and social policy: from exclusion to inclusion. Longman, London

Parsons T 1951 The social system. Free Press, New York

Plummer K 1988 Organizing AIDS. In: Aggleton P, Homans H (eds) Social aspects of AIDS. The Falmer Press, Lewes, p 20–51

Priestley M 1997 Who's *sic* research?: a personal audit. In: Barnes C, Mercer G (eds) Doing disability research. The Disability Press, Leeds, p 88–107

Rosenhan D L 1973 On being sane insane places. Science 179:250–258

Scambler G, Hopkins A 1986 Being epileptic: coming to terms with stigma. Sociology of Health and Illness 8:26–43

Scheff T 1966 Being mentally ill: a sociological theory. Aldine, Chicago

Scullion P A 1999 Conceptualizing disability in nursing: some evidence from students and their teachers. Journal of Advanced Nursing 29 (3):648–657

Sontag S 1991 Illness as metaphor and AIDS and its metaphors. Penguin, London

Thompson K 1998 Moral panics. Routledge, London

Thompson N 1997 Anti-discriminatory practice, 2nd edn. Macmillan, Basingstoke

UPIAS 1976 Fundamental principles of disability. Union of the Physically Impaired Against Segregation, London

Wood P 1980 International Classification of Impairments, Disabilities and Handicaps. WHO, Geneva

World Health Organization 1980 International Classification of Impairments, Disabilities and Handicaps. WHO, Geneva

World Health Organization 2001 International Classification of Functioning, Disability and Health. WHO, Geneva

CHAPTER

15 Death and dying

Hannah Cooke

KEY CONCEPTS

- Arguments for and against the proposition that we have become a 'death-denying' society
- Rationalist and bureaucratic discourses about death
- The 'rediscovery' of death and the hospice movement
- Communication and awareness in care of the dying
- Inequalities of care and the 'disadvantaged dying'

Death is denied

> *'It's not that I'm afraid to die. I just don't want to be there when it happens'. (Woody Allen,* Without Feathers *1976)*

It has become a common belief that death is denied in modern society. Thus according to Corr (1993: 32):

> *'Death is now perceived as socially unacceptable or forbidden. Death is dirty and indecent, an unfair violation of life which should be preventable ... Death is to be removed or hidden from social view. Dying is displaced from the home to institutions ... Mourning is restrained and often almost perfunctory'.*

Yet, according to Simpson (1987), death is a 'badly kept secret'; such an unmentionable topic that there are now thousands of books in print announcing that we are ignoring the subject of death.

> *'The announcements that death is taboo and that our society denies death continue, yet death is more and more talked of'. (Walter 1994: 1)*

How then do we make sense of the persistence of the view that our society is 'death denying' (Becker 1973), and what evidence is there to support such an assertion?

Patterns of mortality have changed as a result of demographic and epidemiological transitions leading to gains in life expectancy in developed countries and a shift from infectious diseases to degenerative diseases as causes of death (Seale 2000). Arguably, this has been a key factor shaping contemporary attitudes to death. In 1955, Gorer wrote a short article entitled the 'Pornography of Death'. In it he argued that death could no longer be discussed openly, it had become as clandestine and secret as sex was to the Victorians. Gorer said that death as a natural process had become unmentionable and yet violent death played an increasing part in the fantasies offered to audiences by the mass media. This 'pornography of death' was the price that our culture paid for distancing itself from natural death.

Gorer's article was followed by many similar arguments, most notably in the work of Aries (1981) who used his historical researches to argue that death had become hidden in contemporary society. According to Aries, the nineteenth century was the 'beginning of the lie' (1981: 561). Prior to this period, everyone died in public and the death of a man 'solemnly altered the space and time of a social group'.

Aries noted with approval, the elaborate mourning rituals that accompanied 'traditional' death and in particular, that women in mourning were 'invisible under their crepe and voluminous black veils'.

In contrast, according to Aries, society now ignores death and:

> '*A new image of death is forming: the ugly and hidden death*'.

Aries can be criticized for his sweeping generalizations about European history and also for the fact that he writes exclusively about the 'dying man'; and the wealthy dying man at that. Traditional society paid little attention to the death of the poor who may be treated with more dignity and respect today (Richardson 2000). Furthermore, traditional mourning practices often confined and segregated widows as Aries approvingly notes. Yet this tells us as much about the subordination of women as about attitudes to death (Hockey 1997).

Writers such as Aries, romanticized premodern death, seeing it as characterized by an openness and emotional accompaniment that has been contrasted with the bleakness and isolation of modern death. Walter (1994) has suggested that this romanticizing of pre-modern death resembles the romanticizing of the 'noble savage'. Similar themes have been evident in the 'natural childbirth' movement.

These ideas about the 'denial of death' provided a rallying cry for movements such as the hospice and palliative care movement which wanted to reform the care of the dying and bereaved. In the nineteenth century, nurse reformers presented the image of the home nurse as a lower class drunkard who was incompetent and dangerous, as we saw in Chapter 9. Dickens immortalized this stereotype with the character of Sairy Gamp in his novel *Martin Chuzzlewit*. The reformers of the day sought to replace her with a sanitized, evangelized and disciplined workforce (Dingwall et al 1988). Thus, they harked back to a mediaeval past in which nursing was a sacred duty in order to justify their reforms. Similarly, many of the reformers that Lofland (1978) has dubbed the 'happy death' movement hark back to an idealized past and contrast it with the horrors of modern death. Aries' work provided the most eloquent example of this narrative. The image of the hospital death, alone, afraid, in pain and surrounded by machinery was contrasted with a traditional and 'natural' death within the bosom of the family.

Contemporary historians have reassessed the myth of Sairy Gamp, arguing that it was a stereotype convenient to the reformers of the time, but not strictly accurate (Dingwall et al 1988). Perhaps the 'denial of death' will be similarly recognized as a myth in years to come. It is important to be aware of the existence of such myths since they can shape the directions that reform movements take.

Certainly, for a 'taboo' subject, death is overwhelmingly present (Walter 1991). Gorer argued that the ever-growing fantasies of death portrayed in the media were pornographic since they were devoid of humanity and emotion. Yet recently, it has become evident that, alongside the fantasy deaths offered up by the entertainment industry, much media coverage of death deals precisely with these emotional issues; offering a commentary on the grief of the dying and bereaved (Walter et al 1995). For example, the death of Diana, Princess of Wales provoked an outpouring of discussions about such feelings within the media (Kear &

Steinberg 1999, Walter 1999). Walter described this media coverage as 'emotional invigilation'. When dealing with death, popular culture is preoccupied with acceptable and unacceptable expressions of suffering and grief. Emotional expression is approved, but not too much, and we must show that we care but we must also be brave. The death of Princess Diana offered enormous scope to the media in their discussions of the proper reactions of the Royal family, politicians, the public and even of their own feelings.

> *'So brave, grief stricken William and Harry hold back the tears'*
>
> *'The Duchess has lost someone she has always considered a sister. There are no words to describe the pain in her heart'*
>
> *'We are a nation today in a state of shock, in mourning, in grief that is so deeply painful for us'*
>
> *'I am crying as I write this ... I cannot believe Diana is dead' (*Daily Mirror *1997)*

According to Walter et al, such preoccupations reflect a new uncertainty about how to act and feel in the face of suffering and death. As our society has become more secular and individualistic, prescribed mourning rituals have largely disappeared leaving us unsure of what to say and do. Their later study of front-page tabloid coverage of violent death also shows the ways in which gender stereotypes continue to dominate media representations of death. They conclude that 'several different discourses of death are being conducted on an almost daily basis' (Pickering et al 1997). This suggests that media representations of death are far more complex and multifaceted than Gorer had suggested.

Recent instances of public mourning, such as the events following the death of Princess Diana (Walter 1999), also suggest that modern 'folk' rituals have arisen to replace the more formal rituals of the past. For example, the laying of mass floral tributes and the creation of roadside shrines at the site of a traumatic death have become familiar occurrences. Thus according to Brennan (2001), the mourning for Diana was both extraordinary and paradoxically 'quite normal after all'.

Blauner (1966) argued that death was both 'present' and 'absent' in modern society. He thus gave a more balanced account than Gorer (1955) had given. He suggested that better life expectancy meant that death in the prime of life had become the exception rather than the rule. Prior to the twentieth century, deaths from infectious diseases were prevalent and death touched the lives of everyone. Social life was threatened by the frequent deaths of younger people who still had important social roles. Thus, mourning rituals were necessary to restore social equilibrium since death regularly disrupted the social order. By contrast, nowadays most people are old when they die. The deaths of the old, according to Blauner, affect far fewer people since the old have already had to relinquish their social roles. The elderly may be dispatched at a perfunctory crematorium service, with only a handful of mourners. For them, mourning rituals have declined and their deaths pass largely unnoticed. However 'untimely' deaths still disrupt the social order and these deaths will be mourned more expressively.

Thus Pickering et al (1997) showed that media representations focus almost exclusively on 'untimely' deaths which threaten the social fabric. The deaths of the old rarely warrant media attention. Within a culture which places a high social value on modernity and change, the skills and knowledge of the old are no longer seen as a valuable resource to be handed on to a younger generation. Instead, too often the old are seen as obsolete and 'past their sell-by date'.

Death illuminates the cultural values within a society. Arguably, the modern management of death shows just how ageist our society has become. Social death occurs when an individual is no longer an 'active agent in the social world' (Mulkay 1993) and comes to be treated as a non-person, someone whose life and concerns are no longer of any value or importance. The old, it is argued, are socially dead before they are biologically dead (Sudnow 1967). They are denied social participation, devalued and institutionally segregated. Even in the contemporary movement to humanize death, the old are notable by their absence. Terminal care services remain largely institutionally separate from care of the elderly and care disproportionately for the younger dying (Seale 1998).

We can conclude therefore that contemporary societal responses to death are complex and that denial is only one of a range of responses. Responses to death reflect societal inequalities and tell us much about contemporary judgements of social worth.

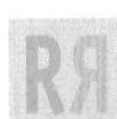

REFLECTION POINT

We have seen that a common theme of much contemporary discussion of death is that death is 'denied' or 'taboo' in contemporary society. This is disputed by some authors and the evidence suggests that contemporary attitudes to death are complex and contradictory. Look at recent reports of deaths in newspapers or on TV. What do they tell you about contemporary attitudes to death?

Death is hidden

In a variation on the argument that we live in a 'death-denying' society some sociologists argue that death is hidden in contemporary society (Mellor & Schilling 1993). It is necessary for all societies to some extent to ignore death in order to commit themselves to everyday life. Death can call into question the world building activities of individuals and a failure to deal with death adequately can threaten our individual and collective sense of meaning. Many contemporary sociologists have suggested that modern societies have particular difficulties dealing with death which both threatens individuals with 'extreme terrors of personal meaningless' and threatens the social order with 'a more widespread attendant loss of meaning and order' (Mellor 1993). This concurs with Berger's (1967) view that every human society is 'in the last resort men (and women) banded together in the face of death'. Berger further explains:

> *'Death radically puts into question the taken-for-granted "business as usual" attitude in which one exists in everyday life'. (Berger 1967: 43)*

We have seen that there are multiple discourses about death in contemporary society. A major concern for some authors is the decline in religious values, which offered a communal response to death. The absence of religious explanations and rituals is said to lead to private anxiety and anomie (however the evidence for the decline of religion is mixed as we saw in Chapter 3). Thus, according to Turner (1991) the death of God has left us 'literally and culturally naked' and...

> *'In a society dominated by the values of youthfulness and vitality, death has become an embarrassment rather than an ever present facet of daily existence'. (Turner 1991: 235)*

Giddens (1991) has noted that a particular feature of contemporary society (an era he describes as 'high modernity') is a concern with self-identity (see Chapter 5 for a summary of Giddens' major ideas). We live in a highly individualistic society obsessed with individual choice and control. A variety of therapies and self-help guides help us to create a positive self image and sense of self. An important part of the cultivation of self-identity is the cultivation of the body. Consumer culture places enormous emphasis on products to enhance the appearance and well being of the body (as we see in the endless 'makeover' shows on TV) and increasing importance is placed on the body as constitutive of the self (Mellor 1993).

Thus, the prospect of death in such a society can threaten the most profound loss of self.

By contrast, death and bodily decay are important symbols in many religious traditions. In these cultures, transcendent values define the self. For example, in Sinhalese society, Buddhists are invited to meditate on the decay of the dead body. This is a religious duty which reminds them of the transience of their earthly existence (Obeyesekere 1989). Similarly in Mediaeval Europe '*memento mori*' (reminders of death) were commonplace in art and artefacts. In high modernity by contrast, bodily fitness is cultivated to ward off thoughts of death and decay; for fear that such thoughts will bring with them what Berger and Luckman (1967) have called the 'onslaught of the nightmare'.

Thus, many contemporary sociologists see European societies building a world of secular meanings in which death is distant, something that happens only to other people. This is in stark contrast to societies in which religious values still dominate. In this new secular world, the dying are isolated and have to face death alone and unsupported. Elias (1985) argues that the 'civilizing processes' that have shaped our society place a high value on privacy and emotional reserve. Thus, it is no longer possible to speak to the aged and dying of their death and they are condemned to extreme loneliness. For Mellor (1993), it is this 'privatization of meaning' which has led to the 'sequestration' of death. He describes the dying as hidden away in institutions and isolated from human contact.

We noted earlier the existence of multiple discourses about death in contemporary society. Thus, it is no surprise that we can find challenges to this account of death as isolated and hidden. Seale (1995a) argues that our society places a high value on emotional accompaniment at the time of death. His study of those who had died alone showed that for survivors, dying alone was seen as a threatening and untoward event for which they had to account and atone. It is common for responsibility for dying alone to be imputed to the dead person; neighbours might express regret or guilt but justify their social distance by describing the deceased as someone who 'kept themselves to themselves'. Media accounts of dying alone universally construct these as 'bad' deaths (Seale 2003). This does not of course mean that such 'bad deaths' do not happen more frequently than we might consider desirable.

Another challenge to Mellor's (1993) thesis is the hospice and palliative care movement which has done much to humanize death and to put care of the dying on the public policy agenda. We can argue that hospices far from 'sequestering' the dying, place a high value on home care. Many patients express a preference for dying at home and meeting patients' preferences regarding place of death has been an important part of the hospice movement's agenda (Grande et al 1998, Thomas et al 2004). However, even within hospices, patients with particularly distressing lingering deaths may be 'sequestered' by staff (Lawton 1998, see also Chapter 8).

REFLECTION POINT

We have seen that some sociologists have argued that the dying are separated (sequestered) from the rest of society. For example in hospital wards, dying patients may be hidden away in side wards. From your own experience, think of any instances that you have encountered that illustrate the 'sequestration' of dying patients.

Death is rationalized

We have seen therefore, that there is an influential argument that death has become hidden and that we have become a death-denying society. This argument remains influential despite evidence that it over-simplifies contemporary responses to death.

An alternative argument suggests that contemporary public discourses about death have not ceased but changed. Since the industrial revolution, we have moved from a religious to a scientific and bureaucratic treatment of death. At the same time as a decline in mourning rituals, the surveillance of death by the state became increasingly important. A new rationalist discourse of death arose leading to a new set of bureaucratic practices for the management of death such as the death certificate, the post-mortem and the coroner's court (Armstrong 1987).

Throughout the nineteenth century, there was a vocal debate on the disposal of the dead and accounting for death became vital to the government of populations (Prior 1989, Richardson 2000). We have noted that societies have to some extent to ignore death in order to function. Modern social institutions also need to control the impact of death by calculating its probability. For example the life insurance industry became an important part of the modern management of death (Seale 1998). An industry of death accounting has thus arisen. Accounting for death became a medico-legal discourse, which located death and disease within the human body. The discipline of pathology looked for explanations of death within the corpse. Physical and individualist explanation of death came to replace social and religious explanations (Prior 1989).

Prior's (1989) study of the certification of death shows how the medico-legal management of death came to individualize explanations of the cause of death. Until the end of the nineteenth century, the vocabulary of causation linked the physical body to the social body. Early reports of coroners and the Registrar General had included reference to the price of food and fuel, levels of pauperism and the climate. In the nineteenth century, you could still officially die of poverty, neglect or 'unskilful medical treatment'. Gradually, social factors and human agency were erased from accounts of death, so that by the late twentieth century, a victim of violence in Belfast was recorded as having died from 'bruising and oedema of the brain associated with fractures of the skull'.

Modern techniques of surveillance of the corpse arose as a result of the change in the medical 'gaze' from the whole person to the bodily organs (Foucault 1973, Jewson 1976). The expansion of anatomical dissections and post-mortem examinations was not achieved without resistance. A belief in the resurrection of the dead led many to oppose the dissection of corpses. Before the 1832 Anatomy Act, dissection was part of the punishment reserved for convicted felons. The rise of modern medicine in the early nineteenth century led to a lucrative trade in corpses. The corpse became a commodity and grave robbers emerged to supply the expanding medical schools with bodies for dissection, since demand outstripped the legal supply of corpses. In order to stamp out grave robbery, the 1832 Anatomy Act created a new supply of corpses by permitting the bodies of paupers to be used for dissection. Thus, it seemed to many that hereafter, poverty rather than crime, was to be punished by dismemberment (Richardson 2000). It is important not to sentimentalize the past. Writers such as Aries (1981) have noted with approval that in Victorian times the corpse remained at home in the front parlour until the funeral. Yet Richardson's (2000) study of the history of dissection showed that the poor often kept the corpse at home until it began to rot in order to ensure that their loved one was in an unfit state for the pathologist's scalpel. Paupers who escaped the pathologist's scalpel were buried with little ceremony in unmarked mass graves.

Richardson has argued that there is a 'fearful symmetry' about past and present and that there are 'alarming parallels' between the procurement of bodies for dissection in the past and the contemporary procurement of organs for transplantation and scientific research. In contemporary society, human organs have a commodity value not unlike the commodity value of the nineteenth-century corpse. Demand continues to outstrip supply. The nineteenth-century market in the dead 'graduated through compulsion, theft, secrecy and dishonesty to burking' (Richardson 2000: 422). (The term 'burking' derives from the nineteenth-century 'body-snatchers' Burke and Hare who murdered their victims and sold their bodies to medical schools). What the nineteenth-century trade in corpses showed most starkly was the inequalities of a society in which the poor were worth more dead than alive. Richardson cites a study of the global traffic in organs by the anthropologist Scheper-Hughes (2000) to argue that global inequalities raise the same fears amongst the poor in some countries today.

Richardson's distrust of the medical management of death reflects a persistent cultural theme. The Western, rationalist ideas, which underpin organ transplantation, are not universally accepted. The concept of 'brain death' marks a radical shift in cultural understandings of death (Ohnuki-Tierney 1994). The idea of 'brain death' causes continued unease and uncertainty about the borderline between life and death in some cultures, since it is a measure of prognosis rather than actual death (Seale 1998). The concept of 'brain death' redefines biological death to bring it in line with social death. In Japan, this concept remains very controversial. For example only one heart transplant had been carried out prior to 1995 and the doctor involved was prosecuted for murder (Lock 1995).

Controversy surrounding the boundaries of life and death is not unique to Japan. In the UK, the recent public outcry about the procurement of organs for research at Alder Hey children's hospital demonstrated the depth of public unease and distrust surrounding the care of the dead. In particular, bereaved parents accused medical institutions of a 'lack of respect' for the dead (Royal Liverpool Children's Inquiry 2001). Such fears are not without foundation. According to Hafferty (1988) the informal culture of medical students abounds with tales in which medical students play pranks with body parts in order to shock outsiders. According to Hafferty (1988) this oral culture reinforces a professional culture which values emotional detachment and may lead to the depersonalized treatment of patients. Interestingly, contemporary artistic representations of death such as the work of Damien Hirst reproduce this dehumanized discourse showing its wider cultural influence on contemporary images of death.

Some sociologists have been highly critical of these dehumanizing discourses about death. For them, such discourse is morally bankrupt. For example both Baumann (1987) and Ritzer (1996) have argued that the scientific rationalist discourse about death found its most complete expression in the Nazi Holocaust. The Nazi death camps were in some ways the most extreme expression of a rationalistic and utilitarian approach to life and death. Death and killing were bureaucratized and medicalized. Doctors and nurses attended the railway sidings at Auschwitz to sort the inmates of incoming trains into those fit to survive and those for disposal in the gas chambers (Seidelman 1991). For them, the Jews had already attained 'thing-like' status; they were socially dead. Thus according to Bauman 1987, the success of the Holocaust was due in part to the 'skilful utilization of "moral sleeping pills" made possible by the Nazis' use of modern technologies and bureaucratic techniques.

Seidelman (1991) has suggested that medicine was founded on a rationalist discourse which seeks to divide those who are fit to live from those who are not and that the activities of Nazi doctors highlighted the moral failings of this discourse. A more recent example of doctors attempting to decide who is fit for life has been the debate over the 'high cost of dying' (Scitovsky 1994). US statistics showing high medical expenditure in the last months of life have led to calls to ration life-saving treatments. This fits the ethos of 'managed care'. Thus, terminal 'care pathways' may be as much about limiting treatment as about providing it. The Canadian Health Services Research Foundation (2004) has argued that the 'high cost of dying' is a powerful myth, which persists despite 30 years of research evidence that contradicts it. Calls to curtail treatment of the dying treat the dying as already socially dead.

REFLECTION POINT

We have seen that sociologists used the concept of 'social death' to describe the depersonalized treatment of people such as the old and dying. How can health professionals avoid giving depersonalized treatment to patients who are near the end of their life?

Similarly, the rationalist discourse about euthanasia can be seen as seeking to hasten biological death, so that is coterminous with social death. Mak et al (2003) found that requests for euthanasia were associated with a disintegrating sense of self associated with unresolved life events and poor social support. Thus according to Seale (1997, 1998), exercising control of the timing of our biological death is one way that contemporary individuals try to avoid the 'lingering dissolution of the social bond'.

McInerney (2000) has suggested that the euthanasia or 'requested death' movement reflects contemporary preoccupations with individual identity and privacy and a rejection of state control over individual lives. Emmanuel (1994) has argued that it is no coincidence that there was a revival of the euthanasia movement in the era of Thatcherism and Reaganism, just as there was in the economic depression of the 1920s. He describes the euthanasia movement as expressing cultural values of 'raw individualism, unfettered capitalistic competition for survival ... and curtailment of social 'safety net' programs for the poor, old and sick'.

Most studies of euthanasia have surveyed the views of healthy members of the public and the patient's voice is seldom heard (Mak et al 2003). Advocates of euthanasia argue that it is the only solution to intractable physical suffering. Seale and Addington-Hall (1998) however, found that fear of dependency or of becoming 'a burden' may be a more important motivation for requests for euthanasia. Their study showed elderly women were least likely to be cared for by someone with an emotional investment in their continued existence; surviving carers were less likely to agree that they were missed and more likely to agree that they should have died sooner. It was these old women who were significantly more likely to have requested euthanasia. Thus, Seale (1998) concluded that there was some support for the argument put forward by the founder of the modern hospice movement:

> *'I do not think any legalised right to die can fail to become, for many vulnerable people a "duty to die" or at best the only option offered'. (Saunders 1992: 3)*

Throughout this book, we have discussed the social inequities that can afflict both death and life. It seems that such social inequalities would also shape the distribution of euthanasia requests.

REFLECTION POINT

We have seen that some sociologists have suggested that a particular set of social conditions have been associated with calls for legalized euthanasia. Calls for euthanasia reflect the high value placed on individual autonomy in contemporary society. Arguments against euthanasia reflect a concern that some individuals will feel under pressure to end their life. Do you agree or disagree with Cicely Saunders suggestion that legalized euthanasia will become a 'duty to die' for many vulnerable people?

Death is humanized

THE 'HAPPY DEATH' MOVEMENT

> *'You matter because you are you. You matter to the last moment of your life'. (Saunders, quoted in Brignall 2003: 1335)*

In contrast to the euthanasia movement, the contemporary hospice movement has argued passionately for society to value lives of the terminally ill and to assist people to live fully until they die. This movement to humanize death was described by Lofland (1978) as the 'happy death' movement. Hospice carers have sought to invest death with new meaning and these values find their expression in the concept of the 'good death'. The 'good death' is one where there is freedom from physical suffering and awareness, acceptance and discussion of death (McNamara 2004). Kubler Ross (1975) thus described dying as the 'final stage of growth'.

Kubler Ross was a pioneer in the field of 'death counselling'. She argued that the dying typically needed to pass through five emotional stages on the journey to death.

- Denial and isolation
- Anger
- Bargaining
- Depression
- Acceptance.

This five-stage model became enormously influential and Seale (1998) has suggested that an orderly classification of dying was appealing to professionals who needed to organize disturbing experiences. The evidence base of Kubler Ross's work has been questioned and a more critical view of her model has developed among some palliative care staff who have argued that there is no 'right' way to die and that professionals need to be responsive to individual differences (Sheldon 1997).

The idea of the 'good death' was part of what Walter (1994) called 'revivalist' discourse. The colonization of care of the dying by psychotherapy reflects the particular approaches to dying of a society which is both secularized and individualized (Walter 2003). Thus, communication and awareness have become central to contemporary approaches to dying.

COMMUNICATION AND AWARENESS OF DYING

An important goal of the hospice movement has been to improve communication with the dying. Studies in this field have criticized communication with dying patients and accused health professionals of a lack of commitment and skill (Ford et al 1996). Hinton for example found that patients were willing to discuss their diagnosis and prognosis but were seldom given the opportunity to talk (Hinton 1967: 1980).

Much of our understanding of communication with the dying has derived from the work of Glaser and Strauss (1965). In their work with the dying in San Francisco hospitals, they found a number of patterns of communication and truth telling which they described as 'awareness contexts'.

- In 'closed awareness', the truth was kept from the patient
- 'Suspicion awareness' existed when the patient tried unsuccessfully to extract the truth from family and carers
- 'Mutual pretence' existed when both sides pretended to be unaware of the truth
- In 'open awareness', the truth was shared between patient, family and staff.

Glaser and Strauss (1965) criticized the high levels of closed awareness in their study associating closed awareness with unhappiness and isolation. Their work has been used widely to argue for more honesty with dying patients and to promote the emotional accompaniment of patients in their journey towards death.

Recent surveys suggest that there is now much more openness on the part of health professionals dealing with the dying. Williams (1989) has suggested that in the USA, it is now the rule to tell patients of their diagnosis rather than the exception. In the UK, the approach has been rather more cautious with doctors emphasizing the patient's wish to know as a deciding factor. Seale (1991) found that the increased openness with patients was largely found in the treatment of cancer patients. Cancer patients are much more likely to be told the truth than patients dying of other conditions. This does not necessarily reflect the certainty of their prognosis since patients dying of other conditions were often not told, even when death was expected.

There have been a number of criticisms of the concept of 'awareness contexts', perhaps most importantly, they imply that doctors have certain knowledge that they can choose to impart to the patient or not. This underestimates the uncertainty of diagnosis and prognosis in many conditions. Schou (1993) suggests that dying is an ambiguous concept and that 'there is no facile boundary between the end of mainstream treatment and the beginning of dying'. In her study of oncology units, there was a general preference for openness with patients, yet this sat uncomfortably with the orientation of these units towards curative treatment. Oncology units tried to promote an upbeat image in which the battle against cancer was one that they could be seen to be winning and yet most patients receiving active treatment in her particular study had scant chance of a cure.

Timmermans (1994) suggests that uncertainty may be a strategy used by patients and staff alike to maintain hope. Seale (1998) suggests that some people may prefer what he calls 'disregarded dying'. They will hold on to hope by maintaining 'business as usual' (as we saw described earlier by Berger 1967) by ignoring death for as long as possible. By contrast, in critical care Harvey (1996) found that staff constantly struggled to achieve certainty and control in what were often highly unpredictable situations. The belief that open awareness is the most desirable communication pattern in care of the dying has gained widespread acceptance, yet in some situations it is clearly neither feasible nor appropriate.

REFLECTION POINT

We have seen that the sociological concept of 'awareness contexts' has helped health professionals to think about how to improve communication with the dying. There is an extensive literature which has criticized health professionals' communication with the dying. Reflect on your own experience and think of examples of good and less good communication with patients with life threatening illness. How could communication be improved?

NURSING THE DYING

As we have noted in earlier chapters, nurses have viewed communicating with patients as central to their role. Nurses caring for dying patients have talked at length about their role in communicating with the dying (May 1992). Field (1989) found that communication between nurses and dying patients varied according to setting and was often poor. Seale (1991) however, found that patients saw doctors as the most important source of information and family and friends as the most important source of emotional support. Mayer (1987) reported that cancer patients rated technical competence as the most important component of nursing whereas nurses rated expressive activities more highly. James (1992) in a study of hospice nursing found that nursing care was composed of physical labour, emotional labour and organization. It may be that patients are telling us that physical and emotional labour are inseparable and that we should not privilege communication above giving physical care. According to Seymour (2004) good palliative care nursing links emotional labour to 'painstaking physical care giving'.

REFLECTION POINT

We have seen that nurses place a high value on delivering psychological care to people with life-threatening illnesses. However, we have seen that patients also place a high value on competent physical care. Seymour suggests that good palliative care also involves 'painstaking physical care'. From your own experience, reflect on examples of good and less good physical care of people near the end of their life. How could such care be improved?

THE FUTURE FOR PALLIATIVE CARE

We have seen that the hospice move has changed attitudes to the dying in recent times, particularly in relation to the care of cancer patients. The rationalization of death tended to remove death from the care and control of the family and community to bureaucratic institutions and according to Adams (1993) represented a 'defeminization' of death. Seale (1995b) suggests that the new discourses about death promoted by the hospice movement present death as an emotional and spiritual journey and offer a new form of 'heroic death' in which the individual can demonstrate courage and a 'beatific state' in the face of death. This, says Seale, represents a particularly feminine heroics with its emphasis on emotional expression and self-sacrifice.

The growth of the modern hospice movement in the UK owed much to the leadership of one charismatic individual, Dame Cicely Saunders.

BIOGRAPHY

Cicely Saunders (1918–2005)

Cicely Saunders was born in Hertfordshire and qualified as a nurse in 1944. However, a back problem forced her to retrain as a medical social worker, qualifying in 1947. During her work as a social worker, she had an intense spiritual relationship with a dying Polish man and they discussed the idea that she might found a home where dying people might find peace in their final days. He left her £500 so that he could be 'a window' in her home. Saunders was advised to train as a doctor if she wanted to achieve her goal and after qualifying, she studied pain management and terminal care. She finally founded St Christopher's Hospice in 1967 and it has led the field in the development of hospice and palliative care. Saunders introduced the concept of 'total pain'; that is pain which has physical, emotional, social and spiritual dimensions and thought hospice care should address all aspects of pain. Her book *Living with Dying* (1983) is the classic statement of the principles of hospice care.

James and Field (1992) have suggested that the early ideals of the hospice movement have been eroded, as it has become increasingly routinized and bureaucratized. Its dependence on the state for financial support has led to a pressure to conform to bureaucratic procedures such as quantitative audit. There is a danger therefore that the 'softer' aspects of care which were believed to be so important to the early leaders of the hospice movement are overlooked as hospice is increasingly managerialized. Palliative care may then become just another medical speciality concerned only with the measurable control of symptoms. There is considerable debate within the hospice movement as to how much routinization and bureaucratization have taken place. There has also been debate as to just how much these trends compromise the ideals of hospice care (Clark 2002, Clark & Seymour 1999).

DISADVANTAGED DYING

Positive though the humanization of death may be, we must note that the hospice movement has had a limited reach. The 'heroic script' is most available to younger patients dying from cancer and AIDS. The hospice movement has had little impact on those dying from other conditions. Furthermore, there are marked social inequalities in hospice and palliative care provision and it is less freely available to disadvantaged groups such as ethnic minorities and the less affluent (Koffman & Camps 2004). Although there are limitations to the extent to which we have become a 'death denying' society there are still some people whose deaths we choose to ignore. A particular change noted in Seale's study has been the increasing numbers of elderly people dying in private residential homes where palliative care and emotional accompaniment in the journey towards death are often unattainable. For these people, death has not been humanized. These are some of the 'disadvantaged dying'. According to Seale (1995b: 613):

> *'Those who are in extreme old age ... the demented and the institutionalized, have much less opportunity to strike an heroic pose, but are more frequently portrayed as dribbling, undignified figures, waiting for death as a release from life. The lives and deaths of these individuals have become the horror stories of our time'.*

Thus, even at the hour of our death, social inequalities continue to shape our fate. Until we recognize our responsibility to all those who are dying the 'happy death' movement will be unable to claim that it has fully humanized death.

Discussion points

1. How have social attitudes to death changed in the last 100 years?
2. What social changes do you think would improve the quality of life of people nearing death?
3. What changes in healthcare and nursing would improve the care of people who are dying?
4. Do you think that the legalization of euthanasia would improve the quality of life of the terminally ill?

CHAPTER SUMMARY

This chapter began by looking at social attitudes to death. It considered the argument that death had become a taboo subject in contemporary society. It also considered the opposing arguments that death was a 'badly kept secret' which was still a very central preoccupation in the media and public life. It reviewed studies of media representations of death which suggested that there is a new uncertainty about how to behave in the face of death.

The chapter also reviewed arguments that dying people themselves had become 'sequestered', i.e. hidden away and separated from mainstream society. Here, again there is a mixed picture. New forms of support have developed such as the hospice movement but some dying people (particularly the elderly) face loneliness and isolation. There is some evidence that the scientific and bureaucratic management of death can lead to depersonalized treatment of people who suffer life threatening illness. You were asked to think about the ways in which nurses could improve the care of people nearing the end of their life. The concept of 'social death' was introduced which describes the ways in which people such as the elderly are treated as if they were no longer a member of human society. The contribution of this concept to debates about euthanasia and the costs of terminal care was discussed and you were encouraged to think about your own views on this issue. Throughout this book, we have considered the impact of inequality on care. In this final chapter, we considered the ways in which inequalities shape the experience of care at the end of life.

FURTHER READING

Walter T 1994 The revival of death. London, Routledge

Seale C 1998 Constructing death: the sociology of dying and bereavement. Cambridge University Press, Cambridge

The two books above are useful on the sociology of death.

Glaser B, Strauss A 1965 Awareness of dying. Aldine, Chicago

Glaser and Strauss still provide the classic study of communication in care of the dying.

Saunders C, Baines M 1983 Living with dying: The management of terminal disease. Oxford University Press, Oxford

Cicely Saunders' work gives a classic statement of the ideals of the hospice movement.

REFERENCES

Adams S 1993 A gendered history of the social management of death in Foleshill, Coventry, during the inter-war years. In: Clark D (ed.) The sociology of death: theory, culture, practice. Blackwell, Cambridge, p 149–168

Aries P 1981 The hour of our death. Allen Lane, London
Armstrong D 1987 Silence and truth in death and dying. Social Science and Medicine 8:651–657
Baumann Z 1987 Modernity and the holocaust. Polity, Oxford
Becker E 1973 The denial of death. Free Press, New York
Berger P 1967 The sacred canopy: Elements of a sociological theory of religion. Doubleday, New York
Blauner R 1966 Death and social structure. Psychiatry 29:378–394
Brennan M 2001 Towards a sociology of (public) mourning. Sociology 35(1):205–212
Brignall I 2003 You matter to the last moment of your life. British Medical Journal 326:1335
Canadian Health Services Research Foundation 2004 Mythbusters: The cost of dying is an increasing strain on the healthcare system. Journal of Health Service Research and Policy 9(4):254–255
Clark D 2002 Between hope and acceptance: the medicalization of dying. British Medical Journal 324:905–907
Clark D, Seymour J 1999 Reflections on palliative care. Open University Press, Buckingham
Corr C 1993 Death in modern society. In: Doyle D (ed.) Oxford textbook of palliative medicine. Oxford University Press, Oxford, p 28–35
Dingwall R, Rafferty A, Webster C 1988 An introduction of the social history of nursing. Routledge, London
Elias N 1985 The loneliness of the dying. Routledge, London
Emmanuel E 1994 The history of euthanasia debates in the United States and Britain. Annals of Internal Medicine 121:793–802
Field D 1989 Nursing the dying. Tavistock, London
Ford S, Fallowfield L, Lewis S 1996 Doctor patient interactions in oncology. Social Science & Medicine 42(11):1511–1519
Foucault M 1973 Birth of the clinic. Tavistock, London
Giddens A 1991 Modernity and Self Identity. Polity, Oxford
Glaser B, Strauss A 1965 Awareness of dying. Aldine, Chicago
Gorer G 1955 The pornography of death. Encounter 5:49–52
Grande G, Addington-Hall J, Todd C 1998 Place of death and access to home care services; are certain patient groups at a disadvantage? Social Science and Medicine 47(5):565–579
Hafferty F 1988 Cadaver stories and the emotional socialization of medical students. Journal of Health and Social Behaviour 29:344–356
Harvey J 1996 Achieving the indeterminate: Accomplishing degrees of certainty in life and death situations. The Sociological Review 44:78–98
Hinton J 1967 Dying. Penguin, Harmondsworth
Hinton J 1980 Whom do dying patients tell? British Medical Journal 281:1328–1330
Hockey J 1997 Women in grief: cultural representations and social practice. In: Field D, Hockey J, Small N (eds) Death, gender and ethnicity. London, Routledge, p 129–148
James N 1992 Care=organization+physical labour +emotional labour. Sociology of Health and Illness 14(4):488–509
James N, Field D 1992 The routinization of hospice: charisma and bureaucratization. Social Science and Medicine 34(12):1363–1375
Jewson N 1976 The disappearance of the sick man from medical cosmology. Sociology 10:224–244
Kear A, Steinberg D 1999 (eds) Mourning Diana: Nation, culture and the performance of grief. Routledge, London
Koffman J, Camps M 2004 No way in: Including the excluded at the end of life. In: Payne S et al (eds) Palliative care nursing principles and evidence for practice. Open University Press, Buckingham, p 364–384
Kubler Ross E 1975 Death the final stage of growth. Prentice Hall, New Jersey
Lawton J 1998 Contemporary hospice care; the sequestration of the unbounded body and ‘dirty dying’. Sociology of Health and Illness 20 (2):121–143
Lock M 1995 Contesting the natural in Japan: moral dilemmas and technologies of dying. Culture Medicine and Society 19:1–38
Lofland L 1978 The craft of dying: the modern face of death. Sage, Beverley Hills
Mak Y, Elwyn G, Finlay I 2003 Patients voices are needed in debate on euthanasia. British Medical Journal 327:213–215
May C 1992 Nursing work, nursing knowledge and the subjectification of the patient. Sociology of Health and Illness 14: 472–488
Mayer D 1987 Oncology nurses’ versus cancer patients’ perceptions of nurse caring behaviours: a replication. Oncology Nurses Forum 14(3):48–52
McInerney F 2000 Requested death: a new social movement. Social Science and Medicine 50:137–154

McNamara B 2004 Good enough death: autonomy and choice in Australian palliative care. Social Science and Medicine 58(2):929–938
Mellor P 1993 Death in high modernity: The contemporary presence and absence of death. In: Clark D (ed.) The sociology of death: Theory, culture, practice. Blackwell, Cambridge, p 11–30
Mellor P, Schilling C 1993 Modernity, self identity and the sequestration of death. Sociology 27(3) 411–431
Mulkay M 1993 Social death in Britain. In: Clark D (ed.) The sociology of death: Theory, culture, practice. Blackwell, Cambridge, p 31–49
Obeyesekere G 1989 Despair and recovery: Sinhala medicine and religion. An anthropologist's meditations. In: Sullivan L E (ed.) Healing and restoring: Health and medicine in the world's religious traditions. Macmillan, New York, p 127–148
Ohnuki-Tierney E 1994 Brain death and organ transplantation. Current Anthropology 35(3): 233–254
Pickering M, Littlewood J, Walter T 1997 Beauty and the beast: sex and death in the tabloid press. In: Field D, Hockey J, Small, N (eds) Death, gender & ethnicity. Routledge, London, p 124–141
Prior L 1989 The social organization of death: Medical discourse and social practices in Belfast. Macmillan, London
Richardson R 2000 Death, dissection and the destitute. University of Chicago Press, Chicago
Ritzer G 1996 The McDonaldization of society. Pine Forge Press, California
Royal Liverpool Children's Inquiry 2001 Report of the Royal Liverpool Children's Inquiry. HMSO, London
Saunders C 1992 Voluntary euthanasia. Palliative Medicine 6:1–5
Scheper-Hughes N 2000 The global traffic in human organs. Current Anthropology 41(2):32
Schou K 1993 Awareness contexts and the construction of dying in the cancer treatment setting: 'micro' and 'macro' levels in narrative analysis. In: Clark D (ed.) The sociology of death: Theory, culture, practice. Blackwell, Cambridge, p 238–263
Scitovsky A 1994 The 'high cost of dying' revisited. Milbank Memorial Fund Quarterly 72(4):561–591
Seale C 1991 Communication and awareness about death: A study of a random sample of dying people. Social Science and Medicine 32(8):943–952
Seale C 1995a Dying alone. Sociology of Health and Illness 17(3):376–392
Seale C 1995b Heroic death. Sociology 29(4):597–613
Seale C 2000 Changing patterns of death and dying. Social Science and Medicine 51(6):917–930
Seale C 1997 Social and ethical aspects of euthanasia: a review. Progress in Palliative Care 5:141–146
Seale C 1998 Constructing death: the sociology of dying and bereavement. Cambridge University Press, Cambridge
Seale C 2003 Media constructions of dying alone: a form of 'bad death'. Social Science and Medicine 58 (5)967–974
Seale C, Addington-Hall J 1998 Dying at the best time. Social Science and Medicine 45:477–484
Seidelman, W 1991 Medical selection: Auschwitz antecedents and effluent. International Journal of Health Services 21(3):401–415
Seymour J 2004 What's in a name A concept analysis of key terms in palliative care nursing. In: Payne S et al (eds) Palliative care: nursing principles and evidence for practice. Open University Press, Buckingham, p 55–74
Sheldon F 1997 Psychosocial palliative care. Stanley Thornes, Cheltenham
Simpson M 1987 Dying, death and grief: A critical bibliography. University of Philadelphia Press, Philadelphia
Sudnow D 1967 Passing on: the social organization of dying. Prentice Hall, New Jersey
Thomas C, Morris S M, Clark D 2004 Place of death: preferences among cancer patients and their carers. Social Science and Medicine 58(12):2431–2444
Timmermans S 1994 Dying of awareness: the theory of awareness contexts revisited. Sociology of Health and Illness 16(3):322–339
Turner B 1991 Religion and social theory. Sage, London
Walter T 1991 Modern death – taboo or not taboo. Sociology 22(2):293–310
Walter T 1994 The revival of death. Routledge, London
Walter T 1994–5 Natural death and the noble savage. Omega 30(4):37–48
Walter T 1999, ed. The mourning for Diana. Berg, Oxford
Walter T 2003 Historical and cultural variants on the good death. British Medical Journal 327:218–220
Walter T, Littlewood J, Pickering M 1995 Death in the News: the public invigilation of private emotion. Sociology 29(4):579–596
Williams R 1989 Awareness and control of dying: Some paradoxical trends in public opinion. Sociology of Health and Illness 11(3):201–212

Index

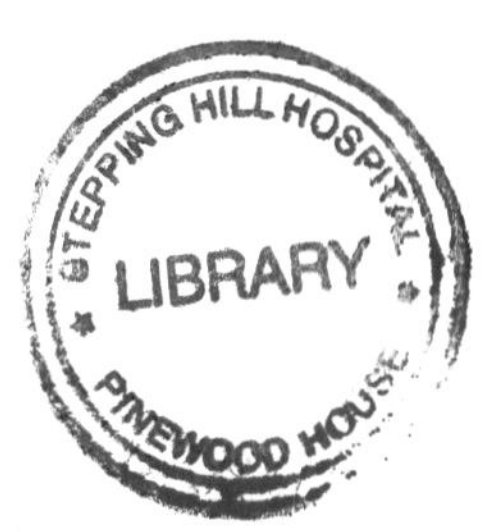